Critical Issues in Reproductive Health

THE SPRINGER SERIES ON

DEMOGRAPHIC METHODS AND POPULATION ANALYSIS

Series Editor

KENNETH C. LAND

Duke University

In recent decades, there has been a rapid development of demographic models and methods and an explosive growth in the range of applications of population analysis. This series seeks to provide a publication outlet both for high-quality textual and expository books on modern techniques of demographic analysis and for works that present exemplary applications of such techniques to various aspects of population analysis.

Topics appropriate for the series include:

- General demographic methods
- Techniques of standardization
- Life table models and methods
- Multistate and multiregional life tables, analyses and projections
- Demographic aspects of biostatistics and epidemiology
- Stable population theory and its extensions
- Methods of indirect estimation
- Stochastic population models
- Event history analysis, duration analysis, and hazard regression models
- Demographic projection methods and population forecasts
- Techniques of applied demographic analysis, regional and local population estimates and projections
- Methods of estimation and projection for business and health care applications
- Methods and estimates for unique populations such as schools and students

Volumes in the series are of interest to researchers, professionals, and students in demography, sociology, economics, statistics, geography and regional science, public health and health care management, epidemiology, biostatistics, actuarial science, business, and related fields.

For further volumes:
http://www.springer.com/series/6449

Andrzej Kulczycki

Editor

Critical Issues in Reproductive Health

Springer

Editor
Andrzej Kulczycki
Associate Professor
Department of Health Care Organization and Policy
University of Alabama at Birmingham
Birmingham
Alabama, USA

ISSN 1389-6784
ISBN 978-94-007-6721-8   ISBN 978-94-007-6722-5 (eBook)
DOI 10.1007/978-94-007-6722-5
Springer Dordrecht Heidelberg New York London

Library of Congress Control Number: 2013945923

Printed on acid-free paper

Springer is part of Springer Science+Business Media (www.springer.com)

Contents

List of Abbreviations

AGWG	Adolescent Girls Working Group (Liberia)
AIDS	Acquired immunodeficiency syndrome
ANC	Antenatal care
API	Active pharmaceutical ingredient
APROFAM	Asociación Pro-Bienestar de la Familia de Guatemala
ART	Assisted reproductive technology
ARV	Antiretroviral (drug therapy)
ASRM	American Society for Reproductive Medicine
CBA	Community-based adaptation
CBD	Community-based distribution
CDC	Centers for Disease Control and Prevention (USA)
CEO	Chief executive officer
CHFP	Community Health and Family Planning Project (Ghana)
CHPS	Community-based Health Planning and Services program (Ghana)
CHO	Community health officer (Ghana)
CHW	Community health worker
COP	Conference of the Parties
CO_2	Carbon dioxide
CRM	Coastal resources management project (Philippines)
DAC	Development Assistance Committee (of the OECD)
DAH	Development assistance for health
DALY	Disability-adjusted life year
DFID	Department for International Development (United Kingdom)
DHS	Demographic and Health Surveys
DMPA	Depot medroxyprogesterone acetate (also known as Depo-Provera)
EC	Emergency contraception
ECP	Emergency contraceptive pills
EDH	Egyptian Demographic and Health Survey
EIM	European IVF Monitoring Program
EMA	European Medicines Agency
EPAG	Economic Empowerment of Adolescent Girls (Liberia)

EPF	European Parliamentary Forum on Population and Development
ESHRE	European Society for Human Reproduction and Embryology
EU	European Union
FHI	Family Health International (now known as FHI 360)
FIGO	International Federation of Gynecology and Obstetrics
FP	Family planning
GDM	Gestational diabetes mellitus
GHI	Global Health Initiative (United States)
GIFT	Gamete intrafallopian transfer
GMP	Good manufacturing practice
GNI	Gross national income
HIV	Human immunodeficiency virus
HPV	Human papillomavirus
HSA	Health surveillance assistant (Malawi)
ICPD	International Conference on Population and Development
ICSI	Intracytoplasmic sperm induction
ICU	Intensive care unit
IMCI	Integrated Management of Childhood Illnesses
IMF	International Monetary Fund
IPCC	Intergovernmental Panel on Climate Change
IPPF	International Planned Parenthood Federation
IPV	Intimate partner violence
IUD	Intrauterine device
IUI	Intrauterine insemination
IVF	In-vitro fertilization
LA/PM	Long-acting and permanent method
LARC	Long-acting reversible contraceptive
LBW	Low birthweight
LISGIS	Liberian Institute of Statistics and Geo-Information Services
LNG	Levonorgestrel
LNG-IUS	Levonorgestrel releasing-intrauterine system
MCH	Maternal and child health
MDG	Millennium Development Goal
MENA	Middle East and North Africa
MEP	Member of the European Parliament
MMR	Maternal mortality ratio
MOH	Ministry of Health
MSI	Marie Stopes International
MSSL	Marie Stopes Sierra Leone
M&E	Monitoring and evaluation
NAPAs	National Adaptation Programmes of Action
NDSS	Navrongo Demographic Surveillance System (Ghana)
NET-EN	Noristerat (also known as norethindrone (or norethisterone) enanthate
NGO	Non-governmental organization
NICU	Neonatal intensive care unit

NPFPC	National Population and Family Planning Commission (China)
ODA	Official development assistance
OECD	Organisation for Economic Co-operation and Development
PAAL	Pharm Access Africa, Ltd.
PAC	Post abortion care
PEPFAR	President's Emergency Plan for AIDS Relief (United States)
PHE	Population, health and environment
PMTCT	Prevention of mother-to-child transmission of HIV
PID	Pelvic inflammatory disease
PNA	Performance needs assessment
PoA	Programme of Action
PPAL	Planned Parenthood Association of Liberia
PRAMS	Pregnancy Risk Assessment Monitoring System (United States)
PrEP	Pre-exposure prophylaxis
RH	Reproductive health
RTI	Reproductive tract infection
SART	Society for Assisted Reproductive Technology (United States)
SC	Spontaneously (naturally) conceived
SFDA	State Food and Drug Administration (China)
SRH	Sexual and reproductive health
SRHR	Sexual and reproductive health and rights
SRA	Strict regulatory authority
SSA	Sub-Saharan Africa
STD	Sexually transmitted disease
STI	Sexually transmitted infection
TFR	Total fertility rate
THINK	Touching Humans In Need of Kindness (Liberian NGO)
UK	United Kingdom
UN	United Nations
UNAIDS	Joint United Nations Programme on HIV/AIDS
UNDP	United Nations Development Programme
UNFCCC	United Nations Framework Convention on Climate Change
UNFPA	United Nations Population Fund
UNICEF	United Nations Children's Fund
USA	United States of America
USAID	United States Agency for International Development
USFDA	(United States) Food and Drug Administration
WHO	World Health Organization
WIC	Special Supplemental Nutrition Program for Women, Infants and Children (United States)

Chapter 1
Introduction and Overview

Andrzej Kulczycki

Poor reproductive health can have devastating consequences on individuals and families, along with adverse impacts for health care systems, economic well-being and society. Good reproductive health contributes to healthy sexuality, individuals and families, as well as wanted children and more optimal societal and economic outcomes. Although a number of countries had earlier adopted the concept, it was the 1994 International Conference on Population and Development (ICPD) which explicitly recognized sexual and reproductive rights as fundamental to women's health, and gave much momentum to the field. It also moved beyond the confines of traditional family planning approaches, set new goals for reproductive health and rights, and highlighted their importance for policymakers and publics worldwide. However, a political backlash soon ensued, the HIV/AIDS epidemic worsened with no apparent end in sight, and new funding priorities and mechanisms emerged.

The revised international agenda for poverty reduction and development articulated in the Millennium Development Goals (MDGs) adopted in 2000 acknowledged the need to reduce maternal mortality and HIV/AIDS. However, it fell short of more explicitly recognizing the interplay between reproductive health, poverty reduction and development, and largely side-tracked other reproductive health issues. The MDG goal of maternal mortality reduction is the most off-track goal and unmet reproductive health needs remain large, notwithstanding recent progress and a changed international political environment. In 2001, shortages in reproductive and sexual health were estimated to account for nearly one-fifth of illness and preventive death worldwide, and one-third among women of reproductive age. This toll stemmed largely from problems related to pregnancy and to sexually transmitted infections (STIs), notably HIV/AIDS, which are particularly acute in the world's poorest communities. There have been recent significant reductions in the global

A. Kulczycki, Ph.D. (✉)
Associate Professor, Department of Health Care Organization and Policy,
University of Alabama at Birmingham (UAB), Birmingham, AL, USA
e-mail: andrzej@uab.edu

A. Kulczycki (ed.), *Critical Issues in Reproductive Health*, The Springer Series on
Demographic Methods and Population Analysis 33, DOI 10.1007/978-94-007-6722-5_1,
© Springer Science+Business Media Dordrecht 2014

burden of disease from maternal conditions and HIV/AIDS, but with the target dates for realizing the ICPD vision (2014) and MDG goals (2015) imminent, it is clear that much more work is needed on how best to improve reproductive health knowledge, policy and care.

This book presents a set of papers intended to stimulate and advance such research by highlighting various understated and vital cross-cutting themes for the reproductive health field, especially as it looks forward to the next decade. The book attempts to address a number of critical issues in reproductive health, including current debates and controversies; identify research, policy and practice gaps and priorities; and illustrate innovative solutions to addressing some of the multiple challenges in these areas. The book thereby seeks to enhance interest and enlighten scientific, policy and programmatic dialogue on reproductive health. It is intended for health, social, and behavioural scientists and professionals; students in health-related fields, the social sciences, and current affairs; as well as others interested in reproductive health. Addressing reproductive health challenges from a broader interdisciplinary perspective is needed. Contributing authors represent many different disciplines and most are well-established in their respective areas of expertise and known for their scholarly and dispassionate analyses.

The chapters presented here are topical and thought-provoking; they map out ideas for developing, expanding and filling in the research, policy and programmatic agendas, especially on cross-cutting issues about which relatively little has been published. Chapters illustrate a rich and varied set of cases, are comparative in scope, and most use mixed method approaches. Although many major world regions are represented, there is greater focus on sub-Saharan Africa where reproductive health problems are more acute due to such factors as past neglect, weak health services, ingrained gender inequalities, deep poverty, ineffective governance, and global political economic imbalances. In 2010–2012, UN agency reports indicated that sub-Saharan Africa accounted for 12 % of the world's population at the end of 2010, but 57 % of its pregnancy-related deaths, 49 % of its infant mortality, and 67 % of all HIV infections. Nonetheless, recent declines in such deaths suggest improving prospects for sub-Saharan Africa; also, although not entirely peaceful and democratic, after decades of slow economic growth, more countries have seen steady gains in the past decade and the region has a fast-growing middle class. Nevertheless, Africa remains the most important priority in global health.

The book also devotes more attention to emerging issues in family planning because of the topic's centrality to primary and preventive health care needs, especially for women, and its comparative neglect in global health assistance efforts over the past two decades. The timing coincides with the London summit on family planning held in mid-2012, which promised strengthened political commitment and new monies for family planning in poor countries. Inevitably, this volume cannot cover the entire range of reproductive health. Less space is devoted to HIV/AIDS on which numerous books and a greater share of articles have been published recently and which, though a great human tragedy, already commands a disproportionately large share of research and donor efforts. In 2012, there is also growing optimism that the struggle against HIV/AIDS was reaching a tipping point as improved access to highly effective antiretroviral drugs (ARVs) were reaching more people.[1]

The volume is divided into three parts: (1) expanding the research base; (2) advancing policy; and (3) strengthening service and program capacity. This structure mirrors commonly accepted divisions between these three areas of interest, but these are also viewed as interconnected by contributors to this book. Chapters in Part I, for example, seek not only to deepen the research frontier, but also to advance knowledge that informs policy and programming on how to improve reproductive health. This introductory chapter previews some of the major issues raised in the book, sets the frame for the chapters that follow, and highlights some of their important findings.

1.1 Expanding the Research Base

Part I of the book contains five chapters that address key areas of concern including reproductive tract infections (RTIs), the construction of medical and popular knowledge, risk and consequences of spousal violence during pregnancy, reproductive preferences and behaviors, contraceptive method mix and access, emergency contraception and the reduction of unintended pregnancy, infertility treatment use and its potential associated adverse maternal and infant outcomes. Chapters 2, 3, 4, 5 and 6 develop sound evidence to improve the research base and offer a more solid foundation for policies and programs. Such well-grounded studies help point the way to solutions for the dilemmas of addressing reproductive health in diverse communities worldwide.

Women in many societies are loath to discuss reproductive health problems with family members, medical practitioners, and often even with other female friends or peers. This silence is associated with discomfort about the sexual connotations of such problems, such that they are treated as a normal part of life and merely a common expression of having a female body. In Chap. 2, Alaka Malwade Basu draws attention to the much under-studied topic of gynaecological morbidities. She discusses both this reported tendency to normalize reproductive health problems as well as attempts by clinicians and by researchers to overcome the resultant internalized and institutionalized barriers to diagnosing and treating such problems. She also considers whether clinicians and researchers may be swinging the

---

[1] In late 2012, UNAIDS reported that new infections in 25 low- and middle-income countries had dropped by 50 % in recent years, with 13 of those countries located in sub-Saharan Africa, a region where AIDS-related deaths had fallen by over one-third in the last 6 years. This progress helped raise optimism that after 30 years and 30 million deaths, real progress is being made towards an AIDS-free generation. However, in 2011 there were still 2.5 million new infections (down 700,000 from the 2001 figure) and 1.7 million deaths (600,000 fewer than in 2005) due to AIDS-related causes, and HIV/AIDS continues to be the chief cause of death for women of reproductive age worldwide (UNAIDS 2012).

pendulum in the opposite direction in their zeal to identify problems that need biomedical treatments. Diagnostic protocols in many countries could be leading to an undue number of false positives because the language of reproductive health distress may be used to articulate other kinds of physical or mental problems that have no name in these cultures. This chapter does not minimize the problem of reproductive tract infections (RTIs); rather, it suggests that their recent emphasis and, in particular, the construction of associated medical knowledge, clinical and treatment strategies, may lead to wasted resources and may inadvertently mask other important health concerns.

Next, Alaka Basu weighs evidence on discrepancies in reproductive health rates estimated from diverse data sources including surveys, clinical examinations and laboratory diagnoses, primarily in South Asia. The author questions the role of new technologies in detecting, preventing and treating RTIs, including STIs. These technologies have greatly increased the volume of diagnoses but their validity has, in contrast, received inadequate critical examination. Many people have varying definitions and interpretations of reproductive health and its con-stituent parts. Ideally, vernacular, practitioner, and academic terms and under-standings should be more closely aligned.

Intimate partner violence (IPV) is a pervasive problem worldwide, with many negative effects on women's physical and mental health, maternal-fetal and repro-ductive health outcomes. It also hinders progress towards realizing development goals. These issues are the subject of a growing body of research in many countries, although most studies remain rather limited in scope, depth, or quality. For many countries, accurate information on multiple aspects of IPV remains difficult to obtain and persistent methodological limitations restrict the generalizability of find-ings. For the Middle East and North Africa (MENA), IPV is woefully understudied, including that which occurs during pregnancy. Chapter 3 extends work on this topic to Egypt, in the first of the book's two chapters centered on the Arab region's most populous and pivotal country which, as of this writing, faces ongoing turmoil.

Using nationally representative, population-based survey data, Andrzej Kulczycki examines the prevalence, correlates, attitudes and selected health-related outcomes associated with spousal physical violence during pregnancy. This study shows such violence is not uncommon in Egypt, has multiple roots, and constitutes a serious public health problem that demands urgent attention. However, many married women (and men) condone wife beating and few seek help, underscoring the pervasive cul-ture of silence and fatalism that surrounds this issue and which makes addressing its roots very difficult. Results further show that spousal physical violence during preg-nancy is significantly associated with increased risk of STIs/STI symptoms, though not with changes in the likelihood of receiving antenatal care. Research attention needs to focus more on the complex interplay of factors associated with IPV during pregnancy and their health-related dimensions. This chapter adds to the very limited evidence base on the topic for MENA countries, which must be expanded as a matter of priority for building effective interventions and policy.

Currently, some of the lowest contraceptive prevalence rates in the world are found in large swathes of sub-Saharan Africa, making it vital to assess present and future needs in African family planning programs. An unusually rich demographic laboratory for monitoring the impact of health interventions in rural West Africa is afforded by the Navrongo longitudinal demographic surveillance system in the Kassena-Nankana district of northern Ghana (Binka et al. 2007). This is an isolated rural district where health, social and economic problems severely constrain development. Navrongo has also been the site of an ongoing trial of alternative approaches for family planning introduction to address a number of unanswered related research questions.

In rural Sahelian settings, addressing the contraceptive needs of women can precipitate anxiety and opposition among men. The Navrongo Community Health and Family Planning Project (CHFP) addresses the profoundly complex gender challenges of introducing reproductive health services in such a societal setting by developing a multi-faceted approach to outreach and dialogue with chiefs, elders, lineage heads, and male social networks. This outreach was conducted in conjunction with a program of community gatherings in which community leaders were involved in explaining the program to men, thereby raising their awareness and acceptance of family planning. In Chap. 4, Philip B. Adongo, James F. Phillips, and Colin D. Baynes examine the relative impact of contrasting modes of community-based distribution (CBD) program delivery on socio-cultural processes that mediate fertility and contraceptive behavior in a rural African setting. This research attests to the critical importance of mitigating the social costs of family planning to women by addressing the concerns and needs of men. The findings also carry implications on how family planning services should best be made available elsewhere in sub-Saharan Africa.

Emergency contraception[2] has become available in numerous countries over the past decade, but a range of barriers continues to restrict access. Emergency contraception occupies a unique niche among contraceptive users because it offers women a post-coital option and a second chance to avoid unintended pregnancy. This continues to lead to many misperceptions and much confusion. In Chap. 5, Lisa L. Wynn, Hosam Moustafa, and Ahmed Ragab provide an ethnographically informed study on the stalled implementation, social meanings, and marketing of emergency contraception in Egypt. Specifically, they examine why emergency contraception is so little known and used in Egypt, the strategies employed to market emergency contraceptive pills (ECPs) and define its users, and how activists thereby construct a health problem (and its solution) for public consumption.

The chapter situates the status of ECPs in Egypt within the context of Islamic jurisprudence and social concerns about the sexuality of young Egyptians. It stresses the importance of understanding reproductive health activism in terms of the politics of what can and cannot be said about sexuality in a particular society. Wynn and colleagues contend that social expectations surrounding the sexuality of different

---

[2]Emergency contraceptive pills are the most commonly used emergency contraceptive method and may comprise a larger dose of standard combined hormone oral contraceptive pills, progestin-only oral contraceptive pills, or a dedicated progestin-only emergency contraceptive product. The insertion of a copper intrauterine device (IUD) may also provide emergency contraception.

social classes interact with cultural symbolism and religious interpretation to shape Egyptian interpretations of the appropriateness of emergency contraception. As with Chap. 3, the findings apply both to the world's largest Arab population and may also hold relevance to elsewhere in the MENA region. The authors additionally highlight the complex interplay between local and global politics that so often undermine well-intentioned policy initiatives, including one of the first significant attempts to introduce emergency contraception into the Arab world.

Involuntary childlessness can lead to much personal grief, relationship distress and, in many societies, stigma and even persecution. During the last few decades, clinical services for infertile persons have mushroomed in many societies and by 2010, about five million babies had been born worldwide as a result of assisted reproductive technologies (ARTs).[3] However, the high cost of such treatments and the lack of insurance or state support prevent many from being able to access and use them. ARTs also increase preterm and multiple births and have been linked to a range of adverse outcomes, although risks may be attributable to factors other than the ART techniques themselves (Reddy et al. 2007). Research on ARTs and other infertility treatments and their potential adverse maternal and infant outcomes faces multiple methodological challenges. Although regulatory oversight in more countries is leading to a move to transfer single embryos, concerns remain about possible risks for both mother and offspring.

Far less research attention has been paid to less invasive and cheaper technologies, which include fertility drugs such as ovulatory stimulants. Non-ART treatments are now estimated to account for close to 5 % of all U.S. births, or about four times more than the number conceived through ART use (Schieve et al. 2009). In Chap. 6, Suzanne Dhall and Andrzej Kulczycki examine the use of these low tech interventions and their potential risks for a wide range of potential adverse maternal and perinatal outcomes, independent of the effects of plurality and other confounders. They overcome the severe constraints to U.S. published data sources on infertility and its treatment by using a novel data source and comparing findings for women receiving non-ART infertility treatment to those receiving ART treatments, rather than drawing comparisons to women who conceive spontaneously. They examine live birth files for Texas, the second most populous U.S. state that is often said to preview future trends nationally and that has huge disparities in reproductive health, services for which are bitterly contested. They find that infertility treatment seekers have a higher prevalence of prior chronic illnesses and poor pregnancy outcomes, with maternal and perinatal outcomes comparable by treatment type. This is in contrast to the striking differences found in outcomes in either the ART or non-ART

---

[3]As reported in the press release "5 million babies," ESHRE (European Society of Human Reproduction and Embryology), 2 July 2012 (http://www.eshre.eu/ESHRE/English/Press-Room/Press-Releases/Press-releases-2012/5-million-babies/page.aspx/1606). The first 'test tube' baby was born as a result of in vitro fertilization (IVF) in 1978, since when ARTs have become available to ever more would-be mothers and fathers. Success rates from a single fresh treatment cycle of IVF and ICSI appear to be stabilizing at around a 30–32 % pregnancy rate for each embryo transferred.

group women when compared to those who spontaneously conceived, even after controlling for confounders. These results have several clear policy messages, particularly as non-ART treatments are being delivered in a much less controlled process and are not required to be reported.

1.2 Advancing Policy

This section of the book comprises five chapters concerned with advancing reproductive health policy and understanding a range of threats and opportunities to its formulation and implementation. The first four chapters are global in scope, but also embed studies of specific national cases. They emphasize reproductive health policy as a contentious terrain embedded in broader struggles concerning population policy and development, global health, climate change and ideology. All five chapters also consider to a varying degree the political dynamics that shape reproductive health policies and choices. The fifth chapter contains a round-table symposium that seeks to chart more effective paths ahead. Contributors to this chapter have played major leadership roles focused on different aspects of the field in distinct settings, and they continue to make significant efforts. They have been invited here to step back and reflect on the past trajectory and current situation of the field and, in the process, to draw valuable lessons and suggestions for better positioning it in the near future.

International efforts to reduce high levels of fertility and reproductive ill-health in the developing world have long followed a convoluted course. This reflects shifts in the consensus on population and development thinking that evolved in the second half of the twentieth century. The 1994 ICPD re-shaped thinking on population and development and altered the landscape for international population assistance. In Chap. 7, Andrew B. Kantner examines global reproductive health governance and considers how well the ICPD paradigm and women's health outcomes have fared since this seminal event was held. He also discusses prospects for more effectively addressing women's health needs in the future. The chapter first summarizes the path of thinking about population-development and reproductive health interrelations, as well as recent trends and best practices in the major arenas of reproductive health (family planning, maternal mortality and health care, abortion, and STIs/HIV/AIDS).

It is no longer clear whether a broad international consensus currently exists on population and development, even though population dynamics are widely seen as influencing reproductive health and other development outcomes, as reflected in the MDGs crafted by the United Nations (UN). Andrew B. Kantner further discusses the ICPD's disappointing aftermath for many reproductive health program efforts and for the generation of global resources, particularly for family planning, in stark contrast to the progress made regarding HIV/AIDS. He traces commonalities and discontinuities in the implementation of policies by the U.S. government, the largest donor to global reproductive health assistance efforts worldwide. This allows him to distill forgotten lessons and to suggest pointers for more successful implementation of President Obama's ambitious Global Health Initiative announced in 2009 and which, as of this writing, continues to have a protracted and difficult gestation. The author concludes with a review of current prospects for reviving interest in global population issues and for reinvigorating family planning and reproductive health programs. He also discusses how promised new resources might be best allocated and deployed, particularly in light of what is known about past efforts to improve reproductive health outcomes.

In recent decades, many countries have expanded the grounds under which abortion may be legally performed, particularly during early pregnancy. This development has occurred as abortion procedures have become safer, childbearing preferences have fallen, and respect for women's rights and autonomy have increased. Some countries also introduced and supported more permissive abortion laws primarily to control population growth. In contrast to Latin American and African states which overwhelmingly tend to have more restrictive abortion policies (as well as weaker commitments to family planning programs), the world's two demographic giants, China and India, both implemented more liberal abortion policies when their governments began to strongly promote the family planning programs that they had earlier instituted (Kulczycki 1999, 2011). It is not inconceivable that demographic arguments may resume prominence as an underlying rationale behind abortion legislation, and potentially in a more restrictive direction. Those concerned with fostering women's reproductive health and rights may need to monitor closely the interplay between abortion and population policies. In Chap. 8, Dennis Hodgson examines state perceptions and policies on fertility levels alongside recent patterns and changes in abortion legislation.

At the end of the first decade of this century, one-eighth of the world's population lived in the 41 countries that have adopted policies to raise their current fertility level, nearly all in response to recently declining birth rates (UN 2011). The populations of the 33 pronatalist countries with liberal abortion policies tend to have below replacement level fertility and stagnant or even negative annual growth rates. Religious and other opponents of induced abortion and nationalists worried about the debilitating effects of population decline have started to contend that access to abortion has to be restricted if the problematic effects of below replacement fertility on age structure, health care and pension costs, and labor force needs are to be reversed. The author discusses current and future political problems likely to be faced by countries with liberal abortion policies that are adopting increasingly pronatalist strategies; and then asks if these states (including the cases of Russia, Poland and South Korea) may be moving toward restricting access to abortion in future due to growing concerns about the potential effects of below replacement level fertility. Dennis Hodgson also considers this new challenge for reproductive rights movements in several Asian countries with generally larger populations than the numerous, relatively small, European low fertility countries with liberal abortion policies. The resultant pressures on policy makers will constitute a growing threat to reproductive rights, an issue likely to receive greater attention in years to come.

An issue fast assuming great significance concerns the impact of climate change. It is now evident that human-induced changes have started to affect the atmosphere and, in turn, people and the environment. In many countries, shifting temperature and precipitation patterns are already making scarce water supplies even more difficult to manage. Climate change presents one of the most serious health threats facing the world and promises to threaten global sustainable food security, particularly for the most vulnerable. In addition, the fundamental moral and ethical dimensions of global warming call for a re-examination of how we use and share the earth's resources, what we pass on to future generations, and how we live in harmony with the environment. Historically, humanity has accommodated increases in population size through various adaptive mechanisms, but the world's growing population, which surpassed seven billion people in late 2011, will undoubtedly magnify the challenges posed by climate change. Many have questioned drawing linkages between these forces. This is partly because of the difficulties of studying two complicated phenomena and their current and expected effects, as well as fears about the potential for unleashing coercive programming that could violate the rights of individuals and couples to decide freely and responsibly their number and spacing of children. Such controversies have made it more problematic for those in the reproductive health field to advance thinking and programming in this area.

In Chap. 9, Karen Hardee reviews current thinking concerning the role of population and reproductive health in climate change research, discourse and policy discussions, and considers whether this will go beyond previously stalled attempts to consider 'population and environment' linkages in reproductive health and development planning. Hardee discusses current programming on mitigation and adaptation to climate change, how family planning/reproductive health considerations are slowly beginning to be factored into the picture, and how they could be more actively considered in such efforts. She describes nascent approaches to develop reproductive health programming as an integral component of more sustainable environmental practices in areas more vulnerable to climate change. These issues will not recede even if they do not receive the attention they deserve, and most people would rather will them away. The UN's most recent climate change conferences (held in Durban, 2011 and Doha, 2012) further underscored how far world leaders are from making hard decisions and implementing steps even to lower greenhouse gas emissions.

Chapter 10 carries a systematic analysis of international reproductive health aid by Hendrik P. van Dalen and Maja Micevska Scharf. Global aid flows are vital to shaping reproductive health outcomes and are considered here in the context of the global economy and shifting policy approaches to global reproductive rights. The authors review the best available time series data on financial contributions disbursed by governments, NGOs and private institutions, and analyze the shifting landscape of donor policies, programs and financing, as well as their consequences. The authors point to a lack of urgency, insufficient funding, and shifting and diverging priorities, among other factors, in accounting for why the current allocation of aid does not accord well with the plans made at the ICPD in 1994. Development assistance earmarked for reproductive health has come to concentrate on HIV/AIDS at the expense of maternal and child health and family planning. The authors point out that HIV/AIDS programs themselves would profit considerably from a more balanced approach and that the rise in HIV/AIDS funds has disrupted local health care systems, whereas a more balanced investment in reproductive health and HIV/AIDS would make better use of the existing infrastructure. Such needed changes have so far proven very difficult to implement.

Future health needs are difficult to predict, but this analysis also shows how strong the influence of one donor (the United States) is in this setup. Heavily influenced by their support bases, successive U.S. administrations have especially influenced resource flows for reproductive health and its advocacy. The EU has recently become a more important and reliable partner for much of the reproductive health agenda, while private foundations play an increasingly influential source. The landscape of population assistance is a highly volatile one, brought about not only by political issues like the Global Gag Rule[4] and the PEPFAR program,[5] but also by issues of collective action design, as assistance under the heading of the MDGs has crowded out family planning. The analysis further highlights the need for greater efficiency in a time of limited resources and global economic uncertainty, an important argument made also by many donor countries and institutions.

1.3   A Look Back and Push Forward

The final chapter to the second part of the book features a round-table symposium on the past, present and future of reproductive health. This comprises commentaries from five authors who have made distinct contributions to the field's development over their varied careers. Each has been asked by the editor to look

---

[4]The Global Gag Rule has been a recurrent political flashpoint in the U.S. abortion debate ever since it was first announced by U.S. President Ronald Reagan at the time of the 1984 International Conference on Population held in Mexico City (and after which it is also referred to sometimes as the 'Mexico City policy'). The policy required NGOs that receive funds from the United States Agency for International Development (USAID) for international population assistance (notably for family planning) to refrain from using their own, non-USAID funds to provide any activities that perform, counsel, or promote abortion services, even in cases of rape or incest. Successive U.S. Republican administrations have re-imposed the policy and misleadingly presented it as a direct step in defunding abortions conducted overseas, even though the U.S. government has been prohibited from directly funding such services under the 1973 Helms Amendment to the Foreign Assistance Act. Although aimed nominally at abortion, the policy has had multiple negative public health repercussions such as reducing access to family planning, postabortion care, maternal and child health services, and for some time, even to HIV-prevention and AIDS-related services (Crane and Dusenberry 2004; Kulczycki 2007).

[5]The President's Emergency Plan for AIDS Relief (PEPFAR) program was created by in 2003 by President Bush and extended by his successor, President Obama. It authorized large new resource allocations for HIV/AIDS programs in severely affected low-income countries and has expanded the use and availability of anti-retroviral HIV/AIDS drug therapies in such nations, particularly in sub-Saharan Africa.

back critically on where the reproductive field has been in the past and where it is at presently, so as to derive valuable insights and pointers to move the field forward. Each individual contribution to Chap. 11 constitutes a rich set of insights and observations. Collectively, they remind us that the field has made some major gains since it rose to ascendancy on the world stage at the ICPD, and that it has expanded and been enriched in the process. Yet despite these gains, there are still huge deficits in many areas of reproductive health, the promotion of reproductive rights is often problematic, and it remains difficult to raise adequate funds to realize reproductive health and to provide extra services. Each of the contributors stresses the importance of the policy environment for advancing reproductive health science and praxis. They also underscore the need to better advocate for evidence-based policy and the instruments (such as the MDGs) to make it happen.

Daniel Pellegrom takes stock of his career as president of a major international reproductive health organization to discuss the central challenges facing the reproductive health movement. These, he argues, are conceptual and political, rather than technical. The early pioneers of the movements for family planning and women's health in the U.S. and overseas understood that their movements were about social reform, which is inherently controversial. This perspective is often lost on those trained to provide technical expertise and assistance alone. However, reproductive health is about more than providing preventive health care. The field is controversial because, like other humanitarian efforts, it involves providing services to the poor and the most disadvantaged, as well as respecting the most basic and personal decisions, which include those concerning childbearing. Hence, those working in the reproductive health field must be willing to take a stand for social justice and be prepared to challenge traditional notions about gender roles, sex and sexuality.

The second contribution is by Marleen Temmerman, who combines her experience as a gynecologist, reproductive health researcher and politician, and Neil Datta, who helps coordinate the work of European members of parliament concerned with sexual and reproductive health. They consider the contrasting responses of the international community to the exceptionality of both family planning and HIV/AIDS. Advocates concerned with this deeply stigmatized disease have been vastly more effective in securing the public acceptance and political will needed to generate resources and action. The authors argue that better communication of evidence-based facts is critical to depoliticizing family planning (and, more generally, to sexual and reproductive health and rights). This would help advance implementation efforts and overcome inadequate public and political concern with strengthening women's rights and health systems. It could also help moderate cultural, religious, and other interpretations that may deny individuals' rights and harm sexual and reproductive health.

Enormous progress can be made through good science and passionate advocacy. Jill Sheffield underscores this point in the third commentary, where she reflects on her career in advocating for maternal health and for women's health and empowerment more generally, as well as on the success of recent efforts to help put MDG 5 back on the international agenda. This progress has been spurred along by alerting politicians more forcefully to the intersection between maternal health and economic growth, and the multiple returns such investments yield. Making this better business case has had a powerful galvanizing effect (as at the global Women Deliver conferences of 2007, 2010, and 2013, which were well attended by world leaders and covered by its media), although there is a continued need to further substantiate the linkages highlighted and to make sure their benefits are widely shared within society. In contrast, the previous longstanding focus on health or medical outcomes alone was associated with insufficient political will and investment on strategies that work. The author distills eight take-home lessons for future advocacy efforts in this area and for reproductive health more generally.

The contribution by Stan Bernstein draws on his involvement in UN activities concerning the ICPD, the Millennium Project, and the subsequent re-integration of family planning and other reproductive health concerns into the MDGs. Recent discussions of population growth as a driver of global climate change and of political and economic insecurity ignore the need for investments in reproductive health programs that would, inter alia, help implement lower desired family size preferences. (In much the same way, development dialogue on health focuses almost exclusively on the reduction of mortality outcomes, to the neglect of other aspects of health). The author argues that despite the essential focus on individual rights and welfare, reproductive health additionally needs a more instrumental mentality to garner more investments that could help better realize those rights. He sees opportunities to capitalize on new foci that seem likely to emerge in a successor arrangement to the ICPD and MDGs. Other pertinent issues that may win more official recognition include women's empowerment and agency, the social context of unintended pregnancy, intergenerational relations, and health systems strengthening. These potential prospects could help ensure the integration of reproductive health components with other health care delivery.

Lastly, Elizabeth Lule reflects on the large, unfinished reproductive health agenda in her native Uganda, and on her work experiences with major international NGO, bilateral and multilateral institutions. Among other issues, she stresses that the reproductive health field should incorporate social justice and equity considerations with the same passion as it does individual rights. This would allow, for example, more targeted services to underserved, marginalized and vulnerable groups, which could reduce the huge disparities in reproductive health and accelerate progress to achieving the MDGs. The author briefly surveys opportunities and threats within the fragmented and unpredictable global aid architecture, and cautions that we should be mindful of how program planning, implementation, and accountability occur at different levels, and how service integration is attempted, monitored, and evaluated. Bolder thinking on this front may permit the reproductive health field to more effectively embrace new financing mechanisms, instruments, and partnerships, as well as multi-sectoral approaches that are becoming more common across various fields and that could have greater multiplier effects for reproductive health, social and economic outcomes.

1.4 Strengthening Service and Program Capacity

Part III of the book deals with application and presents several innovative strategies for strengthening service and program capacity to deliver reproductive health care in the face of profound health system and programmatic challenges. The four chapters included in Part III emphasize new thinking, best practices and lessons learned about how to transcend programmatic barriers, respond to client needs, and strengthen services and programs. New technologies and other innovations hold much promise to improve health, but inattention to many details of the service context, as well as the economic, social and political systems within which they operate, leads to the widespread failure of many good health technologies to get delivered and used, especially for poor people in poor countries (Frost and Reich 2008). The chapters in this section emphasize the critical importance of bringing technologies and services to those who need them, as well as to more effectively plan for such success and to reduce gaps in access. In response to such prescient needs, increased attention is given here to contraceptive care in sub-Saharan Africa. Contraception is a proven, cost-effective way to reduce mortality substantially as well as to help women and couples plan their families. As indicated in Chaps. 7 and 10 especially, access to family planning has been sorely neglected in development priorities. The need for strengthened reproductive health services, especially family planning, is substantial and urgent, nowhere more so than in sub-Saharan Africa which lags far behind the rest of the world in family planning use.

New business models and strategies for registering and introducing technologies, new and improved contraceptives, and improved modes of service delivery, hold great potential for helping women meet their family planning needs. Many women lack access to long-acting reversible contraceptives (LARCs)[6] such as intrauterine devices (IUDs) and hormonal implants, which tend to be underutilized. These are safe, highly effective, cost-effective, and low-maintenance methods, with the ideal 'forgettable' default state (no regular action by the user and no routine clinical follow-up are required) and rapid reversibility (or return to fertility). The first three chapters in this section discuss efforts to introduce and re-position IUDs, low-cost implants and injectables in the contraceptive method mix. However, the promise of such new and revitalized methods can be dissipated by numerous cultural, economic, social and medical barriers to accessing and using family planning methods. In particular, medical barriers at the national regulatory or policy level (which may impede approval, promotion or advertising of existing or newly developed methods), or at the program or individual provider level, often result in the unnecessary denial or delay of services to women and couples who would like to plan their families and prevent unintended pregnancies (Shelton et al. 1992; Bertrand et al. 1995).

---

[6]The acronym LA/PM (long-acting and permanent method of contraception) is also used to refer to female sterilization and vasectomy, as well as IUDs and hormonal implants. These are all clinical methods of family planning, in contrast to the "re-supply" methods of condoms, pills and injectables. The term 'long-acting' helps focus attention on the method's intrinsic characteristics rather than the length of time a client may actually use the method.

Such barriers need not apply if programs, providers and policymakers are prepared to address these deep-seated obstacles to access.

The chapters in this section emphasize the critical importance of bringing technologies and services to those who need them, as well as to more effectively plan for such success and to reduce gaps in access. The first three chapters document ways to make LARCs and injectables more widely available through national health systems, community-based provision, and other channels. Chapters 12 and 13 use diffusion theory to help inform and account for successful uptake of innovative practices in this endeavour. Increasing access to quality family planning and reproductive health care often depends on understanding how change can be induced in medical settings. These are hierarchical and conservative, with well-established policies and routine practices, and clinical providers acting as gatekeepers to services. In Chap. 12, Roy Jacobstein discusses strategies to accelerate the rate, extent, and sustainability of change in medical care settings, with particular regard to 'jumpstarting' the IUD in sub-Saharan Africa. Worldwide, the IUD is the most popular method of contraception after female sterilization, relied on presently by one in seven women of childbearing age. However, increased options, as well as a set of provider biases and client misperceptions, have led to IUD use falling in many countries, even in African countries with relatively strong family planning programs such as Kenya.

Chapter 12 discusses a holistic programming model, which holds that a coordinated package of programmatic activities among the supply, demand, and policy/advocacy program areas can be not only efficacious, but also mutually reinforcing. This model guided the implementation of a project to "revitalize" IUD use in Kisii District of Kenya's Nyanza Province. The author describes how this approach has reversed the method's fortunes and proved sustainable despite severe jolts to the health system. Particular attention was paid to four important cross-cutting elements in reproductive health programming: the fundamentals of care (safety, quality, and choice); use of local data for decision-making; gender equity; and stakeholder participation. Although modest in size, funding, geographic scope, and duration, this effort demonstrates that gains in IUD uptake and use, along with other positive service changes, can be fostered and sustained long after project activities have ended in medical settings initially resistant to such change and in the resource-strapped public sector. These developments likely also promoted greater use of other reproductive health services and occurred despite district restructuring, transfer of skilled staff, and pervasive misunderstandings about the IUD. Many of the lessons learned may further apply to the levonorgestrel-releasing intrauterine system (LNG-IUS), which is being introduced in more countries. This offers women the same long-acting, low-maintenance protection of the regular copper-IUD with fewer potential side effects of bleeding and cramping, and with added gynecological value.[7]

---

[7]The LNG-IUS offers endometrial health benefits, helps treat menorrhagia and, slightly reduces risk of pelvic inflammatory disease (PID). By reducing heavy menstrual bleeding, the LNG-IUS is also the contraceptive method of choice for most women who are more prone to iron-deficiency anemia (whereas copper-bearing devices tend to reduce hemoglobin).

Contraceptive injectables and implants may be preferable to IUDs for women because they are more readily initiated, requiring no vaginal procedure. Injectables are also among the most effective reversible methods that are independent of intercourse. They are useful when other options are contraindicated or disliked, although they can be associated with menstrual irregularities and weight gain. The injectable most widely used in most countries is Depo-Provera (medroxyprogesterone acetate, DMPA), which prevents pregnancy for up to 3 months with each intramuscular injection.[8] In Chap. 13, John Stanback and Reid Miller chart and account for the recent extraordinary rapid rise of injectable contraceptives as the most common modern method choice in sub-Saharan Africa. He explains this spread in part to the method's intrinsic characteristics (effectiveness, ease of use, and privacy), but more importantly to several other factors specific to the continent. This recent diffusion carries the potential for changing the story of family planning in rural Africa, where clinics are few and far between, and typically offer few contraceptive choices. However, access to injectable contraception in the region has always been over-medicalized, notwithstanding a chronic shortage of health care workers and high levels of unwanted fertility and maternal mortality. The result of the innovation was logical, but radical in the eyes of many local medical authorities and in the context of major vertical health care programs: the provision of the continent's favorite contraceptive by its lowest level health workers and through the under-utilized mechanism of community-based family planning programs.

The author outlines why adoption has stalled so far in Nigeria, why uptake is slow in Kenya, and key reasons for the ongoing successful scale-up of recent small pilot studies in Ethiopia, Madagascar, Malawi, Senegal and Uganda. These programs are demonstrating that community health workers (CHWs) can safely and effectively administer injectables, and that these services should be part of family planning programs in resource-limited settings. Growing international consensus on these matters is helping this practice spread in an increasing number of African countries, a diffusion process fueled by the combination of evidence, advocacy, and the common sense of giving women what they want, where they want it. In the process, the 'radical' notion of community provision of injectables, pioneered three decades ago in Bangladesh, is finally arriving on the continent that needs it most. Moreover, this innovation may spread even faster with the anticipated availability of a new technology that replaces syringes and vials with a simple, new pre-filled injection device called "Uniject."

---

[8]Depo-Provera contains a progestin, a drug very similar to progesterone, the hormone normally produced by the ovaries every month as part of the menstrual cycle. Also known as 'Depo' or simply as 'the shot,' DMPA has been used since the 1960s, although its introduction and acceptance in many parts of the world only occurred after it was approved by the US Food and Drug Administration in 1992. Combined injectable contraceptives are widely used outside the U.S. and include monthly injections of progesterone and estradiol taken to inhibit fertility. Injectables are also convenient, discrete, and have various non-contraceptive health benefits, as well as the possible side-effects noted in the text. There have also been longstanding fears about possible reduction in bone mineral density associated with prolonged DMPA use; and in 2011, a new possible association was reported with HIV acquisition and transmission, although this remains unproven and the evidence (based on an observational study design) is far from persuasive (see also Chap. 13).

Hormone-releasing sub-dermal implants prevent pregnancy for several years after a single administration and have high rates of user satisfaction. However, they have been underutilized due to high cost, a lack of trained providers in some areas, and the flawed experience of Norplant, a five-rod implant in the 1990s (Harrison and Rosenfield 1998). Worldwide use remains low, although implants are more cost-effective in the long term than short-acting methods such as less expensive oral contraceptives and other hormonal methods. Chapter 14 assesses ongoing efforts to construct effective architecture at the global and national levels for the large-scale introduction and diffusion of a low-cost, two-rod, levonorgestrel-releasing implant manufactured in China. Sino-implant (II) has been proven to be similarly effective and safe, and its cost substantially undercuts that of other contraceptive implants on the market and procured by international donors. By 2011, it had already been used by over seven million women in China and Indonesia, and had been registered in 15 countries (mostly African); and in 2012, this growing success pressured other implant manufacturers to lower their prices. Kate Rademacher, Heather Vahdat, Laneta Dorflinger, Derek Owen, and Markus Steiner describe how a new global business model has been pieced together between public, private, and non-governmental organizations to facilitate access to this affordable, high-quality, long-term contraceptive option in resource-constrained countries.

Pharmaceuticals are now made in an increasing number of countries. Contraceptive commodities manufactured in emerging market countries present specific challenges with respect to ensuring product quality and obtaining regulatory approval, issues which are not well understood. The authors outline the development of a strategy coordinated across multiple countries for successful product registration, introduction, and scale-up. These activities have included setting up quality assurance mechanisms to meet international standards; working with distributors to gain national regulatory approval and establish price ceilings; supporting a dossier submission to WHO's prequalification program; conducting post-marketing survelliance studies; and providing technical assistance with introduction activities at the country level. The authors further describe early experiences with product introduction in Sierra Leone and Kenya, the first countries outside of Asia to register Sino-implant (II) under the trade name Zarin. Service statistics and key informant interviews suggest some initial successes and positive client feedback. Findings also indicate the need for increased attention to overcome service delivery and procurement constraints, and to ensure that medical barriers to access are not institutionalized. Nevertheless, initial results suggest that the appropriately phased introduction of contraceptives into reproductive health programs can lead to substantial cost-savings for governments and donors, as well as expanded access to highly effective methods.

The final chapter of this section focuses on adolescents/young adults, who are both our common future and a vulnerable population with unique needs. This hard-to-reach population often receives scant program resources, with more work needed to better understand ways to improve their access to reproductive health care and to simultaneously help them secure livelihoods. The challenges to conducting such work are especially complex in post-conflict and fragile states. Their health systems do not often figure into international health priorities and policies, peace building and stabilization operations, and human rights and governance. In such settings, expanding the evidence-base to deepen understanding of the complex relationship between the well-being of vulnerable youth and a country's development goals is crucial to developing meaningful interventions. Chapter 15 describes the development and application of a new approach for improving access to resources and services for vulnerable young people in post-conflict settings and other fragile states. The steps comprising the approach are not unique, but their integration into a cohesive process bringing evidence more directly into institutional decision-making sets it apart from other needs assessment activities or situation analyses.

Adam Weiner and Andrzej Kulczycki illustrate this approach with an application to marginalized Liberian youth, particularly out-of-school adolescent mothers and young adults. This project sought to combine adolescent sexual and reproductive health with efforts to develop stable employment opportunities by eliciting and making heard the voices of vulnerable communities, and by promoting collaboration between them and local, national and international partner agencies. The methods also involve analyzing data on the coverage of youth services to profile beneficiaries; and disaggregating population-based data to create vulnerability maps and to profile large concentrations of marginalized young people for identifying gaps in service provision. The subsequent linkage of tailored sexual and reproductive health information and services with livelihood programs may expand social capital and employment-based capabilities, and facilitates the design of services that are accessible, geographically targeted and appropriate. The authors discuss how this approach has led to several such improved programs. The efforts of local and international NGOs to expand service delivery, however, have also faced the challenges of shifting institutional priorities, fiscal sustainability, staff changes, and continued lack of impact evaluation. Nevertheless, this systematic process to address the needs of marginalized youth and provide more equitable access to programs and services is also broadly applicable to other resource-poor and fragile states.

Reproductive health is essential for us all. The concept provides a framework for thinking about sex and reproduction, and for highlighting many of its components and interrelations. While the concept seems relatively simple enough, in reality, countless social and other determinants help shape reproductive health and multiple needs are not being met. This book cannot cover all potential topics, but the editor and contributors have sought to address a number of emerging and cross-cutting issues. They have provided a set of informative essays that are comprehensive in scope and which may stimulate and advance work in this vital field. The contents of this book will find different niches among different readers. All will benefit from the insights they will be able to synthesize given the diversity of disciplines, geographic locations, and professional expertise of the authors. My hope is that the reader will use this book either as a beginning or as a resource, but not as an end, to his or her exploration of the subject.

The genesis of this work has multiple roots. In teaching a course on reproductive health for over a decade, I had often sought to steer students to new and emerging critical issues. This also came naturally from working within the field. I began to conceptualize the need and outline for this book. As editor, I had general oversight of the project and steered it along. I corresponded and talked frequently with the authors to help discuss their thoughts and to assure consistent attention to detail, but always allowing them to speak in their own rich and powerful voices. Many thanks go to each author for preparing the manuscripts and sharing their valuable expertise. I also much appreciate helpful comments from Robyn Davis, Suzanne Dhall, Ronnie Johnson, and Cassandra Pappenfuse on various manuscripts in this volume. I would additionally like to extend my gratitude to Evelien Bakker and Bernadette Deelen-Mans of Springer for the encouragement and patience they have shown me in bringing this volume to fruition. Last but not least, thanks to my phenomenal family – my parents, to whom I dedicate this book; my two special daughters, Anna and Izabella; and my great partner and wife, Lucia – thanks for everything you do and for being who you are – simply special.

References

Bertrand, J. T., Hardee, K., Magnani, R. J., & Angle, M. A. (1995). Access, quality of care and medical barriers in family planning programs. *International Family Planning Perspectives, 21*(2), 64–69, 74.

Binka, F. N., Bawah, A. A., Phillips, J. F., Hodgson, A., Adjuik, M., & MacLeod, B. B. (2007). Rapid achievement of the child survival Millennium Development Goal: Evidence from the Navrongo Experiment in northern Ghana. *Tropical Disease and International Health, 12*(5), 578–593.

Crane, B. B., & Dusenberry, J. (2004). Power and politics in international funding for reproductive health: The Global Gag Rule. *Reproductive Health Matters, 12*(24), 128–137.

Frost, L. J., & Reich, M. R. (2008). *Access: How do good health technologies get to poor people in poor countries?* Cambridge, MA: Harvard University Press.

Harrison, P. F., & Rosenfield, A. (Eds.). (1998). *Contraceptive research, introduction, and use: Lessons from Norplant.* New York: National Academy Press.

Kulczycki, A. (1999). *The abortion debate in the world arena.* London/New York: Macmillan/ Routledge.

Kulczycki, A. (2007). Ethics, ideology, and reproductive health policy in the United States. *Studies in Family Planning, 38*(4), 333–351.

Kulczycki, A. (2011). Abortion in Latin America: Changes in practice, growing conflict, and recent policy developments. *Studies in Family Planning, 42*(3), 199–220.

Reddy, U. M., Wapner, R. J., Robert, W., Rebar, R. J., & Tasca, R. J. (2007). Infertility, assisted reproductive technology, and adverse pregnancy outcomes: Executive summary of a National Institute of Child Health and Human Development workshop. *Obstetrics and Gynecology, 109*(4), 967–977.

Schieve, L. A., Devine, O., Boyle, C. A., Petrini, J. R., & Warner, L. (2009). Estimation of the contribution of non-assisted reproductive technology ovulation stimulation fertility treatments to US singleton and multiple births. *American Journal of Epidemiology, 170*(11), 1396–1407.

Shelton, J. D., Angle, M. A., & Jacobstein, R. A. (1992). Medical barriers to access to family planning. *Lancet, 340*(8831), 1334–1335.

UNAIDS (Joint United Nations Programme on HIV/AIDS). (2012). *UNAIDS report on the global AIDS epidemic.* Geneva: UNAIDS. Available at: http://www.unaids.org/en/media/unaids/ contentassets/documents/epidemiology/2012/gr2012/20121120_UNAIDS_Global_ Report_2012_en.pdf. Accessed 30 Nov 2012.

United Nations (UN). (2011). *World population prospects: The 2010 revision.* New York: UN. Available at: http://esa.un.org/unpd/wpp/index.htm

Part I
Expanding the Research Base

Chapter 2
The Vocabulary of Reproductive Health

Alaka Malwade Basu

2.1 Introduction

A Bengali speaking acquaintance who volunteers at a health centre for Bangladeshi immigrants in East London likes to tell the following story. She once explained in great detail the mechanics of taking the contraceptive pill to the wife in a couple that had come to the clinic for birth control help. Several weeks later, the couple was back, greatly upset that the wife was pregnant. When my acquaintance asked if the pill taking instructions had been strictly followed, the husband took umbrage at her suspicious questioning and declared that he had been most particular about taking the pill with breakfast every morning for 3 weeks and beginning the cycle again after a gap of 1 week. In other words, he had manfully assumed that my friend's advice had been meant for him as he was the household head, and that she had been looking at his wife as she spoke only because she was a well-brought up South Asian woman who did not lock eyes with strange men.

Communication is a funny thing. Even when there appears to be a shared meaning attached to specific words and sentences, a meaning that a dictionary of that language specifies, the dictionary may not be the final arbiter. As the controversies in the philosophy of language illustrate, the meaning of a word often resides in the mind of the speaker or the listener, and this meaning may be sometimes identical to, at other times similar to, and sometimes very different from the meaning attached to that word by the language purist. The meaning of a word also depends on the function it is expected to perform in a given context – to inform, to request, to command, or to simply distract or divert.

This chapter is not about miscommunication when two groups speak clearly different languages. Those barriers are obvious, well acknowledged, and need literal

A.M. Basu, M.Sc. (✉)
Department of Developmental Sociology, Cornell University, Ithaca, NY, USA
e-mail: ab54@cornell.edu

A. Kulczycki (ed.), *Critical Issues in Reproductive Health*, The Springer Series on
Demographic Methods and Population Analysis 33, DOI 10.1007/978-94-007-6722-5_2,
© Springer Science+Business Media Dordrecht 2014

translators. Instead, I focus on situations when all sides are ostensibly speaking the same language and share the literal meaning of words, but still use the same words differently and convey meanings that may not be intended, or one side or the other uses words to deliberately confuse or obfuscate meaning. Often, the intent is also to confuse and to obfuscate to oneself.

In the following sections, I illustrate this proposition by reflecting on some of the ways in which the public health community in general and the reproductive health community in particular may miscommunicate with and/or misunderstand the people it seeks to help. This is of more than intellectual interest; it is also of practical policy interest and underlines the value of qualitative, culturally sensitive, anthropological explorations in public health. It also underlines the need for more innovative methods of diagnosis and treatment.

Within public health, language disconnects are present in several health fields, not just in reproductive health. In these other fields, the disconnects are more frequently an outcome of ignorance or a misunderstanding of the modern scientific basis of different illnesses. At other times, they represent folk understandings or observational descriptions of the course of an illness. An example will suffice to elaborate on this point here.

In many of the Indian languages, tetanus is referred to as *athava* or the 'eighth day illness', in reference to its symptoms manifesting themselves after a week (Basu 1992). This can cause some confusion for the outside investigator, but the lay term for tetanus in the English language, lockjaw, is similarly descriptive and is widespread enough not to need scientific explanation. In any case, the medically used word *tetanus* itself does not really deserve approval for any special 'scientific' insights, as it is derived from the Greek *teinein* for 'to stretch', and stretching is as much an observable descriptive event as the '8th day'.

The more interesting examples come from the field of reproductive health. These reflect more than folk understandings or a suspicion of modern medicine. Instead, reproductive health miscommunications often seem almost deliberate – the words used may be plain and non-controversial, but they are anything but plain or non-controversial once one tries to match them with what a language or medical dictionary says. Moreover, the frequent obliqueness or unrelatedness of the reproductive health discourse to actual illness condition has important implications for the diagnosis, treatment and care of a range of reproductive health conditions that appear straightforward to the clinical or laboratory investigator.

The next two sections illustrate what I mean by the proposition that words say more (or less) than they appear to when an underlying reproductive health motif exists. For the sake of convenience, I look at two categories of verbal gymnastics: in the first case, what appears to be a reproductive health vocabulary is actually being used to talk about quite different things, often only tangentially related to reproductive health as we define it in public health. The second set of interesting verbal representations do the opposite: words that seem to have nothing to do with matters of reproductive health are used to talk about reproductive health issues. In both cases, it needs an astute and careful listener to make medical sense of the conversation.

2.2   Reproductive Health Vocabulary as a Metaphor for Other Things

Reproductive health is a fraught subject. In most cultures, matters to do with the sexual and reproductive life of individuals, especially female individuals, evoke both tensions as well as (even if less often) respect. Not only is woman defined as non-man primarily because of her reproductive role, this bounded definition is sustained by the valorization of reproduction (in addition to the valorization of reproduction for the continuation of the species of course). This means that even as it (especially the sexuality that must precede reproductive success) is feared and controlled, the potentially reproductive body is also to be protected and nurtured. Such protection, in turn, means that many cultures have elaborate norms about acknowledging the reproductive potential and expression of women (as seen, for example, in the rituals to mark the onset of menses, or those mother-centric ones surrounding the birth of a child) as well as elaborate ways of dealing with possible reproductive problems. The proliferation of local remedies to ensure fertility is but one example of this valorization of reproductive success.

All this means that problems with the reproductive system are often a legitimate form of complaint by women, in a way in which other kinds of health problems do not merit. Problems with mental and emotional health get particularly short shrift, and perhaps it is not surprising that one way to draw attention to these is for women to frame them in the language of reproductive health.

At the same time, it is also true that these "women's problems" are embarrassing to discuss, especially with an outsider. Such embarrassment is particularly great in the case of reproductive tract infections, because they draw attention to the sexual behavior that often underlies them. Perhaps for this reason, since the 1990s, as the reproductive health paradigm has become the accepted way of addressing questions of population and health concerns, so there has been much speculation, backed up by some empirical evidence, that women in Third World countries have much higher levels of reproductive tract infections (RTIs) and sexually transmitted infections (STIs) than can be inferred from their own reporting of symptoms. This expected underestimation from surveys has been attributed to the fact that many reproductive health problems are asymptomatic, that women see the symptoms as somehow 'normal', and/or that they are culturally unable to freely discuss their symptoms. Such a perspective, together with the expense and difficulty involved in actually testing clinically and in the laboratory for the presence of RTIs, led to the World Health Organization developing what is called the "syndromic" approach to reproductive health, whereby treatment is encouraged after following a series of algorithms or flow charts to diagnose RTIs from preliminary symptoms, especially in low symptomatic patients (World Health Organization 1993, 1995). These algorithms have got increasingly elaborate over time and now include some form of risk assessment to complement the syndromic approach.

There is now a growing body of evidence that this approach has problems; the most important of these being poor 'positive predictive value' (Basu 2006). A large number of studies suggest that the mismatch between self-reporting and clinical or laboratory diagnosis in developing countries is almost always in the direction of clinical examination turning up *less* infection than self-reporting of symptoms, and laboratory testing turning up even less infection than clinical examination. That is, the proportion of cases identified by this method as infected which truly have the disease is low. This kind of over-diagnosis seems to be the most frequent for the most commonly reported reproductive health problem in the developing world – vaginal discharge. In other words, the syndromic approach runs the frequent danger of a high level of false positives. Symptomatic *non*-RTIs and *non*-STIs may be as prevalent or may be even more prevalent than non-symptomatic RTIs and STIs.[1]

However, wondering if many of the self-reported symptoms of RTIs and STIs may represent non-existent 'physical' problems is politically risky business. Thus we have several studies emphasizing the need to probe in greater detail and with greater empathy so that women report their reproductive health symptoms. While this kind of probing is usually motivated by a desire to catch ailments that women might see as 'normal', it runs the very real risk of medicalizing normal physiological states or medicalizing non-physical distress. It would be much more useful to get into the semantics of the survey conversation. What do descriptions of 'weakness' and 'vaginal discharge' and 'lower back pain' represent?

A reading of the anthropological literature and especially the literature on the emotions suggests that the high levels of reporting of particular kinds of apparently reproductive health problems (vaginal discharge in particular, but also lower back pain and generalized 'weakness') is at least partly related to the rules about emotional 'expression' in many cultures, whereby emotional states like sadness, grieving and stress are expressed in the language of physical rather than psychic ailments. These ailments are no less real for being emotional rather than physiological; indeed they are distinct problems of reproductive health given the current definition of reproductive health to include all forms (physical, mental, psychological) of well-being on matters related to sexuality, pregnancy, deliveries and the organs involved in these, but they need another kind of cultural understanding, not antibiotics.

The most frequently cited example in anthropology of emotional states being expressed in bodily language is perhaps the practice of Tahitians describing sadness in terms of fatigue of the body (Levy 1984). In India, women often claim symptoms of vaginal discharge as a proxy for mental depression (Patel and Oomman 1999). Nichter (1981) describes the common constellation of symptoms of vaginal discharge, dizziness, backache and weakness as the "bodily idiom of distress".

Indeed, as Trollope-Kumar reports, in the past (that is, before, reproductive health became an 'official' public health concern), experienced gynecologists would prescribe iron, vitamins, calcium and nutrition, food and rest for many of these symptoms. All this is not to suggest that reproductive tract infections are

---

[1]For growing evidence of this possible overestimation, see Oomman (1996) and Prasad et al. (1999), on India; Zurayk et al. (1995), on Egypt; Bulut et al. (1997), on Turkey; Lien at al (2002), on Vietnam; Nayab (2004), on Pakistan, Pepin et al. (2004), on West Africa, Hawkes et al. (1999), on Bangladesh.

not important in the developing world; of course they are, even if it is difficult to estimate prevalence rates from clinical studies that are based on self-selected groups (as Ramasubban 2000, for example underscores in her review – except that this review assumes that prevalence levels must be much higher than clinically reported levels). It is merely to caution against assuming that the popular discourse, as well as women's self-reports to sufficiently interested and probing medical practitioners, automatically imply that women are plagued by infections that need 'medical' treatment.

The reproductive health implications of such emotional stress are especially important in the early years of marriage in conservative societies, when sometimes painful or otherwise unsatisfactory sexual relations may lead to unspecific health problems and an over-reporting of reproductive tract problems, vaginal discharge being the most commonly reported (Osella and Osella 2002; Obeyesekere 1976; Trollope-Kumar 1999). Such emotional underpinning of supposedly physical reproductive health is still poorly researched in the public health literature; but it illustrates excellently how language can mislead. In turn, correct diagnosis and effective treatment are hampered without ways of overcoming these semantic obstacles. One therefore needs to devise alternative routes to identify and deal with reproductive health issues in the developing world. One such way to better predict and confirm STIs in women might be to exploit the fact that symptoms of such infections in women are much more non-specific than they are in men. And given the constraints on female sexual activity in the South Asian region (that means that women are likely to be getting such infections from their husbands than the other way around), it may be more cost effective as well as medically wise to focus on the diagnosis of STIs in men and then to track the partners/wives of infected men (see Hawkes 1998; Collumbien et al. 1999).

While such a focus makes sense, the problem is that men are also often as unable as women to differentiate the symptoms of STIs from general problems related to the sexual organs and sexual functioning. Thus, when pressed to report possible STIs, they tend to come up with a list of symptoms that could be ascribed to sexually transmitted infection, but could just as likely be problems associated with the reproductive tract (or, as the biosocial literature ominously calls it, the 'nether regions'), like genital itching and rash that are what may be called 'non-contact' related – that is, not acquired through sexual relations (Verma et al. 2001). Or common non-RTI problems like hydrocele and filariasis often get reported as STIs and RTIs (see, for example, Bang and Bang 1997). Moreover, they also often use the medical terminology of STIs and not just the language of STI *symptoms*, to describe non-STI problems of reproductive health. For example, at least partly thanks to public health campaigns, even rural and slum male respondents in different parts of India spout words like 'gonorrhea' and 'syphilis' (more accurately, they spout Indianized pronunciations of these English language words) to interviewers probing reproductive and sexual health (see, among others, Collumbien et al. 1999; Verma et al. 2001).

On the other hand, the last paragraph is not meant to imply that STIs are not a real problem. Indeed, the semantic confusion can lead to underestimation just as it can lead to overestimation in the examples above. For example, Verma et al. (2001) describe how men in their Mumbai slum study ascribe real STI symptoms to non-sexual modes of transmission related to excessive heat in the body generated by wrong diet or too much hard labor. In addition, like women, men often seem to use the language of STIs to express other anxieties, some of which are decidedly related to sexual matters. For example, in a study in Uttar Pradesh, India, the proportions of men who described what seemed to be symptoms of STIs (difficulty urinating, pain during urination, swollen testes) and who admitted to premarital sexual activity were uncannily similar (both around 13 %). This may suggest that breaking norms about sexual behavior may induce greater worries about contracting messy infections rather than actually producing such infections (Narayana 1996). Similar reporting of the symptoms of STI and RT infections often accompanies guilt about supposedly harmful practices like masturbation. As Hawkes (1998) underlines, many of these self-reported symptoms do not turn out to be indications of STIs on clinical or laboratory testing.

At other times, psychosocial anxieties related to a variety of aspects of life, not all of them sexual or reproductive, get described in bodily terms through male complaints about a constellation of symptoms, most commonly a triumvirate of weakness/tiredness, internal heat and excessive semen loss. At one level these are plausibly symptoms of reproductive system problems (whether contact based or not); but they are often also a way of expressing and/or explaining other kinds of unhappinesses and tensions, and the last thing they need is a medical practitioner who prescribes antibiotics or, even worse, as in Collumbien et al.'s Orissa study, declares the presence of HIV/AIDS, but, mercifully, a case of 'curable' AIDS!

The slowly growing literature on men's perceptions and reporting of reproductive health problems is coming up with conclusions that parallel so closely the conclusions of studies of women's reproductive health problems that one needs to seriously reexamine some of the existing stereotypes in the social science literature on the unidirectional nature of gender inequalities in real and apparent reproductive health. It is increasingly obvious that men's reproductive health issues warrant better understanding for biomedical reasons; what is still not sufficiently acknowledged is that male reproductive health matters also need much more social understanding.

In any case, lay persons are not alone in redefining, renaming and reframing reproductive health problems. The medical fraternity often flounders as well. This is at least partly because biomedical definitions and understandings of illness are far from being as precise as they appear to be, even when they hide behind difficult-to-spell-and-pronounce Greek names. O'Flynn's and Britten (2004) description of primary care practitioners in London grappling with diagnoses of dysmenorrhea and menorrhagia among patients who complained of menstrual disorders illustrates this very well. In this study, the problem seemed to be especially acute for male practitioners; these physicians only had textbooks to turn to, whereas female doctors added to this textbook knowledge the non-scientific but very helpful guidelines from personal menstrual experience! Both sets of physicians may use the Greek words to diagnose these menstrual disorders, but finally find themselves reduced to making subjective evaluations of heavy or painful periods that are not much more 'scientific' than their patients' own evaluations.

Discordance between lay and medical interpretations of reproductive health risk can also occur because the *social* meaning attached to supposedly technical terms can vary widely. Take the question of what demographers and public health specialists call 'unsafe' sex. What they mean by this term is 'unprotected' (another favorite phrase within the DHS discourse) sex; or sex that is practiced without contraception, so that it increases the risk of an unwanted pregnancy, and especially sex that is performed without the use of condoms, so that it increases the risks of both unwanted pregnancies as well as STIs, the most horrifying of these of course being HIV.

On the other hand, the social science literature on young people's romantic and sexual behavior finds that the word 'unsafe' often means something very different. For example, when idle youth engage in sexual activity with steady or casual partners in Abraham's (2002) lower middle class survey in Mumbai, India, safety means secrecy, the ability to have fun or serious sex without getting caught out by those who would disapprove or excommunicate – parents, other elders, competitors, spouses, state-sponsored moral police. In other contexts, medically 'unsafe' sex is emotionally 'safe' sex – it legitimizes the problematic erotic by investing a relationship with an aura of love and romance that could not be sustained if there were awkward insistences on preventing pregnancy or infection – such insistence displays a lack of trust in one's partner as well as a lack of love for one's partner in several studies of adolescent sexual behavior.[2]

2.3   Bypassing the Vocabulary of Reproductive Health to Talk About Reproductive Health

If emotional distress is difficult to express in plain language in many cultures and so must resort to the more acceptable vocabulary of reproductive health, this is not to say that the subject of reproductive health is always easily brought up, especially in conversations with strangers, even white-coated strangers. Indeed, if there is one category of health problems that is shrouded in metaphorical language almost deliberately (however subliminally), then this must be the category of health problems related to the sexual and reproductive systems of individuals. Metaphors that describe illnesses like tetanus or small pox in non-medical terms reflect folk understandings or a sense of fatalism/helplessness in the face of (at least at one time) unconquerable illnesses. The reproductive health case is different – ailments related to it require a language of opacity or ambiguity because they arouse embarrassment, conflicting emotions, or political and religious passion. It is no wonder that in North India sexually transmitted diseases are referred to *gupt rog* or the secret illnesses or

---

[2]See for example, Sobo (1995), Rosenthal et al. (1998), Kirkman et al. (1998), and Smith (2004).

ailments of the secret parts of the body. Talking freely and honestly about sexual and reproductive matters is not easy in any culture; when in addition these matters are the cause of discomfort, pain, or guilt or other kinds of suffering, the conversation has to get even more convoluted.

At times, the intent of misleading language is to score a political point. In the reproductive health field, nothing illustrates this polemical role of language better than self-definitions of U.S. groups for and against abortion. Those against abortion by other women call themselves 'pro-life' and those in favor of allowing it are by their own description 'pro-choice'. These are ironic definitions to say the least. A non-American, unfamiliar with late twentieth-century U.S. politics, might be forgiven for assuming that the pro-lifers were a body of pacifists, opposed to war, military invasions, capital punishment, and private gun ownership. And she would be forgiven for assuming that the pro-choicers (if I may coin such a word) were anarchists against big government, social welfare and progressive tax rates, and in favor of a Walmart in every town.

How wrong this innocent non-American would be. The abortion question has its own vocabulary of political grandstanding, one that uses words to convey moral righteousness by both sides. For which moral being can object to the ideology of either pro-life or pro-choice? That these terms do little to enlighten us about the moral ambiguities inherent in the abortion procedure is clear from the inflexibility of the adherents of each position.

These moral ambiguities are perhaps more deeply felt and expressed in the language and terminology of those who might choose to have an abortion themselves, as opposed to hectoring others about their choices. Some years ago I edited a book on the social and political context of abortion (Basu 2003) in which several authors independently ended up reflecting on the cultural vocabulary of abortion in different parts of the world. Most of these authors are anthropologists, and so they brought to their chapters direct evidence from their field sites, which were scattered all over the world and yet demonstrated very similar kinds of semantic tools to lessen the emotional and physical confusion about the abortion decision, even when it was a common occurrence.

Most of these semantic strategies hinge on the ambiguities surrounding important biological questions; and these ambiguities are not just figments of the lay imagination. These unanswered and probably unanswerable questions relate to uncertainties about timing: When exactly does a delayed menstrual period qualify to be called a pregnancy? When exactly does an established pregnancy acquire 'life'? When exactly does a fetus acquire a 'soul'?

Not only is there much scope for ambiguity in the answers to these questions, cultures can often actively encourage such ambiguity. Broadly, this happens in two ways. One, the restoring of menses is not seen as having anything to do with terminating a pregnancy. Secondly, pregnancies (or rather, delayed menses) are not seen as having a clear relationship with the beginning of life. The presence of a life in the womb is seen as beginning with symptoms and under conditions that are only marginally related to the menstrual cycle. In such understandings, what western medicine may call an "abortion" is not an abortion at all until there is a culturally defined pregnancy and a life that can be aborted.

Thus, under many circumstances, a delayed menstrual period is seen as just that - a delayed menstrual period, which may have nothing to do with pregnancy but is instead a sign of other health problems, problems that may in fact later *prevent* a much-wanted pregnancy. Levin (2003) describes the 'cleaning the belly' that restoring regular, healthy menstrual flow is seen to involve in rural Guinea. Needless to say, this action of restoring menstruation to its regular 'healthy' state is not perceived as having anything to do with abortion, which women, as well as the traditional healers who help them restore menses, are strongly against. In this formulation abortion is not only illegal, it is morally abhorrent and against all societal norms. Renne (2003) provides further illustration of such resort to ambiguous language to legitimize what western medicine sees as an abortion. In her study area in Northern Nigeria, many potential abortifacients are referred to as medicines that 'put a pregnancy to sleep' or 'make a pregnancy lie down', the intent being to later reactivate such a sleeping pregnancy at a more fortuitous time.

Cultural ideas about 'human growth' facilitate abortion even more simply in Stambach's (2003) Tanzanian study. Here, a delayed menstrual period signifies nothing more than a 'grain of sand', which can proceed to a real pregnancy and fetus only with continued nourishment from both parents. The nurture from the male in this framework requires continued intercourse with a socially acceptable genitor, so that the flesh, blood and bones that go to make up a life can be generated. Once this happens, abortion is naturally frowned upon. But as long as all that occupies a womb is a few grains of sand, or even 'nyama' (meat) which does not yet have a sufficient and continuous input from the male, it is hardly a human life that is being destroyed when attempts are made to reinstate regular menses.

Women, or indeed families, are not alone in using language to get around normative, legal or religious proscriptions on abortion. Even while endorsing these proscriptions in principle, service providers, the state, as well as organized religion may, through the right choice of words, make it much easier for women to obtain an abortion than a simple perusal of religious or legal views on abortion would imply. Anarfi (2003), for example, describes a popular selling strategy that bypasses legal prohibitions in Ghana. Herbalists prescribe "tonics" which they warn women "not to take if pregnant" since they may lead to a miscarriage. In plain language what this translates into is of course the advertisement of an abortifacient, and girls and women with unwanted pregnancies interpret this message accordingly.

The state too may sometimes collude with this sleight of hand. Perhaps the best example of such collusion is in the rapid rise of "Menstrual Regulation" as a health service in several parts of the world. Amin (2003) describes the legal and religious ambiguities that help Bangladesh to actively promote what it resolutely calls 'Menstrual Regulation' or, even more neutrally and catchily, MR. As it is, four of the five schools of Islamic jurisprudence do not outrightly forbid abortion in the early stages of a pregnancy, that is, before ensoulment. Moreover, there is not complete agreement on when ensoulment occurs. The leeway that this ambiguity provides has been further strengthened by medical technology. The development of the procedure for menstrual regulation, being relatively safe, easy and inexpensive, has made it easier for the health and family planning program to exploit the ambiguity in the meaning of a missed period by the relatively simple method of not doing a pregnancy test for menses which are delayed by only a few weeks (on MR, see also Islam et al. 2004).

Such seeking of the moral high ground by the state or other authorities can sometimes take comical form. For example, in her review of the 1986 debates in the Indian Parliament on commercial sex workers, Gangoli (2009) reveals the energy and moral posturing expended by some Parliamentarians on the nomenclature of 1956 law regarding prostitution and trafficking. Called *The Immoral Traffic* (*Suppression*) *Act*, this law was abbreviated to SITA in the popular discourse. It therefore had to be amended to be called *The Immoral Traffic* (*Prevention*) *Act* or PITA, so as not to offend the sensibilities of the Hindu goddess Sita when sex workers were tried in court.

Not only does non-threatening or non-offending language make it easier to conduct a discourse (audible or mental) on awkward subjects like reproductive health, the awkwardness reduces further when this language can be drawn from the outside, hitherto unfamiliar but respected modern, scientific, industrialized world (Basu 2005). Thus, as Rele and Kanitkar (1980) discuss with reference to the great popularity of sterilizations among lower middle-class women in urban India in the 1970s and 1980s, even the terminology of modern contraception seems to give these women a sense of well-being and control. Sterilizations are not called sterilizations, tubectomies or vasectomies even when these words have vernacular equivalents; instead they are referred to by the generic English word 'operation' whatever the language of discourse (see also Ramasubban and Rishyaringa 2001), and are seen as belonging to the world of modern medicine and rational behavior to which the modern individual aspires. Moreover, talk of these 'operations' is safe because it does not require any mention of sexual or reproductive parts or activities in the way that 'traditional' methods such as withdrawal or rhythm do (on this, see also Caldwell et al. 1982).

Several other studies describe how the very language of folk understandings of illness gets modified upon contact with the forces of the larger world. Often this happens as a way to assuage the scorn of this outside world for indigenous understandings of illness (see, for example, Singer et al. 1988); just as often, it is also a way of claiming membership of this outside world because this is an anonymous world to which folk representations of shame and embarrassment do not apply. As van der Geest and Whyte (1989) eloquently put it, one of the main reasons that western medicines are so popular in developing countries is because they "allow therapy to be disengaged from its social entanglements".

2.4 Discussion

This chapter is not even remotely about the philosophy of language. Nor is it medical anthropology in any theoretical or abstract sense. All I have tried to do is to draw a little from both of these fields to raise some very practical questions related to the diagnosis and treatment of reproductive health problems in different cultural settings. Communication between patients and health providers is the first and most essential step in such diagnosis and care. It is bad enough when, as often is the case, little or no information on symptoms is forthcoming. However, it can be even worse when there is speech, with words that seem to mean something similar to both parties in the exchange but in fact the conversation is actually concealing or misstating more than it illuminates.

The costs of such miscommunication are real, large and destructive. Under- and over-estimates of illness incidence and prevalence at the population level, as well as under- or over-treatment of illness at the individual level are serious obvious costs. There are less obvious ones as well. For example, a study of 958 low-income patients followed up for 2 years found that patients with inadequate health literacy were nearly twice as likely to have been hospitalized during the previous year (31.5 % versus 14.9 %), a relationship that persisted after adjustment for health status and various socioeconomic indicators (Baker et al. 2002). By 'inadequate health literacy' these authors refer to things like patients' tendency to not explain symptoms clearly, or to not understand or follow provider instructions. But I would include here the tendency of health systems to not understand or speak the language of patients with low health literacy. That is, miscommunication is a two-way street.

How best might the reproductive health research and service community deal with the potential for such miscommunication? Perhaps the first thing to remember is that *all* medical systems are culturally constructed, even when the culture in question happens to be the western 'scientific' one that has created the field of modern biomedicine. This does not mean that all systems of health beliefs need to be accommodated by the practitioner of modern medicine, but it does mean that other ways of thinking, expressing and doing need to be acknowledged and fed into the medical practitioner's role in specific ways.

In the context of language disconnects, what are some of these specific ways? They relate to the public health researcher or service provider being both a listener and a speaker. That is, she needs to be able to make sense of what is said to her, as well as to impart sense or meaning in what she tells the patient in return. Making sense of what is said is a matter of interpretation and what different uses of the same words by speaker and listener does is to hinder correct interpretation. Thus, when Haitian women complain of *pediyson* or loss of blood, it is not simply heavy menstrual bleeding that is being alluded to and which the health provider has to decode in its larger context, in order to know if her patient is suffering from non-specific bleeding, or fibroids, or a miscarriage or even an abortion (Singer et al. 1988), or none of these things. The real issue may be anxiety about infertility, about an uncaring partner, or even about financial strain. Obviously the physician's treatment response will be heavily colored by the interpretation of *pediyson*, and it would be a disservice to either just prescribe something to reduce menstrual flow, or to hector the patient to be more specific about symptoms. By the same token, the complainer of heavy vaginal discharge in India may need something other than antibiotics to treat reproductive tract infections, although she may need these as well. The point that Singer et al. (1988) stress is that symptoms themselves are culturally, socially and politically embedded, not merely physical events that can be classified according to WHO's international classification of diseases.

All this is not to say that the reproductive health provider needs a course in Medical Anthropology (although the reproductive health researcher would certainly benefit from one); however he does need to be aware of his own location in a culturally constructed universe of modern biomedicine in which ordinary words have often been appropriated and given very specific, narrow, technical meanings that may not be shared by those outside that world.

Having understood this limitation and having taken the trouble to correctly diagnose a reproductive health condition, the reproductive health provider now needs to choose between different speech options. There is the correct, medically sound, advice and prescription he can dole out, which may or may not be appreciated; or he can high-handedly decide to first 'educate' the patient in 'correct' recognition and reporting of symptoms; or he can use words strategically rather than literally to convey what he wants to convey, rather than what he might end up conveying if he is fussy about the exact meaning of words. For, as already said, meaning lies in the mind of the speaker and the listener, and just as the patient can and does often mold his language to suit what he thinks is the language of the listener, so the health provider can and must speak in language that is conscious of the possible absence of shared meaning, even when there is, superficially, a shared language.

The point here is that language is performance. It is rarely neutral. Meaning is intended, the effect on listeners is intended. In that case, common ground and common frameworks of understanding have to be created. They can be created by patronizingly converting your listener to your terminology, or by doing a bit of give and take that adopts some of the word meanings of the listener. That, to me, seems to be a much more reasonable position for health providers in the field to take than the one taken by the abstract philosopher of language, Hilary Putnam (1975) in his famous paper on "The Meaning of Meaning." Putnam refuses to give the label 'water' to the substance on a hypothetical Twin Earth that mimics the qualities of what we in our world know to be water, but which has the chemical formula XYZ rather than H_2O. This philosophy is a form of 'semantic externalism', or to put it more simply, "meaning just ain't in the head." But that is the opposite of the lesson to take away from this chapter.

References

Abraham, L. (2002). Bhai-behen, true love, time pass: Friendships and sexual partnerships among Youth in an Indian Metropolis. *Culture, Health and Sexuality, 4*(3), 337–353.
Amin, S. (2003). Menstrual regulation in Bangladesh. In A. M. Basu (Ed.), *The sociocultural and political aspects of abortion* (pp. 153–166). Westport: Greenwood Press.
Anarfi, J. (2003). The role of local herbs in the recent fertility decline in Ghana: Contraceptives or abortifacients? In A. B. Basu (Ed.), *The sociocultural and political aspects of abortion* (pp. 139–152). Westport: Greenwood Press.

Baker, D. W., Gazmararian, J. A., Scott, T., Parker, R. M., Ren, D. J., & Peel, J. (2002). Functional health literacy and the risk of hospital admission among Medicare managed care enrollees. *American Journal of Public Health, 92*(8), 1278–1283.

Bang, A., & Bang, R. (1997). *Findings on reproductive tract infections among males presented based on a study in progress at Gadchiroli in a workshop on involving men in a reproductive health program.* Cited in Verma et al. (1999).

Basu, A. M. (1992). *Culture, the status of women and demographic behavior: Illustrated with the case of India.* Oxford: Clarendon Press.

Basu, A. M. (Ed.). (2003). *The social and political context of abortion.* Westport: Greenwood Press.

Basu, A. M. (2005). Ultramodern contraception: Social class and family planning in India. *Asian Population Studies, 1*(3), 303–323.

Basu, A. M. (2006). The emotions and reproductive health. *Population and Development Review, 32*(1), 107–121.

Bulut, A., et al. (1997). Contraceptive choice and reproductive morbidity in Istanbul. *Studies in Family Planning, 28*(1), 35–43.

Caldwell, J. C., Reddy, P. H., & Caldwell, P. (1982). The causes of demographic change in rural South India: A micro approach. *Population and Development Review, 8*(4), 689–727.

Collumbien, M., Bohidar, N., Das, R., Das, B., & Pelto, P. (1999). *Male sexual health concerns in Orissa – An emic perspective.* Paper presented at the Seminar on Social Categories in Population Health, organised by the Committee on Anthropological Demography of the International Union for the Scientific Study of Population, Cairo.

Gangoli, G. (2009). Indian feminisms: Issues of sexuality and representations. In K. M. Gokulsing & W. Dissanayake (Eds.), *Popular culture in a globalized India* (pp. 53–65). Oxford: Routledge.

Hawkes, S. (1998). Why include men? Establishing sexual health clinics for men in Rural Bangladesh. *Health Policy and Planning, 13*, 121–130.

Hawkes, S., et al. (1999). Reproductive tract infections in women in low-income, low prevalence situations: Assessment of syndromic management in Matlab, Bangladesh. *Lancet, 354*, 1776–1781.

Islam, M. M., Rob, U., & Chakroborty, N. (2004). Menstrual regulation practices in Bangladesh: An unrecognized form of contraception. *Asia-Pacific Population Journal, 19*(4), 75–99.

Kirkman, M., Rosenthal, D., & Smith, A. M. (1998). Adolescent sex and the romantic narrative: Why some young heterosexuals use condoms to prevent pregnancy but not disease. *Psychology, Health & Medicine, 3*(4), 355–370.

Levin, E. (2003). Cleaning the belly: Managing menstrual health in Guinea, West Africa. In A. M. Basu (Ed.), *The sociocultural and political aspects of abortion* (pp. 103–118). Westport: Greenwood Press.

Levy, R. (1984). Emotion, knowing, and culture. In R. Shweder & R. LeVine (Eds.), *Culture theory: Essays on mind, self, and emotion* (pp. 214–237). Cambridge: Cambridge University Press.

Lien, P. T., et al. (2002). The prevalence of reproductive tract infections in Hue, Vietnam. *Studies in Family Planning, 33*(3), 217–226.

Narayana, G. (1996, June). *Family violence, sex and reproductive health behaviour among men in Uttar Pradesh, India* (unpublished). Cited in Verma et al. (2001).

Nayab, D. (2004). *Women's ability to identify and address reproductive tract infections: A case study in Pakistan.* Ph.D. thesis submitted to the Demography and Sociology Program, Australian National University, Acton.

Nichter, M. (1981). Idioms of distress: Alternatives in the expression of psychosocial distress: A case study from South India. *Culture, Medicine and Psychiatry, 5*, 379–408.

Obeyesekere, G. (1976). The impact of Ayurvedic ideas on the culture and the individual in Sri Lanka. In C. Leslie (Ed.), *Asian medical system.* Berkeley: University of California Press.

O'Flynn, N., & Britten, N. (2004). Diagnosing menstrual disorders: A qualitative study of the approach of primary care professionals. *British Journal of General Practice, 54*, 353–358.

Oomman, N. (1996). *Poverty and pathology: Comparing rural Rajasthani women's ethnomedical models with biomedical models of reproductive morbidity: Implications for women's health in*

India. Dissertation submitted to the School of Hygiene and Public Health, Johns Hopkins University, Baltimore.

Osella, C., & Osella, F. (2002). Contextualizing sexuality: Young men in Kerala, South India. In L. Manderson & P. Liamputton (Eds.), *Coming of age in South and Southeast Asia*. Richmond: Curzon Press.

Patel, V., & Oomman, N. (1999). Mental health matters too: Gynecological symptoms and depression in South Asia. *Reproductive Health Matters, 7*(14), 30–39.

Pepin, J. S., et al. (2004). Low prevalence of cervical infections in women with vaginal discharge in West Africa: Implications for syndromic management. *Sexually Transmitted Infections, 80*, 230–235.

Prasad, J. H. et al. (1999). *Prevalence of reproductive tract infections among adolescents in a rural community in Tamil Nadu* (unpublished paper). Cited in Oomman (2000).

Putnam, H. (1975). The meaning of 'meaning'. *Minnesota Studies in the Philosophy of Science, 7*, 131–193.

Ramasubban, R. (2000). Women's vulnerability: The recent evidence on STIs. In R. Ramasubban & S. J. Jejeebhoy (Eds.), *Women's reproductive health in India*. Jaipur/New Delhi: Rawat Publications.

Ramasubban, R., & Rishyaringa, B. (2001). Weakness ('*ashaktapana*') and reproductive health among women in a slum population in Mumbai. In C. M. Obermeyer (Ed.), *Cultural perspectives on reproductive health* (pp. 13–37). Oxford: Oxford University Press.

Rele, J. R., & Kanitkar, T. (1980). *Fertility and family planning in greater Bombay*. Bombay: Popular Prakasan.

Renne, E. P. (2003). Changing assessments of abortion in a Northern Nigerian town. In A. M. Basu (Ed.), *The sociocultural and political aspects of abortion: Global perspectives* (pp. 119–138). Westport: Greenwood Press.

Rosenthal, D., Gifford, S., & Moore, S. (1998). Safe sex or safe love: Competing discourses? *AIDS Care, 10*(1), 35–47.

Singer, M., Davison, L., & Gerdes, G. (1988). Culture, critical theory and reproductive illness behavior in Haiti. *Medical Anthropology Quarterly, New Series, 2*(4), 270–285.

Smith, D. J. (2004, April). *Premarital sex, procreation and problems of HIV risk in Nigeria*. Paper presented at the Annual meeting of the Population Association of America, Boston.

Sobo, E. J. (1995). Finance, romance, social support, and condom use among impoverished inner-city women. *Human Organization, 54*(2), 115–128.

Stambach, A. (2003). Kutoa Mimba: Debates about schoolgirl abortion in Machame, Tanzania. In A. M. Basu (Ed.), *The sociocultural and political aspects of abortion* (pp. 79–102). Westport: Greenwood Press.

Trollope-Kumar, K. (1999). Symptoms of reproductive tract infection – Not all that they seem to be. *The Lancet, 354*, 1745–1746.

van der Geest, S., & Whyte, R. R. (1989). The charms of medicines: Metaphors and metonyms. *Medical Anthropology Quarterly, New Series, 3*(4), 345–367.

Verma, R. K., Rangaiyan, G., Singh, R., Sharma, S., & Pelto, P. J. (2001). A study of male sexual health problems in a Mumbai Slum population. *Culture, Health and Sexuality, 3*(3), 339–352.

World Health Organization. (1993). *Recommendations for the management of sexually transmitted diseases* (WHO Global Program on AIDS/STD93.1). Geneva: WHO.

World Health Organization. (1995). *STD Case management workbooks, Modules 1–7*. Geneva: WHO.

Zurayk, H., Khattab, H., Younis, N., Kamal, O., & Wl-Helw, M. (1995). Comparing women's reports with medical diagnosis of reproductive morbidity conditions in rural Egypt. *Studies in Family Planning, 26*(1), 14–21.

Chapter 3
Prevalence, Attitudes, Risk Factors, and Selected Health-Related Outcomes Associated with Spousal Physical Violence During Pregnancy in Egypt

Andrzej Kulczycki

Violence against women is often referred to as gender-based based violence because of its association with the subordinate status of women in many societies. It includes intimate partner violence (IPV), a term often used interchangeably with spousal violence. This may comprise physical violence, the most common form of IPV, as well as sexual, emotional and financial abuse.[1] Husbands are more often the perpetrators and women bear the heavy burden of such abuse. IPV is a serious, costly and widespread problem. It has multiple adverse physical, mental and social impacts for women, children and families, communities and societies (Campbell 2002; Coker et al. 2000, 2002; Ellsberg et al. 2008; Garcia-Moreno et al. 2006; Watts and Zimmerman 2002). The reproductive health consequences may often include unintended pregnancies and poor pregnancy outcomes, as well as more hospitalizations, greater use of outpatient care for acute problems, and less preventive care (Cronholm et al. 2011). Physical violence has also been associated with a range of common gynecological disorders such as fibroids, decreased libido, chronic pelvic pain, pain on intercourse, urinary tract, vaginal, and sexually transmitted infections (STIs) (Letourneau et al. 1999).

In ten non-Western nations, reported lifetime prevalence rates of physical and sexual partner violence have been estimated to range from 15 to 71 % (Garcia-Moreno et al. 2006). U.S. and Canadian population-based surveys indicate 8–14 % of women of all ages report physical assault in the past year by a husband or sexual intimate, and 25–30 % have experienced such abuse during their adult lives (Campbell 2002; Daoud et al. 2012; Tjaden and Thoennes 2000). Violence against

---

[1] In addition to physical abuse, other types of IPV are sexual violence (including sexual harassment and rape), emotional violence (including insults, shouts, intimidation, and restrictions on contacts with family and friends), and economic violence (including being forced to borrow money, to work, or to give income to someone else).

A. Kulczycki, Ph.D. (✉)
Associate Professor, Department of Health Care Organization and Policy,
University of Alabama at Birmingham (UAB), Birmingham, AL, USA
e-mail: andrzej@uab.edu

A. Kulczycki (ed.), *Critical Issues in Reproductive Health*, The Springer Series on Demographic Methods and Population Analysis 33, DOI 10.1007/978-94-007-6722-5_3, © Springer Science+Business Media Dordrecht 2014

pregnant women may adversely affect fetal and birth outcomes, infant and child health, future fertility, as well as other aspects of women's physical and mental health (Bohn et al. 2004; Campbell et al. 2004; Ellsberg et al. 2008; Janssen et al. 2003; Mullick et al. 2005). It affects somewhere between 4 and 8 % of U.S. women (Gazmararian et al. 1996, 2000; Saltzman et al. 2003), with comparable or higher levels of abuse reported in Canada and European countries (Campbell 2002; Daoud et al. 2012). Higher prevalence rates tend to be associated with more inclusive definitions of abuse and low income of respondents.

Despite an increase in research and discussion about the prevalence, determinants, and impacts of IPV in many countries, there is a dearth of studies conducted in the Middle East and North Africa (MENA). However, the limited regional literature shows that IPV is common, severe, widely justified, and chronically underreported (Boy and Kulczycki 2008). It also occurs in all age and social strata. In Egypt and Jordan, the only two Arab countries with nationally representative data, about one–third of ever-married women have reported being beaten at least once by their husbands since marriage, and most ever-married women accepted at least one posited reason for wife-beating (Boy and Kulczycki 2008).

The present study seeks to extend the limited body of research on spousal violence in the MENA region by specifically examining this phenomenon during pregnancy. The chapter investigates prevalence, risk factors, victim characteristics, as well as some salient health-related outcomes and attitudes associated with spousal physical violence during pregnancy. The article compares victims of pregnancy violence to women not subjected to such abuse. It further investigates how marital violence during pregnancy is associated with receipt of antenatal (ANC) care, as well as with STI acquisition. Our application is to Egypt, the most populous nation in the MENA region and of the world's 22 Arabic-speaking countries. Egypt is broadly reflective of all their major trends and, additionally, is known to have high prevalence and acceptance of wife beating as compared to countries elsewhere which have collected comparable population-based survey data (Boy and Kulczycki 2008; Hindin et al. 2008; Kishor and Johnson 2004). IPV remains under-researched in Egypt and in the broader region, however, with especially little known about spousal violence during pregnancy.

3.1 Women's Status and Reproductive Health in Egypt and Arab Countries

Women suffer deep-seated discrimination across the MENA region, holding back economic and social development (Nazir 2005; UNDP 2006). Despite recent gains in life expectancy, maternal health and educational attainment, Arab women are less socially, economically and politically empowered than are women in other regions of the world (with the possible exceptions of South Asia and sub-Saharan Africa). Egyptian women have low decision making power and high illiteracy rates; for example, the 2005 Egyptian Demographic and Health Survey (EDHS) showed that only

59 % of ever-married women were literate, 35 % had never attended school, and 11 % had less than a primary education (El-Zanaty and Way 2006). Like most MENA societies, Egypt retains rigid gender stratification systems, with laws and customs that reinforce the subordinate position of women. Although the status of women has improved somewhat across the region, violence against women remains a major problem (Boy and Kulczycki 2008; Freedom House 2005; Kulczycki and Windle 2011).

Egypt's population was estimated at 81 million in 2010, with 21.1 million women aged 15–49 (UN 2011). The level of economic development remains low, particularly in Upper (southern) Egypt. Female labor force participation rates have risen but as for Arab countries more generally, they remain lower than for any other major world region (Kulczycki and Juárez 2003; UNDP 2011). They are also reinforced by persistent beliefs in the complementarity of the sexes (Hoodfar 1997) and the relatively early age at marriage, moderately high fertility, and low educational levels of many women, who remain socially and economically dependent on marriage. There are few legal protections against IPV and divorce laws invariably grant custody of children to husbands, so that female victims typically stay in their dysfunctional marriages to keep close contact with children (Human Rights Watch 2004). Islamic laws governing inheritance also favor men, husbands, and sons over women, wives, and daughters (An-Na'im 2002). The confluence of these factors may increase tolerance of spousal abuse.

Childbearing patterns have changed dramatically throughout the MENA region, such that women overall now have only about three lifetime births, down from about seven children in 1960. Egypt's trajectory is representative. Over 1960–2008, its total fertility rate (TFR) fell from 7.1 to 3.0 and its contraceptive prevalence rose from a very low base to 60 %, with 58 % of currently married women aged 15–49 using modern methods (although significant differentials in contraceptive use are observed, as for the age at marriage and age at first birth). Coverage of maternity care services has improved but remains inadequate. The 1995 EDHS showed that only 39 % of pregnant women benefited from ANC by a physician, midwife, or nurse, whereas the 2005 EDHS reported that women received ANC in the case of 70 % of births and saw a health care professional for the WHO recommended minimum number of four ANC visits in 59 % of births. Improvements in contraceptive use and health care have contributed to major gains in maternal health. Pregnancy-related deaths were estimated to have fallen by 63 % over 1990–2008 to 82 per 100,000 live births, or a lifetime risk of maternal death of 1 in 380, putting Egypt on track to achieve MDG 5 (WHO et al. 2010). However, these health gains were threatened by the political, economic and societal turmoil following the 2010 revolution. Also, early marriage remains common and carries attendant physical, social and economic costs. In 2005, the median age at first marriage for Egyptian women ages 25–29 still stood at 21.3 years, with 23 % of 19-year-old women already mothers or pregnant.[2]

---

[2] In the MENA region, only Yemeni women are more likely to marry at a younger age and to have higher adolescent fertility. In 1997, their median age at first marriage was as low as 16.0 years and as many as 39 % of women had started childbearing by age 19 (Sunil and Pillai 2010).

In Egypt as throughout the Arab world, there persist many cultural sensitivities and taboos surrounding multiple aspects of sexuality and reproductive health. The prevalence of STIs is unknown because surveillance activities are lacking and very few studies have been conducted. However, STIs are common worldwide and the small number of cases treated in Egypt and regionally most likely severely underestimates true incidence (Mabry et al. 2007; Madani 2006; Sallam et al. 2001). STIs can have serious health consequences for women and men, reducing the quality of life and productivity of those affected; they can also cause irreversible damage to fetuses or infants (Gross and Tyring 2011; Mullick et al. 2005). This makes the recognition, diagnosis and treatment of STIs and, more broadly, of reproductive tract infections (RTIs), a vital issue.

Denial, stigma, and discrimination further impede regional efforts to combat STIs and HIV/AIDS, although conservative social and cultural values which discourage premarital sex likewise underpin the relatively low HIV prevalence rates, as do nearly universal male circumcision rates. In Egypt, strong beliefs also make it more challenging to reduce the nearly universal practice of female genital cutting,[3] which is very rare in other MENA countries. Most Egyptian women still support continuation of the practice, even though it carries multiple obstetric risks and was finally outlawed in 2007 (Banks et al. 2006; Boyle 2002). EDHS data show that female genital cutting occurs at about 10 years on average, making it a customary practice for girls and, possibly, fostering increased tolerance of gender-based violence at a later stage.

Honor crimes, the most extreme form of gender-based violence, also occur in Egypt as elsewhere in the region. A recent systematic review of the research literature on honor killings in MENA countries confirmed a paucity of studies relative to the presumed magnitude of the problem. Most victims are young females murdered by their male kin; and unambiguous evidence of a decline in tolerance of honor killings remains elusive (Kulczycki and Windle 2011). In addition, little is known about IPV in the Middle East and North Africa, but the limited empirical research confirms that spousal abuse is frequent and widely condoned by most women and men. A recent systematic review identified 59 studies, only 21 of which reported data on the prevalence of such violence or on beliefs regarding its justification (Boy and Kulczycki 2008). These covered just nine countries, with most of this research limited in scope, depth, or quality. Only eight studies reported prevalence rates of ever experiencing IPV, with seven indicating lifetime prevalence rates in excess of 20 %.

---

[3]In 2005, 96 % of ever-married women age 15–49 were circumcised. Six in ten ever-married Egyptian women ages 15–49 believed that female circumcision is required by religious precepts and that the husband prefers the wife to be circumcised, and over half thought that it prevented adultery. Few women recognize potential adverse consequences; only 13 % perceived that circumcision makes childbirth more difficult (El-Zanaty and Way 2006). The 2008 EDHS indicated declines in female circumcision rates among the youngest women ages 15–19 and in support for the practice among ever-married women. Beyond Egypt, female genital cutting is common in parts of western, eastern, and north-eastern Africa; in parts of Arabian Peninsula; and among migrants from these areas.

The limited database shows that IPV victims are of all ages and are more likely to be rural and less educated (Boy and Kulczycki 2008).

These prevalence rates, including the above cited national estimates for Egypt and Jordan, fall within the international range. The 1995 EDHS indicated that 34 % of ever-married women aged 15–49 had been physically abused by their husbands (Diop-Sidobe et al. 2006; El-Zanaty et al. 1996). Comparison to the 2005 EDHS shows the 12-month prevalence of wife beating was approximately stable at 16–19 %, but differences in the way questions were asked make it impossible to directly compare findings and to distinguish between changes in reporting and in actual prevalence of wife beating over time (Akmatov et al. 2008). Moreover, IPV may be underreported in Arab countries due to strong cultural emphases on female modesty, reputation (honor), and family solidarity. These attributes render disclosure and discussion of the problem more problematic because it may be viewed as a form of family betrayal.

An updated review conducted for this analysis identified seven studies that presented self-reported prevalence rates of physical abuse during pregnancy for MENA countries. The estimates range from 5 to 33 % and are based on hospital and clinic studies (Anson and Sagy 1995; Clark et al. 2009; Faramarzi et al. 2005; Fisher et al. 2003; Khawaja and Tewtel-Salem 2004; Rachana et al. 2002; Sahin and Sahin 2003). A large hospital-based report of pregnant women in Saudi Arabia, for example, found that victims were more likely to be treated for preterm labor, placental abruption, and kidney infections, as well as to experience fetal distress and to have cesarean births (Rachana et al. 2002). However, myriad study design features, definitional and time frame differences render it difficult to compare prevalence rates across these studies and restrict their generalizability. The only nationally representative data come from Egypt. The 1995 EDHS suggested that of ever-married Egyptian women who reported having ever been beaten since their first marriage and who were either parous or currently pregnant, almost one in three (32 %) had been beaten during pregnancy (El-Zanaty et al. 1996). The more detailed 2005 data are the subject of this study.

3.2 Conceptual Framework

This is the first study of IPV during pregnancy in the MENA region to use nationally representative data. It also explores the role of community-level variables by adopting the basic tenets of ecological theory to consider multiple influences on IPV, which may operate at different interdependent levels (Bronfenbrenner 1979). It is hypothesized that a set of demographic, social, economic, and attitudinal factors at the individual and household levels, as well as the community context, will be directly associated with a woman's risk of experiencing IPV. Data from the 2005 EDHS are analyzed for ever-married women aged 15–49, with a particular focus on the experience of physical violence during pregnancy. Several outcome variables are considered, as explained below. The study further evaluates the association of the set of covariates and the main independent variable (experience of spousal physical violence during pregnancy) with receiving ANC from a health care professional and with experiencing STIs/STI symptoms.

The socio-demographic factors investigated are treated essentially as control variables, because literature exists on the impacts of these individual character-istics. Women's empowerment has received much attention as a significant factor in explaining a range of demographic, socio-economic, and health behaviors. This nexus of factors is particularly pertinent in societies such as Egypt, where gendered inequities and the status of women are strongly contested. Empowerment is a multi-faceted construct and includes elements of agency and the resources needed to exercise life choices. Important dimensions of empowerment assessed here include women's educational attainment, cash earnings for those with recent work experience, and a composite indicator of women's participation in house-hold decision-making.

The broader community context can further protect or enhance the risk of IPV, as well as the likelihood of receiving ANC or acquiring STIs. For example, community economic deprivation may be associated with fewer opportunities for education, work, and capital accumulation. Men may find it very difficult to fulfill their role as economic provider for the family, which may condition people to become more tolerant of community violence and more violent themselves. Various indices of household socioeconomic status have been negatively associated with physical abuse of wives in different contexts (e.g. Koenig et al. 2003). This study uses a score based on average household standard of living to test the hypothesis that community inequalities may be associated with such violence. Social norms about the roles and opportunities of women are tested through their level of educational attainment. Specifically, ever-married women with limited educational attainment may have fewer resources, poor prospects for work outside marriage, and perceive few alter-natives to marriage, all of which may lead them to be more tolerant of abusive husbands. Also, the geographic concentration of patriarchal attitudes may perpetu-ate norms about the low value of women and justify their poor treatment. An addi-tive 'wife-beating' index is derived to indicate the level of acceptance of community-level attitudes toward spousal violence in different situations.

Accordingly, this study develops and tests several competing hypotheses, namely that the odds of experiencing spousal physical violence during pregnancy are lower for: (1) women living in less economically deprived communities, as measured by higher aggregate household standard of living; (2) women who are less disadvantaged in terms of building up human capital, as characterized by living in areas where levels of female educational attainment tend to be higher; and (3), net of household economic status, women living in less patriarchal com-munities, as measured by lower aggregate level of acceptance of wife-beating. In addition, (4), the effects of community context will operate partly through indi-vidual and household or family variables, such that wife beating during preg-nancy may be expected to be higher among young, poor, less educated, and rural couples. However, IPV likely occurs in all socio-economic groups and across more mature couples as well.

This chapter further explores several health-related outcomes associated with IPV during pregnancy. Existing studies of the association between receipt of ANC from a skilled health provider and IPV tend to be clinic-based, may not be representative of the general population, and may also underestimate the association because beaten wives are often prevented from seeking ANC (Thananowan and Heidrich 2008; O'Campo et al. 1994). This leads to the hypothesis that women beaten during pregnancy by their husbands are somewhat less likely to obtain ANC care than are other ever-pregnant women, although the association may be weak.

STIs and STI symptoms are frequent, enhance transmission of HIV, and constitute a major public health problem in many countries. They are associated with such sequelae as pelvic inflammatory disease (PID), infertility, abortions, and neonatal blindness. In Egypt as throughout the MENA region, STI services are severely lacking even though STI prevention and control is cost-effective. The relationship between women's experience of such gynecological morbidities and spousal physical violence during pregnancy remains unexplored in this region. A weak association is expected between spousal physical violence during pregnancy and STIs/STI symptoms. This is due to the increased physiological vulnerability of young women to many STIs, their economic dependence on men, the stigma and potential social consequences attached to STIs in Arab countries where sanctions against nonmarital sexuality are more extreme for women, and the greater problems they face if they need care for such morbidities.

3.3   Data and Methods

Egypt held six DHS surveys over 1988–2008, with the series disrupted by the 2010–2012 regime changes and civil unrest, and the next survey pending as of this writing. Both the 1995 and 2005 EDHS collected data on IPV from randomly selected subsamples of survey respondents. The 1995 EDHS, the first attempt to collect information on wife beating in the history of DHS, included a single non-standardized question in a module on women's status (Kulczycki and Juárez 2003; Kishor and Johnson 2004). The 2005 EDHS adopted a more detailed methodology to collect spousal violence data. This included a modified version of the Revised Conflict Tactics Scale (CTS2), the most widely used instrument for measuring IPV and which has high cross-cultural validity and reliability (Straus et al. 1996, 2003; Straus 2007). These IPV questions were administered in a one-third sub-sample of interviewed households following established guidelines for IPV research and the protection of human subjects (Ellsberg et al. 2001). To maintain confidentiality, only one ever-married woman aged 15–49 years was selected randomly in each household sampled. Over 98 % of selected women responded to both the main survey questionnaire and the special module on domestic violence. This yielded a sample of 5,613 ever-married women aged 15–49, of whom 5,318 were ever pregnant.

These women were asked about both minor physical violence (being pushed, shaken, or slapped; having had an arm twisted or objects thrown at her) and its severe forms (being punched with a fist or with something that could hurt; being kicked or dragged; being burned or strangled; or being threatened or attacked with a knife, gun, or other weapon). They were also asked about sexual assault (physically forced to have sexual intercourse) committed ever and in the last 12 months by the woman's current/most recent husband.[4] Women who had experienced physical or sexual IPV within the 12-month period before the survey were additionally asked if they had sought any assistance to prevent or stop the violence and, if so, from whom. The EDHS further asked women if they had experienced emotional violence (being humiliated in front of others or threatened with harm), committed ever and in the past year. Lastly, women were asked about physical violence sustained during pregnancy: "Has any one ever hit, slapped, kicked, or done anything else to hurt you physically while you were pregnant?" This yielded binary responses on whether ever-pregnant women were ever beaten during pregnancy by a husband or by someone else.

Additionally, all ever-married women interviewed in the 2005 EDHS (n = 19,474) were asked about their attitudes towards IPV. Specifically, they were asked if they thought a husband was justified in hitting or beating his wife in five posited situations: if she burns the food, if she goes out without telling him, if she neglects the children, if she argues with him, and if she refuses to have sexual relations with him. The beating index derived here (scaled 0–4) includes all these scenarios except for burning the food, which was less often seen as a justification for such behavior.[5]

Questionnaire responses provided data on household and women's characteristics, as well as on IPV. Individual-level characteristics included data on age, marital status, number of living children, the educational levels of the respondent and of her partner, and two categorical socio-demographic variables for working status (whether earning cash for the work they do) and place of residence (rural vs. urban). The household's relative economic status (also known as the wealth index, a proxy score for long-term household standard of living) was derived from questions about the dwelling, its amenities and assets, using established methods (Rutstein and Johnson 2004). The extent of women's participation in household decision-making is measured by an additive index (scaled 0–4) which captures the degree to which the wife can decide herself (1 = wife has the final say or joint decision; 0 = husband or someone else decides) about her own health care, major household purchases, purchases for daily household needs, and visits to her family or other relatives. Also analyzed were two binary outcomes: women's receipt of ANC from a trained health care provider (be it a physician, nurse or midwife) and their self-reported prevalence

---

[4]The 2005 EDHS also collected data about physical violence committed by a non-spouse against the woman since she was 15 years old, but did not collect data on violence committed by women against their husbands.

[5]In total, almost one-fifth (19 %) of all ever-married women interviewed in the survey still thought burning the food is sufficient justification for being hit or beaten by a husband, although this was about half the level of toleration for wife-beating in each of the other situations.

of recent STIs/STI symptoms. Specifically, respondents were asked if they had had a STI, genital sore or ulcer, and any genital discharge in the past 12 months, from which a composite index was computed to indicate the extent of self-reported STIs/STI symptoms.

The three contextual variables were constructed using responses from all eligible respondents or households aggregated to the level of the primary sampling unit (PSU). With all 682 PSUs selected for the 2005 EDHS sample being reasonably homogenous geographic units, each woman could be assigned a value for each of the three contextual variables: the average level of female attainment, which captures an important aspect of female empowerment and opportunity in each PSU; an average score for household standard of living, which captures local economic conditions; and the acceptance of wife-beating (beating index), which captures the local values concerning the general treatment of women, as well as associated norms and practices regarding IPV.

Descriptive statistics were computed for all variables, with potential collinearities among the variables investigated. Chi-square and t-tests were used to explore bivariate associations between wife beating and the other covariates. Multivariate logistic regression analysis was then used to examine the predictors of physical abuse during pregnancy, and the association between such violence and selected health-related outcomes. These analyses were adjusted for individual and partner-level characteristics, household and community-level factors. Data analysis was performed using the statistical program SAS for Windows, version 9.1.

3.4 Results

3.4.1 Prevalence of Abuse and Attitudes About Wife Beating

Nearly every second (47 %) ever-married woman aged 15–49 sampled by the EDHS reported having experienced some form of physical violence since age 15, and 22 % had experienced such abuse in the past year (data not shown). One in three respondents (33 %) had experienced some form of physical violence at the hands of their current or a previous husband. Overall, 71 % of women who reported physical violence identified husbands as responsible for at least one episode of such abuse. Other, less frequent perpetrators of physical violence included (in descending order of importance) the woman's father, her brother, and other females, most often the woman's mother (data not shown).

Every second woman (50 %) justified wife beating in at least one of the four situations explored, with one in four respondents accepting it in all four cases. Two of every five women (40 %) justified wife beating if they went out without telling their husbands or neglected their children. Almost as many (37 %) accepted it if the wife argued with him and one in three (34 %) justified it should she refuse to have sex with him (data not shown).

In all, 6.2 % (n=326) of ever-pregnant women reported having ever experienced physical violence during pregnancy, with 5.1 % (n=264) victimized by their present or former husband (Table 3.1). The focus of this study concerns women physically abused by their intimate partners during pregnancy. Their characteristics are next compared to those for all ever-pregnant women who were not physically abused at the hands of their present or former husband (n=4,896). Far fewer women (n=62) reported experiencing such violence committed by non-intimate partners; this is an insufficient number of cases to permit multivariate analysis by the selected variables and to make definitive statements about these victims.

3.4.2 Characteristics of Victims of Wife Beating During Pregnancy

Abuse victims had a similar age profile as non-victims, but they were significantly more likely to be divorced or separated, to have five or more living children and, along with their husbands, to have received no schooling or primary level education only (Table 3.1). Women who experienced physical violence during pregnancy were also significantly less likely to be in the highest two wealth quintiles. Proportionately more victims were rural dwellers and cash earners, but these differences were non-significant.

The additive 'beating' index shows that victims of physical violence during pregnancy were significantly more likely to agree with at least one justification for wife-beating than women not so abused (62 % vs. 50 %). Women were significantly less likely to be abused in pregnancy if they made decisions jointly with their husbands with respect to their own health care, large household purchases, and visits to family or relatives, although the findings were non-significant in the case of household purchases for daily needs (data not shown). Women whose current/recent husbands typically had the final say alone on such matters were also more likely to be physically abused during pregnancy. Victims are more likely to live in communities that have significantly lower levels of education and more tolerant attitudes toward wife beating.

Victims of spousal abuse in pregnancy were significantly less likely to have ever received antenatal care (31 % vs. 39 %) and delivery care from a trained medical provider (36 % vs. 42 %, not shown). They also reported STI/STI symptoms almost twice as often as did women who were not abused during pregnancy (36 % vs. 20 %; only one woman who reported having been beaten in pregnancy did not respond to this question).

3.4.3 Help-Seeking Behavior

Two of every three women (66 %) abused in pregnancy sought help to deal with the violence, in most cases from relatives (data not shown). Strikingly, not one such woman sought assistance from medical personnel. Women who did not seek help

Table 3.1 Descriptive characteristics of ever-pregnant women ages 15–49 surveyed according to whether they did or did not experience spousal physical violence during pregnancy, Egypt, 2005

Characteristic	Not abused during pregnancy N = 4,896[a] (%)	Abused during pregnancy by present/ former husbands N = 264[a] (%)	p-value
Individual-level variables			
Age			
15–29	35.9	36.4	0.9485
30–39	34.6	33.7	
40–49	29.5	29.9	
Parity			
0–1	18.6	14.4	0.0510
2–4	57.5	56.1	
5+	23.9	29.5	
Marital status			
Married	94.3	82.6	<.0001
Widowed	3.7	3.4	
Divorced/separated	2.0	14.1	
Education			
None	34.1	43.6	<.0001
Primary	15.7	27.7	
Secondary/higher	50.3	28.8	
Working for cash			
Yes	17.4	20.5	0.1991
No	82.6	79.5	
Husband's education[b]			
None	22.9	35.1	<.0001
Primary	19.4	26.4	
Secondary/primary	57.7	38.4	
Household characteristics			
Place of residence			
Urban	42.3	38.6	0.2651
Rural	57.7	61.2	
Household wealth			
Poorest	18.5	26.4	<.0001
Poorer	17.8	24.5	
Middle	20.0	23.3	
Richer	21.9	15.0	
Richest	21.8	10.9	
Women's empowerment			
Decision-making index[c]			
0	12.6	21.2	<.0001
1	8.0	11.3	
2	16.3	17.7	
3	22.9	15.0	
4	40.1	34.7	

(continued)

Table 3.1 (continued)

Characteristic	Not abused during pregnancy N=4,896[a] (%)	Abused during pregnancy by present/ former husbands N=264[a] (%)	p-value
Attitudes towards wife beating[d]			
0 (No to all items)	50.5	38.2	0.0004
1 (Yes to 1 item)	7.6	9.8	
2	7.9	6.9	
3	9.2	14.5	
4	24.8	30.6	
Community-level variables, mean (SD)			
Female education	6.52 (3.1)	6.06 (3.0)	0.0053
Household wealth	3.09 (1.0)	2.97 (1.0)	0.0748
Beating index	1.50 (0.8)	1.63 (0.7)	0.0091
Health-related outcomes			
Prenatal care			
Yes	39.4	31.4	0.0099
No	60.6	68.5	
STI/STI symptoms[b]			
Yes	19.7	36.4	<0.0001
No	80.3	63.4	

[a] Values weighted to be nationally representative

[b] There are 27 missing responses for husband's education and 51 missing responses for STI/STI symptoms

[c] Whether woman has final say or decides jointly with husband in regard to her own health care, making major household purchases, making purchases for daily household needs, and visits to her family or other relatives

[d] Whether respondent believes a husband is justified in beating his wife in regard to four posited scenarios: if she goes out without telling him, if she neglects the children, if she argues with him and if she refuses to have sexual relations with him (based on responses of 0=no (or don't know) and 1=respondent agrees)

stated, in descending order of importance, that they considered the violence not important, a part of life, or that they were embarrassed, afraid, or did not want to disgrace the family. These explanations are indicative of widespread fatalism and resignation in the face of such violence.

3.4.4 Risk Factors for Spousal Physical Violence During Pregnancy

Multivariate results show that of the woman's characteristics, age, parity, and education (of either spouse) were not associated with being beaten during pregnancy. Compared to current wives, divorced or separated women reported a sevenfold

Table 3.2 Multivariate logistic regression analysis of risk of experiencing spousal physical violence during pregnancy among ever-pregnant women ages 15–49 (n=5,265), Egypt, 2005

Variable	Model OR (95 % CI)	Model 2 OR (95 % CI)
Age	0.99 (0.97, 1.01)	0.99 (0.97, 1.01)
Education		
None	1.00 (0.73, 1.37)	0.97 (0.71, 1.39)
Place of residence		
Urban	1.42 (1.04, 1.93)*	0.99 (0.66, 1.49)
Parity		
5+	1.29 (0.92, 1.81)	1.31 (0.93, 1.85)
Marital status		
Divorced/separated	7.28 (4.76, 11.11)***	7.76 (5.04, 11.95)***
Working for cash		
Yes	1.48 (1.07, 2.06)*	1.50 (1.08, 209)*
Husband's education		
None	1.21 (0.89, 1.66)	1.18 (0.86, 1.61)
Household wealth index		
Poorer	1.07 (0.74, 1.54)	1.00 (0.69, 1.46)
Middle	0.84 (0.57, 1.24)	0.76 (0.50, 1.15)
Richer	0.47 (0.29, 0.76)*	0.40 (0.24, 0.67)**
Richest	0.30 (0.17, 0.53)***	0.26 (0.14, 0.48)***
Women's status variables		
Beating index		1.09 (1.00, 1.18)*
Community-level variables		
Beating index		1.15 (0.88, 1.50)
Household wealth		1.81 (1.27, 2.59)*
Female education		0.92 (0.84, 1.00)*

OR odds ratio, *CI* confidence interval
***Significant at <0.0001; **<0.01; *<0.05

increase in risk of experiencing physical violence during pregnancy. Women working for cash and urban dwellers are also significantly more likely to be victims of abuse in pregnancy, whereas living in more affluent households confers a protective effect (Table 3.2)

Inclusion of attitudes toward wife beating[6] and community-level influences in the second multivariate model did not diminish the strength of the covariates identified above except for urban residence, which is no longer predictive of spousal physical violence during pregnancy. Multivariate adjustment shows that divorced or separated women are 7.8 times more likely to be victims of such abuse than are

[6]The index of female participation in household decision-making is not included in the multivariate analysis due to high multicollinearity between predictor variables, especially with the 'beating index.'

currently married women. Those agreeing with at least one or more rationales for wife beating are more likely to report experiencing marital violence during pregnancy, but living in areas where these attitudes are more prevalent is not significantly associated with suffering physical abuse at such times. However, community-level factors are not consistently related to such errant behavior. Women living in communities with relatively high levels of household wealth are significantly more likely to report being beaten by husbands during pregnancy, but the risk is lower for areas with higher levels of female education.

3.4.5 Wife Beating During Pregnancy and Antenatal Care Coverage

Maternal health and birth outcomes depend in part on the care received by women during pregnancy and delivery. We examined the predictors of women's receipt of ANC and, in particular, if women's access to ANC from a health care professional varies by their experience of violence in pregnancy. Inadequate ANC was significantly more prevalent among older, divorced/separated, and uneducated respondents, as well as women whose husbands lacked formal education (Table 3.3). Conversely, women with five or more children and women in households with higher levels of wealth than the poorest quintile were more likely to have obtained ANC.

All these variables were retained in the second model, but multivariate adjustment is seen to reduce the effects of poverty and wealth. Compared to women in the lowest wealth quintile, women who lived in households with above average levels of wealth were almost twice as likely to receive ANC. Further, Model 2 shows that women who agreed with at least one of the four posited reasons for wife beating are significantly less likely to report receiving ANC, but no such associations are found with any of the community-level factors. In addition, spousal physical violence during pregnancy is not significantly associated with the likelihood of obtaining ANC.

3.4.6 Wife Beating During Pregnancy and Experience of Gynecological Morbidities

Multivariate analysis shows that younger women are more likely to report recent gynecological morbidities (Table 3.4). Women from urban households and those with high parity (at least five children) also have higher odds of experiencing STIs/STI symptoms, but women in the second poorest wealth quintile are at lower risk. Marital status, educational attainment, and cash earning status, are not significant in this model.

Table 3.3 Multivariate logistic model assessing likelihood of receiving antenatal care (ANC) from a health care professional for ever-pregnant women ages 15–49, by selected variables, Egypt, 2005

Variable	Model OR (95 % CI)	Model 2 OR (95 % CI)
Age	0.87 (0.86, 0.88)***	0.86 (0.85, 0.87)***
Education		
None	0.58 (0.48, 0.68)***	0.58 (0.49, 0.69)***
Place of residence		
Urban	1.07 (0.91, 1.25)	0.92 (0.75, 1.14)
Parity		
5+	1.58 (1.30, 1.91)***	1.65 (1.35, 2.00)***
Marital status		
Divorced/separated	0.53 (0.33, 0.83)**	0.52 (0.33, 0.83)**
Working for cash		
Yes	1.09 (0.92, 1.30)	1.07 (0.89, 1.28)
Husband's education		
None	0.76 (0.63, 0.92)**	0.73 (0.61, 0.89)*
Household wealth index		
Poorer	1.34 (1.07, 1.68)*	1.22 (0.97, 1.54)
Middle	1.44 (1.15, 180)**	1.263 (0.99. 1.59)
Richer	2.16 (1.70, 2.75)***	1.80 (1.38, 2.35)***
Richest	2.18 (1.67, 2.85)***	1.72 (1.27, 2.35)**
Spousal physical violence during pregnancy		
Yes		0.83 (0.91, 0.99)
Women's status variables		
Beating index		0.95 (0.91, 0.99)*
Community-level variables		
Beating index		0.93 (0.81, 1.07)
Household wealth		1.12 (0.93, 1.35)
Female education		0.99 (0.95, 1.04)

OR odds ratio, *CI* confidence interval
***Significant at <0.0001; **<0.01; *<0.05

The effects of urban residence and age are retained after controlling for confounding factors (Model 2), although the effects of high parity and of poverty are somewhat attenuated. Women who believe wife beating is justified in at least one circumstance are significantly more likely to report acquiring STIs/STI symptoms. So are women living in communities where such attitudes are more prevalent, as are those living in areas with above average levels of household wealth. On the other hand, the average level of educational attainment in the PSU in which a woman lives, net of her own education, does not influence her risk of experiencing gynecological morbidities. Of special note, women abused during pregnancy are 2.4 times more likely to report experiencing STIs/STI symptoms than are women who have not been subjected to such marital violence.

Table 3.4 Multivariate logistic model assessing likelihood of having a sexually transmitted infection (STI) or STI symptoms for ever-pregnant women ages 15–49, Egypt, 2005

Variable	Model OR (95 % CI)	Model 2 OR (95 % CI)
Age	0.97 (0.96, 0.98)***	0.97 (0.96, 0.98)***
Education		
None	0.89 (0.75, 1.07)	0.88 (0.73, 1.06)
Place of residence		
Urban	1.38 (1.17, 1.62)**	1.30 (1.04, 1.62)*
Parity		
5+	1.25 (1.03, 1.52)*	1.21 (0.99, 1.48)
Marital status		
Divorced/separated	1.28 (0.85, 1.94)	1.07 (0.70, 1.65)
Working for cash		
Yes	0.87 (0.72, 1.06)	0.87 (0.72, 1.06)
Husband's education		
None	0.83 (0.69, 1.01)	0.83 (0.68, 1.02)
Household wealth index		
Poorer	0.76 (0.60, 0.96)*	0.79 (0.62, 1.01)
Middle	0.91 (0.72, 1.14)	0.97 (0.76, 1.24)
Richer	0.87 (0.68, 1.12)	0.99 (0.75, 1.30)
Richest	0.83 (0.62, 1.09)	1.01 (0.73, 1.39)
Spousal physical violence during pregnancy		
Yes		2.41 (1.83, 3.16)***
Women's status variables		
Beating index		1.07 (1.02, 1.12)**
Community-level variables		
Beating index		1.39 (1.19, 1.61)***
Household wealth		1.31 (1.08, 1.59)**
Female education		0.98 (0.93, 1.03)

OR odds ratio, *CI* confidence interval
***Significant at <0.0001; ** <0.01; * <0.05

3.5 Discussion

Egypt has high rates of violence against women and of gender stratification in public and family life. According to the 2005 EDHS, one in three ever-married women of childbearing age have been beaten by their husbands. Every second woman agrees that men are justified in beating their wives for at least some reason. In addition, this study confirms that marital violence is not uncommon during pregnancy. It has assessed potential risk factors at multiple levels and several health-related outcomes using nationally representative population-based data, thereby adding to the limited evidence base on the topic in the MENA region.

There are several significant systematic differences between women abused during pregnancy and those who are not. In multivariable logistic regression, some of these differences were reduced, such as those regarding the education of women and their husbands. However, educated women as well as those from lower educational strata continue to face challenges to realizing women's rights and health in Egypt as in other Arabic Islamic countries, and the effects of economic and other factors also play a mediating role. Of the individual, husband, household, and community characteristics studied, working for cash and being no longer married emerge as risk factors for wife beating during pregnancy. Divorce may be a consequence of prior experiences of spousal violence, although the analytic sample included few women who were formerly married at the time of interview. Compared to those in the lowest wealth quintile, women from richer households are less likely to report such abuse. Those who agree that men are justified in beating their wives for at least some reason are more likely than other women to report being victims of pregnancy violence. There is little consistency across community-level variables. The negative association observed between violence during pregnancy and average community levels of female education, however, suggests that increases in human capital and gender equality may help reduce women's risk of experiencing such violence.

After controlling for confounding factors, no association was observed between the likelihood of receiving ANC from a professional health care provider and the experience of IPV during pregnancy. Further exploration of possible protective factors and specific mechanisms is needed, although it is also possible that such women may be prevented from seeking ANC or may otherwise find such care inaccessible. It is perhaps puzzling that no relationship was found between ANC coverage and spousal violence during pregnancy.[7] Egyptian women have tended to receive less ANC than is desirable for monitoring their pregnancies. Findings from the 1995 EDHS showed that ever-beaten Egyptian wives were significantly less likely to visit a skilled ANC provider (Diop et al. 2006). Coverage rates for pregnancy and delivery care improved markedly thereafter. The 2008 EDHS found that trained health professionals administered ANC to 74 % of pregnant women and helped deliver 79 % of live births, up from just 39 and 46 % of cases, respectively, in 1995 (El-Zanaty and Way 2009). However, these gains may have been partly offset by the political and economic instability that followed the 2011 regime change.

The risk of self-reported STIs/STI symptoms is higher among young and urban women, as expected. After adjusting for other explanatory variables, women subjected to violence from their husbands in pregnancy were 2.4 times more likely to acquire STIs/STI symptoms than were other ever-pregnant women. Although this study does not prove causality, the strength of this relationship after controlling for covariates suggests that physical IPV is a risk factor for STI acquisition. Recent studies of female IPV victims in the U.S. and elsewhere also attest to higher self-reported STI prevalence relative to women in non-violent relationships (Hess et al. 2012; Kishor 2012). This study extends such findings to

---

[7]For example, a study of Indian women who experienced such abuse found they were significantly less likely to seek ANC (Ahmed et al. 2006).

IPV during pregnancy. Abused women face heightened risk for STIs and HIV/AIDS because they are less able to prevent and respond to both abuse and sexual risk (Fuentes 2008). More work is needed to better explain the correlation between IPV and STI/STI symptoms risk. Agreement with at least one justification for wife beating, and living in areas marked by its greater acceptance, raised the odds of experiencing STIs/STI symptoms; so did living in communities characterized by relatively more affluent households.

This study has several limitations that need to be considered. First, although the sample size of ever-pregnant women abused in pregnancy is adequate for drawing a number of inferences that can be reliably generalized to the national level, it is not large, limiting our ability to examine fully every characteristic of interest.

Second, the actual level of abuse may be even higher than that reported because the analysis is subject to the limitations of self-reported retrospective accounts. Some respondents may have not reported (or otherwise misreported) the abuse due to fear of isolation, being shunned, or spousal retaliation.[8] IPV is a sensitive issue in Egypt as elsewhere in the MENA region, where women's rights are bitterly contested and legal recourse against such abuse is limited. Few women sought help and even when seeking help from family, the reactions received may be hostile. As in other Arab countries, Egyptian women are generally expected to balance their needs and well-being against loyalty to one's husband and preservation of family reputation and community appearances (Haj-Yahia and Sadan 2008). On the other hand, the data used in this analysis were collected with a reliable, well-validated and widely used instrument for assessing IPV, mitigating concerns about their quality. Also, earlier estimates of IPV derived from the 1995 EDHS data are broadly similar, lending further credence to some of the findings presented here.

Third, the survey did not collect data on women whose abuse was so severe that it ended in their death. In the USA, about 40–60 % of murders of women are committed by their intimate partners (Horon and Cheng 2001; Palladino et al. 2011). The percentages may be even higher in countries such as Egypt where women's status is lower and their opportunities in public life are severely circumscribed. However, data on such deaths are sparse and contested for most countries and, for the MENA region, they are virtually non-existent. The estimates derived here are likely to be reasonably accurate. If they may partly underestimate the true level of spousal physical abuse that women may be exposed to during pregnancy, they at least reflect a minimum bound on the level of such violence. It should additionally be noted that the percentage of missing responses is generally very small for a complex survey and for the covariates considered.

Fourth, the question asked of women experiencing violence during pregnancy only considered physical violence. Accordingly, we could not consider other forms of IPV that may exhibit different patterns of association with these and other

---

[8] Some women may also not report the abuse if they think that they can find a solution to the problem, that it would not happen again, that their husband would abandon them and that they may lose custody of children, or for other reasons.

covariates. On the other hand, sexual and physical violence are often intertwined and both are nearly always accompanied by psychological abuse. Exposure to multiple forms of violence may compound the risk of negative health outcomes or behaviors, but composite indicators including all forms of violence indicate that ever-married women experienced levels of IPV only slightly higher than that from physical abuse alone (El-Zanaty and Way 2006).

A fifth limitation is that the data on wife beating during pregnancy could not be analyzed for the most recent pregnancy, because they were collected for ever-experience of physical violence during a pregnancy. The data on ANC apply to all births during the 5 years prior to the survey, whilst those regarding STIs/STI symptoms relate to the past year. These periods of exposure are not equal and they are not indexed to the pregnancy period in which the abuse occurred. Consequently, the odds ratios must be interpreted as associations rather than as causal effects, with due caution dictated further by the cross-sectional nature of the data. However, the findings on the prevalence of violence during pregnancy are persuasive and within the range of studies conducted in other countries. Also, the association between STIs/STI symptoms and IPV during pregnancy is highly significant and plausible.

These limitations notwithstanding, this study helps enhance understanding of spousal physical violence during pregnancy in Egypt, including its prevalence, risk factors, attitudes, and deleterious health effects. The present analysis has a number of methodological strengths compared to other studies of this issue in the MENA region. It has used a validated research instrument and a nationally representative sample, with the survey well executed. The analysis has considered valid comparison groups to help derive study inferences about the extent to which specific attributes at multiple levels, as well as several health-related outcomes, are associated with IPV during pregnancy.

Responses to survey questions concerning women's attitudes about IPV are also prone to measurement error and difficult to interpret. Beliefs about such violence are poorly understood in the MENA region. However, attitudes condoning marital violence are shockingly pervasive in Egypt and in Jordan where similar questions have been used (Government of Jordan and ORC Macro 2003). These high levels of tolerance make it far more difficult to tackle such behavior.

Important avenues for further research should address substantive issues as well as some of the methodological difficulties of collecting data on spousal violence during pregnancy. Studies could collect data from husbands for men's views and explore other forms of such violence, as well as repeated and severe physical abuse during pregnancy. Additional research could assess and control for other determinants of IPV seen during and beyond pregnancy in other settings, as well as to explore women's opinions about possible preventive steps and to plan interventions accordingly. Qualitative research could examine how husbands, other kin, non-relatives, health care providers, law enforcement authorities consider and treat victims of pregnancy violence. Such work would help validate the findings presented here, offer a more complete understanding of the problem, and enhance the ability to recommend policies and measures to minimize the prevalence and consequences of such violence in Egypt and elsewhere.

The findings have some important practice implications. They confirm that pregnancy is a period of risk for spousal abuse in Egypt that needs to be discussed during visits to health care providers in the preconception and pregnancy periods. Not a single victim of pregnancy violence in the sample sought assistance from a health care provider, emphasizing the scale of obstacles to implementing screening.[9] In the U.S., numerous medical associations, governmental agencies, and advocacy groups recommend routinely screening for IPV during periodic health examination and asking relevant questions when seeing patients with suggestive signs or symptoms (e.g. AAFP 2004; ACOG 2012; Todahl and Walters 2011). However, many physicians do not follow these recommendations due to such factors as limited knowledge, inadequate training, fear of offending patients, and other factors (Jeanjot et al. 2008; Rodríguez et al. 1999). Egypt lacks effective interventions for IPV victims and shelters are almost non-existent. Indeed, a recent review of regional literature concluded that there are very few legal, social service, or health care resources for IPV victims, who are unable or unwilling to seek help from legal authorities or from health care providers (Boy and Kulczycki 2008). Few offenders are ever punished or granted help for such violent behaviors. There is also no societal consensus for action against IPV in other Arab countries.

Change is possible but will require increased research, coalition-building, and intervention efforts (Boy and Kulczycki 2008; Kulczycki and Windle 2011). Community interventions could include public awareness and media campaigns to change knowledge, attitudes, social and behavioral norms. Gains in education for both women and men, improvements in the quality of male–female relationships, and empowerment of women, would help further reduce the incidence and consequences of wife beating in pregnancy (and at other times). Women could be encouraged to seek help from health care providers who, in turn, should provide linkages and referrals to various health and welfare services. These need to be enhanced but oftentimes, they still need to be instituted in societies where a certain amount of violence against women is condoned, or at least tolerated. For now and in the near term, such research as presented here and dissemination of its findings is key to recognizing and addressing the magnitude and public health significance of this problem, its criminal justice and social care dimensions, as well as its roots.

References

AAFP (American Academy of Family Physicians). (2004). *Family and intimate partner violence and abuse* [*policy statement and position paper*]. Available at: http://www.aafp.org/online/en/home/policy/policies/f/familyandintimatepartnerviolenceandabuse.html. Accessed 14 Aug 2012.

---

[9]It has been suggested that many Lebanese women would likely welcome increased involvement of health care providers, such as through offering clinical screening and inquiring about IPV. This could be a "socially accepted way to break the silence," helping to prevent the worst abuses and possibly heralding other improvements in the situation for women (Usta et al. 2012).

ACOG (American College of Obstetricians and Gynecologists). (2012). ACOG Committee Opinion no. 518: Intimate partner violence, Committee Opinion No. 518. *Obstetrics and Gynecology, 119*(2 Pt 1), 412–417.

Ahmed, S., Koenig, M. A., & Stephenson, R. (2006). Effects of domestic violence on perinatal and early childhood mortality: Evidence from North India. *American Journal of Public Health, 96*(8), 1423–1438.

Akmatov, M. K., Mikolajczyk, R. T., Labeeb, S., Dhaher, E., & Khan, M. M. (2008). Factors associated with wife beating in Egypt: Analysis of two surveys (1995 and 2005). *BMC Women's Health, 8*, 15.

An-Na'im, A. A. (2002). *Islamic family law in a changing world: A global resource book.* Zed Books: London.

Anson, O., & Sagy, S. (1995). Marital violence: Comparing women in violent and nonviolent unions. *Human Relations, 48*(3), 285–305.

Banks, E., Meirik, O., Farley, T., Akande, O., Bathija, H., Ali, M., & The WHO study group on female genital mutilation and obstetric outcome. (2006). Female genital mutilation and obstetric outcome: WHO collaborative prospective study in six African countries. *Lancet, 367*(9525), 1835–1841.

Bohn, D., Tebben, J., & Campbell, J. (2004). Influences of income, education, age, and ethnicity on physical abuse before and during pregnancy. *Journal of Obstetric, Gynecologic, and Neonatal Nursing, 33*(5), 561–571.

Boy, A., & Kulczycki, A. (2008). What we know about intimate partner violence in the Middle East and North Africa. *Violence Against Women, 14*(1), 53–70.

Boyle, E. H. (2002). *Female genital cutting: Cultural conflict in the global community.* Baltimore: Johns Hopkins University Press.

Bronfenbrenner, U. (1979). *The ecology of human development: Experiments by nature and design.* Cambridge, MA: Harvard University Press.

Campbell, J. C. (2002). Health consequences of intimate partner violence. *Lancet, 359*(9314), 1331–1336.

Campbell, J. C., Garcia-Moreno, C., & Sharps, P. W. (2004). Abuse during pregnancy in industrialized and developing countries. *Violence Against Women, 10*(7), 770–789.

Clark, C. J., Hill, A., Jabbar, K., & Silverman, J. G. (2009). Violence during pregnancy in Jordan: Its prevalence and associated risk and protective factors. *Violence Against Women, 15*(6), 720–735.

Coker, A. L., Smith, P. H., Bethea, L., King, M. R., & McKeown, R. E. (2000). Physical health consequences of physical and psychological intimate partner violence. *Archives of Family Medicine, 9*(5), 451–457.

Coker, A. L., Davis, K. E., Arias, I., Desai, S., Sanderson, M., Brandt, H. M., & Smith, P. H. (2002). Physical and mental health effects of intimate partner violence for men and women. *American Journal of Preventive Medicine, 23*(4), 260–268.

Cronholm, P. F., Fogarty, C. T., Ambuel, B., & Harrison, S. L. (2011). Intimate partner violence. *American Family Physician, 83*(10), 1165–1172.

Daoud, N., Urquia, M. L., O'Campo, P., Heaman, M., Janssen, P. A., Smylie, J., & Thiessen, K. (2012). Prevalence of abuse and violence before, during, and after pregnancy in a national sample of Canadian women. *American Journal of Public Health, 102*(10), 1893–1901.

Diop-Sidibé, N., Campbell, J. C., & Becker, S. (2006). Domestic violence against women in Egypt–wife beating and health outcomes. *Social Science and Medicine, 62*(5), 1260–1277.

Ellsberg, M., Heise, L., Pena, R., Agurto, S., & Winkvist, A. (2001). Researching domestic violence against women: Methodological and ethical considerations. *Studies in Family Planning, 32*(1), 1–16.

Ellsberg, M., Jansen, H. A., Heise, L., Watts, C. H., Garcia-Moreno, C., & WHO Multi-country Study on Women's Health and Domestic Violence against Women Study Team. (2008). Intimate partner violence and women's physical and mental health in the WHO Multi-country Study on Women's Health and Domestic Violence: An observational study. *Lancet, 371*(9619), 1165–1172.

El-Zanaty, F., & Way, A. A. (2006). *Egypt demographic and health survey 2005.* Cairo/Calverton: Ministry of Health and Population, National Population Council, El-Zanaty and Associates/ORC Macro.

El-Zanaty, F., & Way, A. (2009). *Egypt demographic and health survey 2008*. Cairo: Ministry of Health and Population, National Population Council, El-Zanaty and Associates/ORC Macro.

El-Zanaty, F., Hussein, E. M., Shawky, G. A., Way, A. A., & Kishor, S. (1996). *Egypt demographic and Health survey 1995*. Cairo/Calverton: National Population Council/Macro International.

Faramarzi, M., Esaelzadeh, S., & Mosavi, S. (2005). Prevalence, maternal complications and birth outcome of physical, sexual and emotional domestic violence during pregnancy. *Acta Medica Iranica, 43*, 115–122.

Fisher, M., Yassour-Borochowitz, D., & Neter, E. (2003). Domestic abuse in pregnancy: Results from a phone survey in Northern Israel. *Israel Medical Association Journal (IMAJ), 5*(1), 35–39.

Freedom House. (2005). *Women's rights in the Middle East and North Africa: Citizenship and justice*. New York: Freedom House.

Fuentes, C. M. (2008). Pathways from interpersonal violence to sexually transmitted infections: A mixed-method study of diverse women. *Journal of Women's Health, 17*(10), 1591–1603.

Garcia-Moreno, C., Jansen, H. A., Ellsberg, M., Heise, L., Watts, H. C., on behalf of the WHO Multi-country Study on Women's Health and Domestic Violence against Women Study Team. (2006). Prevalence of intimate partner violence: Findings from the WHO multi-country study on women's health and domestic violence. *Lancet, 368*(9543), 1260–1269.

Gazmararian, J. A., Lazorick, S., Spitz, A. M., Ballard, T. J., Saltzman, L. E., & Marks, J. S. (1996). Prevalence of violence against pregnant women. *JAMA: The Journal of the American Medical Association, 275*(24), 1915–1920.

Gazmararian, J. A., Petersen, R., Spitz, A. M., Goodwin, M. M., Saltzman, L. E., & Marks, J. S. (2000). Violence and reproductive health: Current knowledge and future research directions. *Maternal and Child Health Journal, 4*(2), 79–84.

Government of Jordan and ORC Macro. (2003). *Jordan population and family health survey 2002*. Calverton/Amman: Department of Statistics, Government of Jordan/ORC Macro.

Gross, G., & Tyring, S. K. (Eds.). (2011). *Sexually transmitted infections and sexually transmitted diseases*. New York: Springer.

Haj-Yahia, M. M., & Sadan, E. (2008). Issues in intervention with battered women in collectivist societies. *Journal of Marital and Family Therapy, 34*(1), 1–13.

Hess, K. L., Javanbakht, M., Brown, J. M., Weiss, R. E., Hsu, P., & Gorbach, P. M. (2012). Intimate partner violence and sexually transmitted infections among young adult women. *Sexually Transmitted Diseases, 39*(5), 366–371.

Hindin, M. J., Kishor, S., & Ansara, D. L. (2008). *Intimate partner violence among couples in 10 DHS countries: Predictors and health outcomes* (DHS analytical studies no. 18). Calverton: Macro International Inc.

Hoodfar, H. (1997). *Between marriage and the market: Intimate politics and survival in Cairo*. Berkeley: University of California Press.

Horon, I. L., & Cheng, D. (2001). Enhanced surveillance for pregnancy-associated mortality–Maryland, 1993–1998. *JAMA, 285*(11), 1455–1459.

Human Rights Watch. (2004). *Divorced from justice: Women's unequal access to divorce in Egypt* (Human Rights Watch Report, 16, no. 8(E)). Available at: http://www.hrw.org/sites/default/files/reports/egypt1204.pdf. Accessed 20 Aug 2012.

Janssen, P. A., Holt, V. L., Sugg, N. K., Emanuel, I., Critchlow, C. M., & Henderson, A. D. (2003). Intimate partner violence and adverse pregnancy outcomes: A population-based study. *American Journal of Obstetrics and Gynecology, 188*(5), 1341–1347.

Jeanjot, I., Barlow, P., & Rozenberg, S. (2008). Domestic violence during pregnancy: Survey of patients and healthcare providers. *Journal of Women's Health, 17*(4), 557–567.

Khawaja, M., & Tewtel-Salem, M. (2004). Agreement between husband and wife reports of domestic violence: Evidence from poor refugee communities in Lebanon. *International Journal of Epidemiology, 33*(3), 526–533.

Kishor, S. (2012). Married women's risk of STIs in developing countries: The role of intimate partner violence and partner's infection status. *Violence Against Women, 18*(7), 829–853.

Kishor, S., & Johnson, K. (2004). *Profiling domestic violence: A multi-country study*. Calverton: ORC Macro.

Koenig, M. A., Lutalo, T., Zhao, F., Nalugoda, F., Wabwire-Mangen, F., Kiwanuka, N., Wagman, J., Serwadda, D., Wawer, M., & Gray, R. (2003). Domestic violence in rural Uganda: Evidence from a community-based study. *Bulletin of the World Health Organization, 81*(1), 53–60.

Kulczycki, A., & Juárez, L. (2003). The Influence of female employment and autonomy on reproductive behaviour in Egypt. In R. Anker, B. Garcia, & A. Pinnelli (Eds.), *Women in the labour market in changing economies: Demographic issues* (pp. 314–330). Oxford: Clarendon Press.

Kulczycki, A., & Windle, S. (2011). Honor killings in the Middle East and North Africa: A systematic review of the literature. *Violence Against Women, 17*(11), 1442–1464.

Letourneau, E. J., Holmes, M., & Chasendunn-Roark, J. (1999). Gynecological health consequences to victims of interpersonal violence. *Women's Health Issues, 9*(2), 115–120.

Mabry, R., Al-Riyami, A., & Morsi, M. (2007). The prevalence of and risk factors for reproductive morbidities among women in Oman. *Studies in Family Planning, 38*(2), 121–128.

Madani, T. A. (2006). Sexually transmitted infections in Saudi Arabia. *BMC Infectious Diseases, 6*, 3.

Mullick, S., Watson-Jones, D., Beksinska, M., & Mabey, D. (2005). Sexually transmitted infections in pregnancy: Prevalence, impact on pregnancy outcomes, and approach to treatment in developing countries. *Sexually Transmitted Infections, 81*(4), 294–302.

Nazir, S. (2005). *Women's rights in the Middle East and North Africa: Citizenship and justice.* New York: Freedom House.

O'Campo, P., Gielen, A. C., Faden, R. R., & Kass, N. (1994). Verbal abuse and physical violence among a cohort of low-income pregnant women. *Women's Health Issues, 4*(1), 29–37.

Palladino, C. L., Singh, V., Campbell, J., Flynn, H., & Gold, K. J. (2011). Homicide and suicide during the perinatal period: Findings from the National Violent Death Reporting System. *Obstetrics and Gynecology, 118*(5), 1056–1063.

Rachana, C., Suraiya, K., Hirsham, A., Abdulaziz, A. M., & Haj, A. (2002). Prevalence and complications of physical violence during pregnancy. *European Journal of Obstetrics, Gynecology, and Reproductive Biology, 103*(1), 26–29.

Rodríguez, M. A., Bauer, H. M., McLoughlin, E., & Grumbach, K. (1999). Screening and intervention for intimate partner abuse: Practices and attitudes of primary care physicians. *Journal of the American Medical Association, 282*(5), 468–474.

Rutstein, S. O., & Johnson, K. (2004). *The DHS wealth index* (DHS comparative reports no. 6). Calverton: ORC Macro.

Sahin, H. A., & Sahin, H. G. (2003). An unaddressed issue: Domestic violence and unplanned pregnancies among pregnant women in Turkey. *The European Journal of Contraception & Reproductive Health Care, 8*(2), 93–98.

Sallam, S. A., Mahfouz, A. A., Dabbous, N. I., El-Barrawy, M., & El-Said, M. M. (2001). Reproductive tract infections among married women in Upper Egypt. *Eastern Mediterranean Health Journal, 7*(1–2), 139–146.

Saltzman, L., Johnson, C., Gilbert, B., & Goodwin, M. (2003). Physical abuse around the time of pregnancy: An examination of prevalence and risk factors in 16 states. *Maternal and Child Health Journal, 7*(1), 31–43.

Straus, M. A. (2007). Conflict tactics scales. In N. A. Jackson (Ed.), *Encyclopedia of domestic violence* (p. 19). New York/London: Routledge.

Straus, M. A., Hamby, S. L., Boney-McCoy, S., & Sugarman, D. B. (1996). The revised Conflict Tactics Scales (CTS2). Development and preliminary psychometric data. *Journal of Family Issues, 17*(3), 283–316.

Straus, M. A., Hamby, S. L., & Warren, W. L. (2003). *The conflict tactics scales handbook: Revised conflict tactics scales (CTS2) CTS: Parent–child version (CTSPC).* Los Angeles: Western Psychological Services.

Sunil, T. S., & Pillai, V. (2010). *Women's reproductive health in Yemen.* Amherst: Cambria Press.

Thananowan, N., & Heidrich, S. M. (2008). Intimate partner violence among pregnant Thai women. *Violence Against Women, 14*(5), 509–527.

Tjaden, P., & Thoennes, N. (2000). *Extent, nature, and consequences of intimate partner violence* . Washington, DC: U.S. Department of Justice, National Institute of Justice.

Todahl, J., & Walters, E. (2011). Universal screening for intimate partner violence: A systematic review. *Journal of Marital and Family Therapy, 37*(3), 355–369.

UN. (2011). *World population prospects: The 2010 revision.* New York: United Nations.

UNDP. (2006). *Arab human development report 2006: Towards the rise of women in the Arab world.* New York: United Nations Development Programme. Available at: http://www.arab-hdr.org/contents/index.aspx?rid=4. Accessed 28 July 2012.

UNDP. (2011). *Human development report 2011.* New York: Palgrave Macmillan, published for the United Nations Development Programm.

Usta, A. J., Ambuel, B., & Khawaja, M. (2012). Involving the health care system in domestic violence: What women want. *Annals of Family Medicine, 10*(3), 213–220.

Watts, C., & Zimmerman, C. (2002). Violence against women: Global scope and magnitude. *Lancet, 359*(9313), 1232–1237.

WHO, UNICEF, UNFPA, & World Bank. (2010). *Trends in maternal mortality: 1990–2008.* Geneva: World Health Organization.

Chapter 4
Addressing Men's Concerns About Reproductive Health Services and Fertility Regulation in a Rural Sahelian Setting of Northern Ghana: The *"Zurugelu Approach"*

Philip Baba Adongo, James F. Phillips, and Colin D. Baynes

4.1 Introduction

Convenient, nonclinical, community-based services that use community organization, structure and institutions has emerged as the core strategy to expand access to contraceptive technologies in sub-Saharan Africa (Kols and Wawer 1982). Lessons from experimental projects, first in Asia and Latin America, revealed that this approach, collectively termed "community-based distribution" (CBD), can enhance the quality, appropriateness and impact of family planning programs (Foreit et al. 1978; Freedman 1987). Widespread commitment to the CBD approach ensued, and with it, the proliferation of analogous programs in Africa. It was assumed that CBD implementation would expand the acceptability and convenience of contraception and reduce costs, thereby extending use among clientele who seek contraceptives but would not use services that are confined to clinical settings (Ross and Frankenberg 1993). The lack of convenient access to contraceptives was viewed as the primary barrier to the practice of family planning rather than cultural and societal barriers.

In Africa, the proliferation of CBD programs with contrasting operational designs challenged the view that CBD implementation would have uniform consequences. Throughout the region, CBD typically focused on the provision of oral contraceptives, foam tablets, and condoms. Some programs promoted the concept of dual protection against unwanted pregnancy and sexually transmitted infections including HIV/AIDS (e.g. Musau 1997; d'Cruz-Grote 1996). Other CBD initiatives integrated

P.B. Adongo, Ph.D. (✉)
Department of Social and Behavioral Sciences, School of Public Health,
University of Ghana, Legon, Accra, Ghana
e-mail: adongophilip@yahoo.com

J.F. Phillips, Ph.D. • C.D. Baynes, MPH
Heilbrunn Department of Population and Family Health, Columbia University,
Mailman School of Public Health, New York, NY, USA
e-mail: james.phillips@columbia.edu

A. Kulczycki (ed.), *Critical Issues in Reproductive Health*, The Springer Series on
Demographic Methods and Population Analysis 33, DOI 10.1007/978-94-007-6722-5_4,
© Springer Science+Business Media Dordrecht 2014

family planning services with child health and welfare services (e.g. Nicholas 1978; Ringheim et al. 2011). Some CBD projects emphasized the advantages of deploying local volunteers to make family planning supplies and information readily available (Bertrand et al. 1986; Ross et al. 1987), while other programs employed salaried paramedical workers to visit households and provide condom and oral pill supplies (e.g. Zinanga 1990; Munyakazi 1989). Alternatively, CBD agents were engaged in the commercial sales of contraceptives in traditional markets or in conjunction with social marketing efforts (e.g. Bertrand et al. 1993).

Although the various CBD strategies that proliferated in Africa during the 1980s–1990s were shown to contribute to increasing contraceptive adoption (e.g. Goldberg et al. 1989; Dube et al. 1998), research yielded little evidence that they reduced fertility (Phillips et al. 1999). In Africa, where post-partum abstinence customs often substantially reduce fertility, adoption of modern family planning methods can substitute for such birth spacing behaviors, fostering debate about the relevance of CBD to demographic change in the region.

The absence of impact in Africa has been attributed to the persistence of socio-cultural constraints, most prominently gender stratification and inequality. Studies have associated CBD with both decreases in unmet need (Luck et al. 2000) and increases in unmet need (Debpuur et al. 2002) for contraceptives, but the mechanisms through which it attains such effects remain unclear. Several analysts have shown that gender inequity, spousal dynamics, and norms that value large families in male-dominated lineages play a greater role in determining unmet need in Africa than does access (Bongaarts and Bruce 1995; Rutenberg and Watkins 1997). Few studies (e.g. Doctor 2010) have connected CBD inputs with mediating variables, such as spousal communication and fertility preference outcomes. Other studies (e.g. Bawah et al. 1999) connect spousal communication with increases in contraceptive use. Nevertheless, because this evidence lacks sufficient coherence, the policy implications of the effect of CBD strategies on gender dynamics and contraceptive ideational change remain poorly understood.

This chapter assesses the relative impact of contrasting CBD programs on socio-cultural processes that mediate fertility and contraceptive behaviour in a socially and culturally adverse setting in Africa. It uses mixed methods to test the hypothesis that these contrasting operational designs have differential fertility effects. We consider the example of Kassena-Nankana District in northern Ghana, an impoverished rural area characterized by subsistence farming, the persistence of traditional social institutions, and bride-wealth traditions which regard women as property of male-dominated lineages for ensuring reproduction. The people of the locality are predominantly peasant farmers for whom traditional beliefs and ancestral allegiance inform their way of life. Women are allowed very little autonomy, a situation that is reinforced by their low levels of literacy and limited mobility. Owing to dispersed settlements that lack modern economic or communication systems, women are isolated from new institutions, ideas and practices (Doctor et al. 2009). Maternal health seeking has historically been governed by local traditional, poverty and male-dominated gate-keeping systems (Adongo et al. 1997). In this context, family planning services challenge ingrained norms of male prerogative over reproduction.

This chapter uses data from the Navrongo Demographic Surveillance System (NDSS), fertility determinants results from panel surveys, and qualitative interviews to assess the relationship between CBD program strategies and fertility. The Community Health and Family Planning Project (CHFP) in Navrongo combines the challenges of implementing family planning services in an impoverished and traditional Sahelian setting with the opportunity to test hypotheses with excellent longitudinal demographic data that can be interpreted with guidance from qualitative research.

4.2 Cells of the Experimental Design

In 1994 the Navrongo Health Research Center launched a three village pilot project for developing and refining operational strategies for community-based health and family planning services (Nazzar et al. 1995). In 1996, the pilot was scaled up to a district-wide test of the hypothesis that improving family planning services could have demographic effects among the Kassena-Nankana (Binka et al. 1995). The CHFP combined formative, operations and experimental research on a test of the relative effects of alternative service strategies on child mortality and fertility. Each strategy was integrated into a modified regimen of an approach to primary health care known as the "Integrated Management of Childhood Illnesses" (IMCI). As indicated in Fig. 4.1, two arms of the experiment corresponded to four competing policy positions regarding optimal ways to add family planning to IMCI[1]:

Community Health Officers in Village	Mobilizing traditional community organization with the "Zurugelu Approach":	
	No	Yes
No	Comparison (Cell 4)	Zurugelu System only (Cell 1)
Yes	Community Health Officers only (Cell 2)	Combined: Community Health Officers with the Zurugelu system (Cell 3)

Fig. 4.1 Cells in the experimental design

---

[1]The "Integrated Management of Childhood Illness (IMCI)" approach was intended to improve health by training workers to recognize treatment needs of a wide range of health problems and engage parents and communities in improving recognition of illness and appropriate actions (see WHO (2008)).

4.2.1   Cell 1: The Zurugelu System

One set of activities marshalled traditional social institutions for community leadership and participation, with the aim of building male involvement and understanding of the program.[2] The program trained male volunteers to sensitize men to gender and reproductive health issues, address their informational needs, challenge prevailing views on reproduction and promote the use of condoms. Equipped with discussion themes that were developed in focus groups, volunteers targeted opinion leaders, such as chiefs and elders, and used traditional forums, namely durbars, to convene men and disseminate messages.[3] This approach advanced women's position by linking them to leadership opportunities in durbars and outreach events, and involved them in planning and directing events that had been the sole prerogative of chiefs and elders. This arm of the study was termed the "*Zurugelu*" component, which in the local language connotes togetherness for the common good. Family planning services in Cell 1 were delivered through Ministry of Health clinical activities.

4.2.2   Cell 2: Community Health Officers

Cell 2 of the CHFP represents the CBD condition. An existing cadre of Community Health Nurses were trained in community liaison and organizational methods and re-located from sub-district clinics to village-based locations.[4] These retrained workers were termed "Community Health Officers (CHO)." These nurses were based at health posts and equipped to conduct household service outreach, but there were no *Zurugelu* activities. Community leaders were convened and invited to construct, with local volunteer labor and resources, a temporary structure where these nurses could live and work. Over time, Ghana Health Service resources have been used to convert temporary community constructed facilities into permanent health posts known as "Community Health Compounds." In all, 16 Cell 2 and 3 communities took up this challenge, comprising the CHO dimension of the CHFP design.

---

[2]Community engagement components of the Zurugelu approach were designed to sustain access to basic pharmaceutical supplies. Volunteer recruitment and management procedures were adapted from the recommendations of the UNICEF sponsored "Bamako Initiative" which sought to translate social institutions into resources that organize primary healthcare (Knippenberg et al. 1990). Family planning themes and activities were added to Bamako mandated health service strategies.

[3]The term "durbar" refers to an event, convened by chiefs and elders, to assemble family heads for making announcements, building consensus, and gauging community reactions to some event or activity of collective interest. Employed extensively in northern Ghana as an important mechanism for community governance, durbars were utilized in the CHFP to promote health awareness and build understanding of project activities (Tindana et al. 2007).

[4]This approach represented the view promoted by the World Bank at the time which advocated the use of paid, professional nurses to improve the range and coverage of community health care (World Bank 2003).

4.2.3   Cell 3: The Combined Condition

Communities in this cell were exposed to a combination of both the *Zurugelu* and CHO interventions. As in Cell 2, community leaders were invited to convene meetings for the purpose of discussing health problems and feasible means of developing community support for service delivery. Also, as in Cell 2, particular emphasis was focused on discussing the health service capabilities of CHO and health care that could be provided if community members volunteered to construct health posts where nurses could reside and provide services. With guidance from the project, facilities were developed with traditional construction methods and materials, and nurses were posted with a mandate to provide care at these facilities, visit households, promote childhood vaccination, and make family planning available. After the nurses were assigned to village health posts, volunteers were recruited, trained, and deployed to implement the male-focused *Zurugelu* approach to family planning promotion and also support the organizational requirements of CHO services such as the childhood vaccination program, health referral, and community outreach.

4.2.4   Cell 4: The Comparison Area

In Cell 4, usual Ministry of Health clinical and outreach services were conducted with staff densities equivalent to the staffing patterns of the treatment cells. It lacked the community-based service experimental activities of Cells 1, 2 and 3. Though no new technologies were tested in this cell, none of the existing health services were withdrawn either.

4.3   Analytical Framework

The CHFP was designed to address debate about the demographic significance of family planning programs in Africa. By the 1990s, the literature on contraceptive introduction in rural African settings portrayed access to supplies as the main barrier to use, under the assumption that increased availability of services in convenient rural locations offset unmet need for family planning by addressing logistical constraints (Robey et al. 1993; National Population Council 1994; Ghana Statistical Service and Macro International 1994). This "supply-side" perspective is illustrated in Fig. 4.2 by pathways labelled "A."[5] Demand for fertility regulation was deemed to be "latent," owing to social, monetary, and logistical costs associated

---

[5]Figure 4.2 is adapted from the "Easterlin Synthesis Framework" (Easterlin and Crimmins 1985; Easterlin et al. 1988).

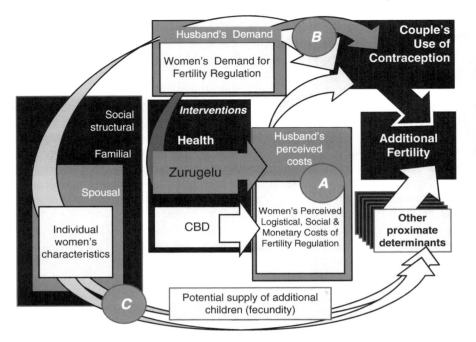

Fig. 4.2 A framework for the determinants of additional fertility (Source: Adapted from Easterlin and Crimmins (1985) and Easterlin et al. (1988))

with contraception. Mitigating these costs, through CBD, was posited to be a viable mechanism for serving the needs of women, and reducing excess fertility.

At the outset of the Navrongo Project, however, the impact of these contraceptive distribution schemes in Africa was unknown and their efficacy the subject of discussion and debate (e.g. Caldwell and Caldwell 1988). Demand-side perspectives in this debate are illustrated by the pathways labelled "B" in Fig. 4.2. In this view, socio-structural factors associated with the corporate community, extended family, and institutions of marriage maintain high fertility norms and motives (illustrated with the exogenous determinants leading to B in Fig. 4.2). Africa, it was argued, is a uniquely unfavourable context for developing CBD supply-side strategies, since the motivation to regulate fertility was negligible (e.g. Frank and McNicoll 1987).

Studies of birth interval dynamics showed that fertility regulation in Africa is often the consequence of cultural practices that profoundly affect birth spacing, even in the absence of contraception (e.g. Shoenmaecker et al. 1981). Shown in Fig. 4.2 as pathway C, cultural practices that sustain post-partum abstinence can be substituted with temporary use of contraception, without affecting fertility levels (Bledsoe et al. 1998). Evidence that CBD can increase contraceptive use does not necessarily mean that CBD reduces fertility.

The framework proposed in this analysis reflects a review of these perspectives and their relative explanatory power vis-a-vis the fertility changes observed over the course of the CHFP. Along with analyses of panel data showing that these patterns evolved over time, qualitative studies were also used to inform the design of the CHFP and assess community reactions during implementation. Analyzed together they reflect the gender context of the project, and each pathway in Fig. 4.2 is delineated by gender, illustrating the consequences of gender stratification, male pronatalist reproductive motives, and the constrained autonomy of women. Men and their motives define the context for women to implement their reproductive preferences. In this context, neither purely socio-structural or cultural climate for contraceptive demand, nor simple efforts to increase access to services, defines the demand for children and motivation to adopt family planning. Based on these findings, it was reasonable to posit that the CHFP could be fully realized without a combined services condition, Cell 3, which addressed the need for strategies that would impact both pathways A and B in Fig. 4.2. To assess the merit of this hypothesis, cell specification of the service delivery approach and concurrent evaluation was required. The following account tells this story and reviews its implications for policy and program action.

4.4 Methods

Since July, 1993, the NDSS has conducted continuous monitoring of health and demographic events such as marital changes, births, deaths, migrations into and out of households on a population of approximately 143,000 individuals and 43,000 women of reproductive age (Binka et al. 1999, 2007; Phillips et al. 2000; Ngom et al. 2001). Beginning in 1993 and ending in 2003, the CHFP augmented the NDSS with a yearly panel survey to collect detailed information on socio-demographic characteristics, reproductive preferences and behaviour, health seeking behaviour, and other topics. A randomized cluster sample of approximately 18 % of 12,000 extended family "compounds" of Kassena-Nankana District was drawn from the NDSS population. All women aged 15–49 and their co-resident spouses were interviewed at the time of each survey, with questionnaire instruments that were designed to maximize comparison with national Demographic and Health Survey modules for reproductive health and family planning (Debpuur et al. 2002).

Qualitative data were compiled at the onset of pilot activities and again in 1996, 2 years after the project had been launched, with the goal of gauging community reactions to the general CHFP. All data used for the present analysis were compiled in 1996. The present analysis thus aims to ascertain the possible predictive value of themes from an early period in the project that could explain long term demographic trends. The 1996 sessions were convened with a special emphasis on fostering discussion of how reactions may have differed by cell. In each cell of the experiment, eight focus group discussions (FGDs) involving men were held with 8–12 men in each group. Half of the sessions were with men under 35 years of age; half were with older men under age 50. These sessions were balanced by gender so that two complete sets of discussions were held in each Cell – one exclusively with men and the other with women. Only married individuals were selected for group discussions. In addition, participants were purposively selected to reflect both men and women who were currently using, those who had ever used, and those who had never used contraceptives. The age of the female participants ranged from 20 to 38 years, and that of the males ranged from 28 to 45 years.

Four individuals with experience in moderating FGDs were recruited and divided into two teams, each comprised of a moderator and a facilitator. Assistance was sought from key informants to help identify and recruit participants from the community for the interviews. Information about the objectives of the discussion and the purpose of the overall study were provided to each potential participant. Confidentiality with regard to their participation and anonymity with regard to their stored data were assured, and each participant was asked for his or her verbal consent to participate in the interview or FGD. Permission to audio-record the discussions was also sought and obtained.

All interviews were tape recorded in Kassim and/or Nankam, the two main dialects of the area. The recordings were then transcribed into English and analysed according to principal themes in an effort to assess the extent of the community's response to program activities. Unique words and phrases or those that were difficult to translate remaining in the local language were left untranslated. Data were analysed using a grounded theory approach which generalised views and perceptions of the various themes (Kruger 1988).

4.4.1   The Fertility Impact of the CHFP

Figure 4.3 presents total fertility rates (TFR) and age-specific fertility rates by cell and project years, respectively. As the figure shows, the TFR declined gradually in all study areas over the 1994–2003 period. Modest fertility declines in Cells 1, 2, and 3 prior to scale-up suggest that access to contraception may have had an impact, although the decline was statistically significant in Cell 3 alone. Where nurses and volunteers worked in combination, fertility declined by one half a birth prior to 2003 (Debpuur et al. 2002; Phillips et al. 2006) and an additional half birth after scale-up by the year 2010.

In all cells, fertility increased in 2000, most prominently in Cell 3. This may have been the consequence of a general operational problem that affected all four areas. In 1999, the Ministry of Health imposed a scheme for the provision of essential drugs that was known as the "Exemption Scheme." All under-5 children were to be provided with cost-free access to essential drugs. But, the central supply of drugs was unsustainable, stockouts were common, and community nurse operations were dramatically curtailed. This disruption in primary health care indirectly affected the provision of contraceptive services. By 2000, project supported changes provided a basis for the Exemption Scheme to function. This restored essential operations,

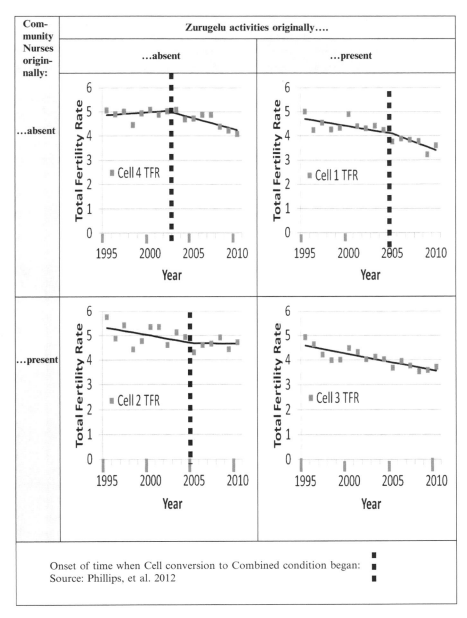

Fig. 4.3 Total fertility rate (TFR) trends in original project cells as defined in 1995 with corresponding post-project trends to 2010 (Source: Phillips et al. (2012))

although the 1999 disruption was associated with widespread discontinuation of contraceptive use in all experimental cells.

Other operational changes in 2000 affected the supply on family planning services. Beginning in 2000, communities of the *Zurugelu* Cell 1 and Comparison Cell 4 were provided with nurses on the CHO Cell 2 model. This change in the design was gradual, with implementation constrained by the pace of construction of community health posts. Nevertheless, the gradual conversion of experimental operations had discernible fertility implications that are illustrated by the trends in Fig. 4.3. Linear spline regression is employed to test the proposition that the scaling-up process was associated with a disjuncture in the TFR time trend for the subsequent period.

It is appropriate to note, however, that expansion of the CHFP followed operational activities that essentially abandoned the *Zurugelu* approach to addressing "social costs" constraints to family planning. Although volunteer operations were developed in the post-CHFP period, the scaling-up process was gradual and centered on the promotion of IMCI and other priority child survival initiatives of the new UNICEF program that focused on volunteer mobilization for accelerating improvement in child health. Since the *Zurugelu* reproductive health emphasis of the CHFP was not scaled up in Cells 2 and 4, "scaling-up" was tantamount to converting Cell 1 to a Cell 3 design while Cell 2 was converted to an approach that was never tested in the experiment: the combination of community nursing with volunteer activities that lacked a family planning focus. Perhaps as a result of this lack of focus on family planning, the post-scale up fertility trend in Cell 2 was unaffected by change and Cell 4 was gradually converted to a Cell 2 design as health posts were constructed and nurses assigned to village locations. Thus, in Cells 2 and 4, *Zurugelu* family planning activities were lacking even though volunteers were deployed for health promotion.

The changes introduced convenient access to comprehensive doorstep health services provided by nurses, but sustained operational variance in the family planning component of community health care. Most importantly, the prior existence of *Zurugelu* activities in Cell 1 led to significant fertility decline when community-based nursing services were instituted in that context, as suggested by the post scale-up slope in Cell 1 that is identical to the slope of Cell 3 in the corresponding period. Conversely, the absence of a male-focused *Zurugelu* strategy in Cell 2 was associated with an insignificant fertility impact of the post-CHFP design of the scale up. Where doorstep family planning was never a focus of the original CHFP – the scale-up of CHFP services in Cell 4 communities had the effect of developing doorstep health services without the provision of correspondingly intense *Zurugelu* family planning activities for men that could offset the social costs of family planning. As a consequence, the phasing in of community-based services had no apparent fertility impact, even though mortality effects of the post-CHFP approach were sufficient to sustain the health and survival impact of the original CHFP operational design. Findings thus suggest that developing family planning access, in the absence of strategies for mitigating social costs, had little discernible impact.

4.4.2   Qualitative Appraisal of Men's Reactions to the CHFP

Qualitative research, conducted early in the CHFP exposure period, provide explanatory data for interpreting the fertility trends in the years that followed. FGDs with male members of the study population in 1996 in each cell revealed that reactions and attitudes formed in response to CBD differed according to delivery strategy. The areas in which differences emerged most prominently involved men's reproductive preferences, acceptance of contraceptive use, views toward women's reproductive autonomy and, lastly, recourse to gender-based violence.

4.4.3   Reproductive Preferences

Contrary to initial evidence of pervasive male misgivings and fears about family planning, many men subsequently expressed the view that family planning can have positive benefits, suggesting that initial project activities were already impacting reproductive preferences. The discussion of reproductive preferences in all experimental cells suggested that the desire to have a large number of children was decreasing even by 1996. A common theme of respondents, in all cells of the project, was the view that the current generation has faced unprecedented agricultural adversity. Given pervasive poverty, men in particular, often expressed the view that having fewer children was more desirable now than had been the case for the previous generation. Several men suggested that parents should respond to adversity by having smaller families so that their limited resources could have a greater impact on the health, educational and professional development of their children. Discussion thus suggested that generalized social change was emerging from recent decades of agricultural adversity, even at the onset of the CHFP.

However, subtle distinctions between cells are evident. Whereas economic and agricultural pressures were salient across cells, attitudes toward decreasing the number of children a family has, nevertheless, varied according to exposure to health service orientation. The shift towards preferences for fewer children, which was most prominent in *Zurugelu* communities, may have been influenced by community gatherings (referred to as "durbars") and the social interaction among peers that such events catalyze. The program appears to have contributed to a transition away from strong pronatalist values by fostering open discussion of the link between family planning and the growing poverty-led demand for spacing and limiting births. As two male respondents exposed to *Zurugelu* activities in Cell 1 stated:

> I think it will be good to have few children. If my father had a small family, I think I should have been able to attend school to a higher level than I have. But because we were many, my father was not able to take care of our school needs and as a result we had to stop schooling at a very low level.

> Those who have never heard it and have now got the message should try and practice it. You have two children now, and there is no food for them to eat yet in the night you won't allow your wife to sleep, two or three days you will have many children crying for food and health care, something you cannot provide.

In Cell 1, these and other responses suggest childhood educational attainment is both increasingly important and unaffordable, given the intensifying economic pressures arising from diminishing agricultural productivity. In Cell 3 where these sentiments were also common, parental costs of child bearing were linked with a perception that family planning was an appropriate response of men to family economic problems, as indicated by the following responses from the men:

> What I have to say is that, in the past when we farmed, we got enough food to take care of our children so that they will be strong and healthy. Now… it is difficult to feed your children, take them to hospital and clothe them. Those who understand the current economic situation will try family planning.

> If you have so many children and they are sick, you cannot cater for them. Here, we want our children to be farmers, but if you have one child at school and two children at home and the one in school comes home asking for school fees, which are now high, and the others are also sick, you will not be able to meet their needs.

Commentary from men in this experimental area not only connects the utility of family planning to mitigate economic pressures by limiting family size, but also the mutually reinforcing link between family planning and child health and care-seeking. The combined approach of Cell 3, including household promotion of child health and management of common illnesses, alleviated men's widespread perception that large families were an essential response to the likelihood that many would die from disease during infancy and early childhood. This view was sustained by the ongoing provision of child health promotion and services in households – improved access to live saving care entrenched the belief that families could succeed in keeping children alive if family size remained within manageable limits. Additional views that figured prominently in discussions with men from Cell 3 included increased practice of birth spacing discussions within couples, increased value attached to women's preferences, a stronger sense of personal commitment to child spacing through family planning specifically, and engagement with the health system more broadly.

Men in households only exposed to the community-health officer (CHO) piece of the intervention expressed views only marginally affected by increased accessed to family planning. Comments made by male community members from Cell 2 regarding the utility of contraception illustrate this effect:

> Women need to be educated well on family planning use. I'm saying this because some women use family planning when they have not given birth, even for the first time, and sometimes not at all [without ever having given birth]. Family planning use is good when a woman has given birth to three or so babies.

> It is good to have a large family because our great grandparents have an adage that 'two heads are better than one.' So if you have two children struggling to make life worthwhile, it is better than having just one child. Man will never eat grass, he shall always survive (man will always live above waters).

Though male participants had become open to family planning, its use was deemed as appropriate only after minimum fertility desires had been attained, at which point spacing though contraceptive uptake could commence. This preference was, in turn, perpetuated by ongoing adherence to traditional, pronatalist norms which, in Cell 2, remained unquestioned in the absence of *Zurugelu* activities.

Those interviewed in Cell 4, where men were neither exposed to *Zurugelu* activities nor services provided by a CHO, maintained typically traditional reproductive preferences owing to the belief that some children are likely to die from disease during their first years. Also emerging saliently in the discussions was a general ambivalence toward the suggestion of smaller family sizes. This is highlighted in the following quotes from male participants in cell 4:

> Family planning is good but the fact is that whenever there is an outbreak of measles, it can kill as many as six or seven children of a single couple, so if you have four children and this happens, it means you have no child. If you can help us with a method that would prevent our children from dying, we can practice family planning.

> Some women cannot even have more than four children so such women's families have been planned by God. Some of us even wish our wives who have just one or two children to have more but we cannot, so how do we practice family planning?

Among those exposed to neither experimental service orientation, attitudes remained closed to the notion of striving for a smaller family size, owing to the inaccessibility of services that could spare children from the scourge of disease. Though men recognized economic and other pressures imposed by rearing many children, they maintained traditional positions resting on the utility of children to "fend for themselves" on farms. Pregnancy and pregnancy outcomes were viewed in largely fatalistic terms – renouncing a couple's right to regulate fertility in defence of God's will. Throughout discussions the problem of infertility or challenges to have enough children emerged almost as commonly as the challenge of rearing many children. Families should focus on meeting their needs for both sons and daughters before any means to plan family size be taken into consideration.

In general, discussions suggest that *zurugelu* activities had attitudinal effects that interacted with the provision of convenient family planning services. Male-focused community outreach resonated with economic conditions that were fostering social change. Supported by the social and economic changes occurring in this setting, men were prompted to increasingly view children as costly rather than as signs of abundance that would contribute to agrarian wealth. In communities where family planning was accessible, emerging views interacted with reproductive health messages and discussions in ways that enabled women to convert their reproductive preferences into spousal discussion of family planning and actual contraceptive use.

4.4.4 Contraceptive Acceptability

Men's attitudes towards implementing reproductive preferences mirrored their expressed attitudes regarding an ideal family size. In the *Zurugelu*-only Cell 1, men seemed conflicted expressing support for family planning, while also expressing discord and mistrust about family planning services. Here also, child survival emerged as a concern of men:

We have actually heard about family planning, but some of us do not want to practice it for fear that our children may all die. My mother gave birth to fifteen of us, but I am now her only child surviving. If she had given birth to two children she would have been childless now. That is why even though we want to practice family planning, on second thought we discard the idea.

One bad thing about [contraceptive use] is that some of the women do it without informing their husbands… [the women] do not respect their husbands… there are women who used to give birth so often, we can see that they allow longer time between their children. We think that these women are practicing family planning, but the fact is that they will not inform you before doing it.

As with reproductive preferences, men not exposed to household child survival services remain inclined to reject family planning, despite the understanding of it generated through *Zurugelu* outreach. Emphasis on maintaining a strong lineage through offspring takes priority over expanding couples' underlying reproductive desires through contraceptives use. Spousal communication is highlighted and valued among participants, at least conceptually, but, in practice, the adoption of contraceptive methods occurs distantly from the household domain. This undermines longstanding male gate-keeping practices and stirs spousal mistrust and a search for clandestine services, ultimately exacerbating traditionally loose conjugal bonds.

Feedback from men exposed to both *Zurugelu* and CHO activities in Cell 3 bore similarities to responses heard in Cell 1; however, men conveyed greater openness to women's use of modern methods, mostly as a function of the increased availability of services that promoted child survival. Family planning in this setting was discussed not simply as a service for women to access in secret, but rather as an opportunity for couples to achieve fertility aims together. The following quotes by men in cell 3 clarify these points:

Our fathers used to have so many children because measles could kill all of them. In their time there was nothing like a clinic or even vaccines against all these diseases but we have been immunizing our children against measles now and for some years now, even though there is normally an outbreak of measles, it is not able to kill the children. In my opinion, family planning is good… we have changed our attitude towards family planning, but health as well.

The contraceptives really help and we are not against the use of these methods but if a woman comes to the clinic without the husband, insist that she brings the husband. These women are trying to take control of our homes as decision makers…. You have to organize a meeting like this one, talk to the women about family planning and tell them to come along with their husbands if they want to adopt a method.

Attitudinal changes may have been fostered by the combination of doorstep prevention and management of childhood illness with volunteer outreach and family planning service delivery from nurses, since health outreach fostered the belief that childhood mortality risks were reduced. Men still believed that they were the appropriate gate-keeper for decisions about contraception, but where *Zurugelu* activities took place, they were better informed and more inclined to discuss reproduction with wives. In this climate of conflict-free dialogue, women's desires could ultimately carry more weight than had previously been the case.

In contrast, men in Cell 2 – where only the Community Health Nurses were operating – tended to believe that women had taken full control of the decision to use contraception. Although they supported the general concept and purpose of family planning, these men lamented their lack of understanding and education about contraceptive methods. This perpetuated myths and misunderstanding of contraceptive side-effects that, in turn, led to reservations and discontinuation of method use. The way in which service delivery targeted only women introduced marital tensions that propagated male aversion to method use, despite their vague agreement with the idea of family planning:

> Family planning makes women become flirts, because they are practicing family planning and they know they will not get pregnant again, they go after men outside their marriages… that it will prevent your wife from getting unwanted pregnancies is good. But we do not know what we can do about the women going outside their marriages to look for men when they are practicing family planning."

Such expressions of spousal mistrust regarding contraceptive use were a source of male anxiety in all cells, particularly in those without exposure to *Zurugelu* activities. Family planning was portrayed as emasculating for men and potentially sterilizing among women. Lack of understanding of contraception in Cell 2, and the need for more education and communication, provided men with misconceptions that were embedded in discussions of this mistrust:

> The problem we have with family planning is that we are not properly educated about it. The women go and they just mix drugs anyhow for them and so some of them can't give birth after taking the drugs. I have a number of sisters who are victims of this. Now they can no longer give birth. You don't educate the women properly.

In Cell 4, where the population was neither exposed to the *Zurugelu* activities nor the CHO, men expressed a sense of helplessness with respect to the concept of family planning in general. Although they had heard of contraceptives and thought that they could be useful, poverty and limited educational opportunities gave rise to the belief that they particularly could not benefit from family planning. These views are highlighted in the following statements made by men from cell 4:

> We have heard about family planning but we have not practiced it. This is because we have not understood it. A husband or a wife may therefore want to practice it but because his or her partner does not understand it, he or she may not agree to do it… some couples practice the methods yet their women still get pregnant. I therefore think we need education on the methods.

> Some people do not have money to practice these methods and a result they always see them as unnecessary. Three years ago, they used to give the pill and the loop to people free of charge in this area. Of late, they do not do that again and people are forced to buy from the drug stores but the prices of these things in the stores are very high that some of us cannot afford them.

In this case, the emasculating effects of introducing family planning did not take effect due to the more fundamental barriers to services that this population faced: knowledge, access and perceived "social costs." Though the monetary cost of contraceptives was the same across cells, the absence of sensitization, outreach and doorstep services in Cell 4 precluded men in this setting from making a cost-benefit decision which would be well-informed, involves spousal communication, and is unencumbered from the opportunity costs and stigma attached to active care-seeking.

4.4.5 Women's Reproductive Autonomy

The CHFP has had a significant impact on shifting gender roles in the exposed communities. As the project progressed, women increasingly took control of their reproductive decision-making, and in response, men gradually learned to accept this fundamental change. Family planning adoption was perceived to be tantamount to women's assertions of autonomy, precipitating concern and anxiety among men across all experimental cells. However, early in the experimental period, there emerged discernable cell variation in male tolerance of women's family planning decision-making. Men in Cell 1 (where *Zurugelu* activities were carried out without the CHO) openly communicated about family planning, but linked the practice to spousal sexual mistrust:

> Some of the women do not feel free to discuss family planning issues with their fellow women because if they discuss it with them and they are not in support, they may go out to talk about them. They may even think that those who want to do it are women who like flirting with men, that is why they want to do that.

> Even if it is that the women see them practicing the family planning, then they will snicker and say the women is flirting and maybe moving outside the house to be away from the husband. So for this she may not decide to discuss with some of the women.

Whereas openness to women's reproductive freedom appears to have been an early response to CHFP activities in Cell 3, the lack of direct services constrained reproductive autonomy. Nonetheless, some men expressed a willingness to take action to mitigate the effects of stigma on service-seeking. In this sense, men in cell 3 seemed not simply supportive of the idea of women's autonomy; they were also involved in putting the concept into practice:

> Some couples do discuss family planning, and when they are all convinced that family planning is good, the man gives the wife the go ahead to use it. Even if it gets to a situation that the woman goes to the nurse and she asks her for her husband to come, the man goes with his wife.

Exposure to the actual service itself, together with the effects of sensitization and communication activities, enabled men to either accompany their wives to a service point or concur with their mobility without undo concern about ostracism from other men. In Cell 3, women's autonomy may have been enhanced more generally, enabling women to participate in village governance:

> There are great changes. If there are meetings, we come out just like today. The men also attend their meeting. In the past when they call meetings and women attend, it is a problem in the house, but now women are free to attend meetings just as men. (Female community member, Cell 3).

In Cell 2, where Community Health Nurses were deployed without supporting *Zurugelu* activities, study participants reported relatively severe social constraints to the practice of women's autonomy. These constraints included male spousal mistrust and recourse to violence with concomitant reluctance among women to discuss family planning with their husbands. In expressing this sentiment, a man noted:

> Some women are aware that their husbands know that they flirt with other men outside their marriages. Such women may therefore not feel free to discuss family planning with their husbands. This may bring a conflict between the man and the woman who has discussed it with the man's wife.

> ... the reason why I will beat my wife if she tells me that she wants to use family planning is that if I have only two children, both of them can die overnight. I can also die as well; so if I allow my wife to use family planning for five years and my children die, one day what will I do if Addah's [referring to a fellow participant] children come to attack my house? That is why I will not let her do it. If I see her using it, I will beat her.

Where services were provided without outreach to men, activities heightened male suspicion that they were excluded from reproductive decision-making, reducing their authority and status in the family. Similar perspectives were expressed by men in Cell 4, where women often sought services clandestinely, and incurring spousal discord in the process:

> Most women do family planning without the knowledge of their husbands. The man may want to have children, but the woman may not be ready at that time and she can't explain that to her husband. So she simply hides and goes to the nurse for the family planning and you will not be aware, and you continue to have sex without the woman becoming pregnant.

Spousal divisions and conflict are increased by the limited male engagement and spousal communication, as well as by the inaccessibility of facility-based family planning services. Men may intensify their gate-keeping activities because they fear the humiliation and disrespect that occurs when women secretly violate reproductive responsibilities and adopt a contraceptive method. Thus, women's autonomy is constrained due to the threat of marital discord and violence which could occur if their facility visits are witnessed and their secret is discovered.

4.4.6 Gender-Based Violence

Male attitudes regarding gender-based violence were a major constraint on women's contraceptive adoption. Acceptance of such violence, and implicit threats that such behavior was related to women's use of family planning, was greater in cells that were never exposed to the male-focused outreach and communication activities characteristic of the *Zurugelu* approach. For example, men from Cell 1 described violence against spouses as a relic of the past, mostly in terms of the concurrent religious transition which took place across study areas from traditional forms of worship to Christianity:

> As for me, I will say [gender violence] has become less common because Christianity was not common here at the time it was high. We had our own way of worshiping before Christianity and Islam came. Our way of marriage is different from Christians and Muslims. ……..after I wed my wife, I have taken a vow never to subject her to any violence treatment. So religion has brought down the level of violence against women in this community.

Although men in Cell 3 – where both experimental arms were implemented – often discussed gender-based violence in terms of forcing their spouses to have sex, the practice was reported as something other men do or something that was reportedly on the decline:

> In this community some men force their wives to have sex with them. It happens that the man is in the mood and a woman is not in agreement. As for me, I don't force my wife to have sex. (Male community member, Cell 3).

With the availability of convenient community-based family planning services, men resort less to forcing sex upon their wives who no longer have to abstain in order to avert unwanted pregnancy. Having been sensitized to pursue spousal communication and consensus, these men tended to discuss marital relations in terms of forming an agreement rather than imposing their will.

In Cell 2 communities, where nurses provided family planning without the support of male-focused volunteers, gender-based violence was also discussed as a reaction to family planning more frequently than in any of the other cells. As one woman noted:

> Men force their wives into sex, especially deep in the night when the whole place is silent. Most quarrels in the dead of night is as a result forced sex. There is the saying that nobody separate fight or quarrels in the dead of the night, so the man will definitely prevail over the women.

Violence in this case was often justified by male respondents as a legitimate response to perceived women's disobedience and disrespect that is implicit in any decision to regulate fertility. Nurse provided services that ignored male concerns, invoked these sensitivities by giving women an avenue to pursue their reproductive freedom in defiance of patriarchal norms. Worries and concerns were most prominent in Cell 2, but in Cell 4 similar responses arose:

> When a man wants to have sex with his wife and she refuses, the man will beat her. The man will say what did I marry for and you're refusing me sex. It is possible that there is something wrong with the woman but the man will not understand her. At times men refuse their wives food stuff like millet for the reason that she is misusing it, but it is because of sex which is not good.

Where men were exposed to *Zurugelu* activities without CHO services, they were more supportive of the of reproductive health services that the project provided. Nevertheless, in the absence of the actual community-based provision of child health services, these supporting attitudes were often unaccompanied by adoption of family planning– an action that men perceived to be a woman's thing. Moreover, motivation to regulate fertility in Cell 1 was offset by concerns about high childhood mortality risks, as illustrated by the following sequential exchange among a panel of older men:

Respondent 1: *The family planning is good [for some people] but rather not good to practice here. This is because if you restrict yourself to about three children and fewer which is very common here, [and death] happens to take two, what do you do again?*

Respondent 2: *The bad effect of family planning is if you restrict yourself to about two children and death happens to take away one.*

Respondent 3: *Among us Kassena people, you may give birth to ten children and they will all be suffering. The eleventh child may be the one who will come to save all the ten others from their suffering.*

Respondent 4: *Quite apart, death is very common among children in this community. So, even though your idea is good, we will give birth to many children so that even if there is death, some will still be left.*

These concerns were less prominent in Cell 3, however, where both arms were deployed. Men could understand the rationale for the concept of family planning without expressing undue concerns that children would not survive. Moreover, where Zurugelu activities engaged with male networks in ways that diffused ideas about the relevance and acceptability of contraception, the program not only expanded the accessibility of family planning services for women, but also enhanced the acceptability of the practice among men.

4.5 Discussion

Recent reviews have expressed renewed concerns that high fertility constrains economic progress in poor countries, and enhanced commitment to family planning programs represents a sound approach to fostering reproductive change (DasGupta et al. 2011; Bongaarts and Sinding 2009). The results of this analysis lend support to the hypothesis that family planning services can have fertility effects even in a profoundly gender-stratified patriarchal setting. However, results bring into question perspectives that focus solely on the provision of contraceptive supplies. The CHFP shows that convenient community-based services are essential but insufficient to achieving fertility impact. In this project, the provision of accessible family planning services, delivered without open advocacy of family planning among men, had no discernable impact. Additional community-based organizational services are required for offsetting male attitudes that elevate the social costs of contraception. Preliminary dialogue with community members suggested to project planners that the CHFP focus on child health services was crucial to achieving fertility impact, but the focus on accessibility and health services was insufficient for sustaining fertility effects. In the post-CHFP era, expansion of the coverage of community-based nursing services, without attention to the social development needs of men, may have led to pronounced benefits for the health and survival of children without having corresponding effects on fertility. The acceptability of fertility regulation was enhanced when child health services suggested to men that child survival had improved, obviating the rationale for large families. Addressing other patriarchal concerns by means of direct dialogue to groups of men and their traditional leaders provided social mechanisms for alleviating tension, misunderstanding, and discord.

Moreover, appropriate engagement with men can introduce direct benefits to the reproductive and social autonomy of women that extend beyond the practice of family planning. Activities that reached men with information, networking, and social support not only offset the social costs of contraception, but also enhanced women's autonomy, facilitating petty trading, fostering social networking and eroding the influence of social institutions that constrain mobility. Nonetheless, men and women have contrasting perceptions about the extent to which gender relations have changed during the initial years of the CHFP. While men expressed the view that gender relations are improving, women often reported the contrary. Social discord that can arise with the introduction of family planning requires sustained and carefully planned programmatic engagement. There is a need to regularly review program strategies, with a particular focus on promoting gender development.

For several decades, proponents of integrated health and family planning programs have advocated service delivery models that expose couples to comprehensive primary healthcare services which include family planning.[6] The success of the *Zurugelu* approach attests to the value of a somewhat broader approach to integration. This includes gender strategies and components that combine services with culturally appropriate forms of outreach that facilitate spousal communication in support of adoption and enactment of appropriate reproductive and child health behaviours. Supply-focused services can precipitate social and household tensions that constrain positive reproductive health results. Supply- and demand-focus strategies are thus mutually reinforcing components of program success.

Demographic results from the post-experimental period attest to the importance of sustaining *Zurugelu* activities. The family planning impact of the Navrongo project was dissipated with the termination of its *Zurugelu* component in 2003 and the launching of a UNICEF sponsored program known as "High Impact Rapid Delivery" that focused on health to the near exclusion of family planning and reproductive health.[7] Nurses assigned to communities in the post-experimental era sustained childhood mortality decline, but no fertility impact was realized. Findings thus attest to the importance of focusing family planning strategies on the needs and concerns of men. Once family planning was openly promoted among men, spousal communication about contraception could be pursued by women without anxiety

---

[6] See for example, Taylor et al. (1976) and Ringheim et al. (2011).

The High Impact Rapid Delivery program was launched in the Upper East Region of Ghana in 2003 as a follow-on to the UNICEF Accelerated Child Survival Program. Although the official aims and clinical components of both programs were similar to CHFP, these initiatives did not provide for the posting of nurses to communities and family planning was not a focus of volunteer training and deployment (Nakamura et al. 2011). Ghana Health Service progress reports on the High Impact Rapid Delivery program make no mention of family planning (see, for example, Ghana Health Service 2010).

about ensuing discord. Without this essential commitment to male mobilization, community-based primary health care will fail to address women's reproductive aspirations and service delivery needs.

4.6   Conclusion

The CHFP was launched in the mid-1990s to address themes in global and national population policy debates. Many observers thought that pervasive poverty, widespread adversity and continuing traditionalism structured high fertility and constrained prospects for family planning programs to succeed in such settings. To others, such constraints signalled the need for a bold, supply-side approach to family planning. Discussion on how best to make services available focused on whether to rely on clinical services and their extension to community locations, or to pursue a more complex approach involving the mobilization of community social institutions and volunteerism. Debate also focused on the relative merits of programs that depended upon paid professional nurses providing care in communities, versus approaches that deployed unpaid volunteers as health promoters. The role of men in family planning services did not originally factor into these discussions, but as evidence was gathered to guide decision-making, gender stratification and related social costs of contraception assumed prominence in strategic planning.

The long term results presented in Fig. 4.3 substantiate the initial findings represented by the supply-side pathway A portrayed in Fig. 4.2 (Debpuur et al. 2002). This chapter has also examined archival qualitative data to explain fertility trends that arose after the project "combined cell" was scaled-up in the study areas. Data compiled after the project not only provide insights into the original results, but may also explain why national CHPS scale-up has had less impact on reducing fertility than anticipated. The long-term demographic data are consistent with findings from the qualitative data compiled early in the project and show that addressing the socio-structural and cultural determinants (represented by pathway B in Fig. 4.2) has been crucial to the success of the project. However, post-experimental trends in Cells 2 and 4 are inconsistent with expectations: scale-up in Cell 2 failed to replicate trends originally observed in Cell 3, while post scale-up trends in Cell 1 replicated the Cell 3 trajectory of fertility decline. Also, scale-up in Cell 4 failed to replicate the Cell 3 trend until 2007.

The inconsistency of post-project scale-up results by cell suggests that the impact of the project was conditional on the degree of post-scale-up operational fidelity to the original model. Field investigation and worker interviews suggest that the operational focus of the *zurugelu* approach on family planning, men, and social mobilization atrophied in the post-project era. Further investigation is being conducted to examine the *zurugelu* atrophy hypothesis. Male volunteers were trained to promote family planning, provide outreach to men, and convene public events to discuss family planning, whereas post-project volunteers were focused on the organization of IMCI and other health priorities. Absent effective means of addressing the social costs of family planning, demand-side perspectives in pathway B predominate. Even if CBD is implemented, unmet need for family planning predominates. As Fig. 4.2 illustrates, fertility determinants among women are embedded in the context of corresponding determinants among men. In the absence of strategies for addressing this stratification, male views predominate and spousal reproductive communication languishes.

Thus, the failure of the scale-up of the project in Cells 2 and 4 to replicate Cell 3 effects following the addition of volunteers attests to the importance of a sustained focus on building support for the program among men. To succeed, programs must create a climate for spousal communication that is free of conflict and allows women to solicit help. The open discussion of family planning enabled women to implement their reproductive preferences, but catalysing conflict-free spousal discussion required enabling strategies from the CHFP. These strategies included the development and delivery of services that reached groups of men through networks and leadership systems that they respected and embraced as their own. The newly trained volunteers added to the project in the post-experimental period may have lacked this focus on family planning. Without the provision of information, avenues for open discussion, and ways to reach men outspoken in their opposition to their wives' reproductive aspirations, the scale-up of project operations lacked fidelity to the original design. The result was a program that failed to utilize patriarchal traditions of communication, networks, and leadership for organizing outreach that would enhance the reproductive autonomy of women. But in Cell 1, where men were involved in operations through the zurugelu approach, the addition of nurses had a pronounced impact, quite possibly because community mobilization generated perceived need for family planning before nurses were readily available to provide convenient care. The end result was a program that had a social impact on demand for family planning that preceded change in actual practice.

The success of *Zurugelu* volunteers cannot be extrapolated to all volunteer-based strategies, however. The CHFP had no discernible fertility effects unless the family planning focus of the *zurugelu* approach was sustained. Moreover, *zurugelu* strategies pursued in isolation of nurse outreach also failed to have fertility effects. *Zurugelu* activities are effective mechanisms for introducing and sustaining ideational change, but without convenient services for women, community mobilization and male outreach was an insufficient strategy for introducing behavioral change. The combination of *zurugelu* activities with CHO services led to a greater and more sustained uptake of contraceptive services than where such activities lacked supporting CBD. It can be concluded that combining CBD with male-focused *zurugelu* activities introduced sustained and significant reproductive change among the Kassena-Nankana of northern Ghana.

Acknowledgements This research was funded by grants to the Mailman School of Public Health, Columbia University from the William and Flora Hewlett Foundation and the Doris Duke Charitable Foundation. The Navrongo Community Health and Family Planning Project was supported by grants to the Population Council from the United States Agency for International Development, the Finnish International Development Agency, and the Mellon Foundation. The Navrongo Demographic Surveillance System was supported by grants to the Ghana Health Service from the Rockefeller Foundation.

References

Adongo, P. B., Phillips, J. F., Kajihara, B., Debpuur, C., & Binka, F. N. (1997). Cultural factors constraining the introduction of family planning among the Kassena-Nankana of northern Ghana. *Social Science & Medicine, 45*(12), 1789–1804.

Akazili, James et al. 2003. *Panel survey report. Community health and family planning project (CHFP). Documentation note 48.* Navrongo, Ghana.

Bawah, A. A., Akweongo, P., Phillips, J. F., & Simmons, R. (1999). Women's fears and men's anxieties: The social impact of family planning in northern Ghana. *Studies in Family Planning, 30*(1), 54–66.

Bertrand, J. T., Mangani, N., Mansilu, M., McBride, M. E., & Tharp, J. L. (1986). Strategies for family planning service delivery in Bas Zaire. *International Family Planning Perspectives, 12*(4), 108–115.

Bertrand, J. T., McBride, M. E., Mangani, N., Baughman, N. C., & Kinuani, M. (1993). Community-based distribution of contraceptives in Zaire. *International Family Planning Perspectives, 19*(3), 84–91.

Binka, F. N., Nazzar, A., & Phillips, J. F. (1995). The Navrongo community health and family planning project. *Studies in Family Planning, 26*(3), 121–139.

Binka, F. N., Ngom, P., Phillips, J. F., Adazu, K., & MacLeod, B. B. (1999). Assessing population dynamics in a rural African society: The Navrongo Demographic Surveillance System. *Journal of Biosocial Science, 31*, 373–391.

Binka, F. N., Bawah, A. A., Phillips, J. F., Hodgson, A., Adjuik, M., & MacLeod, B. (2007). Rapid achievement of the child survival Millennium Development Goal: Evidence from the Navrongo Experiment in northern Ghana. *Tropical Disease and International Health, 12*(5), 578–593.

Bledsoe, C. H., Banja, F., & Hill, A. G. (1998). Reproductive mishaps and Western contraception: An African challenge to fertility theory. *Population and Development Review, 24*(1), 15–47.

Bongaarts, J., & Bruce, J. (1995). The causes of unmet need for contraception and the social content of services. *Studies in Family Planning, 26*(2), 57–75.

Bongaarts, J., & Sinding, S. W. (2009). A response to critics of family planning programs. *International Perspectives on Sexual and Reproductive Health, 35*(1), 39–44.

Caldwell, J. C., & Caldwell, P. (1988). Is the Asian family planning program model suited to Africa? *Studies in Family Planning, 19*(1), 19–28.

d'Cruz-Grote, D. (1996). Prevention of HIV infection in developing countries. *Lancet, 348*(9034), 1071–1074. Retrieved June 12, 2013, from http://www.thelancet.com/journals/a/article/PIIS0140-6736(95)11031-3/fulltext

Dasgupta, M., Bongaarts, J., & Cleland, J. (2011, June 1). *Population, poverty, and sustainable development: A review of the evidence* (Policy Research Working Paper No. 5719). Washington, DC: World Bank.

Debpuur, C., Phillips, J. F., Jackson, E. F., Nazzar, A. K., Ngom, P., & Binka, F. N. (2002). The impact of the Navrongo project on contraceptive knowledge and use, reproductive preferences, and fertility. *Studies in Family Planning, 33*(2), 141–164.

Doctor, H. V. (2010). Has the Navrongo Project in northern Ghana been successful in altering fertility preferences? *African Population Studies, 22*(1), 88–106.

Doctor, H. V., Phillips, J. F., & Sakeah, E. (2009). The influence of changes in women's religious affiliation on contraceptive use and fertility among the Kassena-Nankana of northern Ghana. *Studies in Family Planning, 40*(2), 113–122.

Dube, H. M. B., Marangwanda, C. S., & Ndhlovu, L. (1998). An assessment of the Zimbabwe family planning programme: Results from the 1996 Situation Analysis Study. Harare: Zimbabwe National Family Planning Council and Nairobi: Africa Operations Research and Technical Assistance Project II, The Population Council. Unpublished report.

Easterlin, R. A., & Crimmins, E. M. (1985). *The fertility revolution: A supply–demand analysis.* Chicago: University of Chicago Press.

Easterlin, R. A., Wongboonsin, K., & Ahmed, M. A. (1988). The demand for family planning: A new approach. *Studies in Family Planning, 19*(5), 257–269.

Foreit, J. R., Gorosh, M. E., Gillespie, D. G., & Gary Merritt, C. (1978). Community-based and commercial contraceptive distribution: An inventory and appraisal. *Population Reports. Series J, 19*(March), 1–29.

Frank, O., & McNicoll, G. (1987). An interpretation of fertility and population policy in Kenya. *Population and Development Review, 13*(2), 209–243.

Freedman, R. A. (1987). The contribution of social science research to population policy and family planning program effectiveness. *Studies in Family Planning, 18*(2), 57–82.

Ghana Health Service Regional Health Directorate, Upper East Region. (2010, January–June). *High impact rapid delivery progress report.* Bolgatanga: Regional Health Administration, Ghana Health Service. Unpublished report.

Ghana Statistical Service (GSS), & Macro International. (1994). *Ghana demographic and health survey, 1993.* Calverton: Macro International.

Ghana Health Service. (2010). *High impact rapid delivery progress report.* Bolgatanga, Ghana.

Goldberg, H. I., McNeil, M., & Spitz, A. (1989). Contraceptive use and fertility decline in Chogoria, Kenya. *Studies in Family Planning, 20*(1), 17–25.

Knippenberg, R., et al. (1990). The Bamako initiative: Primary health care experience. Children in the tropics: Review of the International Children's Centre. *Children in the Tropics.* Retrieved June 14, 2013, from http://www.eric.ed.gov/ERICWebPortal/search/detailmini.jsp?_nfpb=true&_&ERICExtSearch_SearchValue_0=ED319533&ERICExtSearch_SearchType_0=no&accno=ED319533

Kols, A. J., & Wawer, M. J. (1982, November–December). Community-based health and family planning. *Population Reports. Series L, 3*(10), L77–L111.

Kruger, R. A. (1988). *Focus groups: A practical guide for applied research.* Beverly Hills, CA: Sage.

Luck, M., Jarju, E., Nell, M. D., & George, M. O. (2000). Mobilizing demand for contraception in rural Gambia. *Studies in Family Planning, 31*(4), 325–335. Retrieved June 12, 2013, from http://doi.wiley.com/10.1111/j.1728-4465.2000.00325.x

Munyakazi, A. (1989). L'experience des abakangurambaga en communes Gatonde et Kihado de la préfecture Ruhengeri. [The experience of the abakanguambaga in Gatonde communities of Ruhengeri prefecture] *Imborezamuryango*, Office National de la Population (Rwanda No. 15, August 14–20). Unpublished report.

Musau, S. N. (1997, January). *Family life education project, Busoga Diocese, Uganda: Cost analysis report.* Arlington: Partnership for Child Health Care, BASICS. Unpublished report.

Nakamura, H., Ikeda, N., Stickley, A., Mori, R., & Shibuya, K. (2011). Achieving MDG 4 in Sub-Saharan Africa: What has contributed to the accelerated child mortality decline in Ghana? *PLoS One, 6*(3), e17774. doi:10.1371/journal.pone.0017774.

National Population Council. (1994). *A draft population policy.* Accra: Ministry of Finance and Planning.

Nazzar, A., Adongo, P. B., Binka, F. N., Phillips, J. F., & Debpuur, C. (1995). Developing a culturally appropriate family planning program for the Navrongo Experiment. *Studies in Family Planning, 26*(6), 307–324.

Ngom, P., Binka, F. N., Phillips, J. F., Pence, B., & MacLeod, B. (2001). Demographic surveillance and health equity in sub-Saharan Africa. *Health Policy and Planning, 16*(4), 337–344.

Nicholas, D. D. (1978, October 16). *The Danfa family planning program.* Paper presented at the 106th annual meeting of the American Public Health Association, Los Angeles.

Phillips, J. F., Greene, W. L., & Jackson, E. F. (1999). *Lessons from community-based distribution of family planning in Africa.* New York: The Population Council.

Phillips, J. F., MacLeod, B. B., & Pence, B. (2000). The Household Registration System: Computer software for the rapid dissemination of demographic surveillance systems. In: *Demographic research* (Vols. 2–6). Rostock: Max Planck Institute for Demographic Research. http://www.demographic-research.org/volumes/vol2/6/default.htm

Phillips, J. F., Bawah, A. A., & Binka, F. N. (2006). Accelerating reproductive and child health programme impact with community-based services: The Navrongo experiment in Ghana. *Bulletin of the World Health Organization, 84*(12), 949–955. Retrieved http://www.pubmed-central.nih.gov/articlerender.fcgi?artid=2627578&tool=pmcentrez&rendertype=abstract

Phillips, J. F., Jackson, E. F., Bawah, A. A., MacLeod, B., Adongo, P., Baynes, C., & Williams, J. (2012). The long term fertility impact of the Navrongo Experiment in rural northern Ghana. *Studies in Family Planning, 43*(3), 175–190.

Ringheim, K., Gribble, J., & Foreman, M. (2011). *Integrating family planning and maternal and child health care: Saving lives, money, and time*. Washington, DC: Population Reference Bureau.

Robey, B., Rutstein, S. O., & Morris, L. (1993). The fertility decline in developing countries. *Scientific American, 269*(6), 60–67.

Ross, J. A., & Frankenberg, E. (1993). *Findings from two decades of family planning research*. New York: Population Council.

Ross, J. A., Lauro, D. J., Wray, J. D., & Rosenfield, A. G. (1987). Community based distribution. In R. J. Lapham & G. B. Simmons (Eds.), *Organizing for effective family planning programs*. Washington, DC: National Academy Press.

Rutenberg, N., & Watkins, S. C. (1997). The buzz outside the clinics: Conversation and contraception in Nyanza Province, Kenya. *Studies in Family Planning, 28*(4), 290–307.

Shoenmaecker, R. I., Lesthaeghe, R., & Tambashe, O. (1981). The child-spacing patterns and the postpartum taboos in tropical Africa. In H. Page & R. Lesthaeghe (Eds.), *Child-spacing in tropical Africa-traditions and change* (pp. 25–72). London: Academy Press.

Taylor, C. E., Newman, J. S., & Kelly, N. U. (1976). The child survival hypothesis. *Population Studies, 30*(2), 263–278.

Tindana, P. O., Singh, J. A., Tracy, C. S., Upshur, R. E. G., Daar, A. S., Singer, P. A., Frohlich, J., & Lavery, J. V. (2007). Grand challenges in global health: Community engagement in research in developing countries. *PLoS Medicine, 4*(9), e273. doi:10.1371/journal.pmed.0040273.

World Bank. (2003). *Making services work for poor people, The 2004 world development report*. New York: Oxford University Press.

World Health Organization. (2008). *A systematic review of the effectiveness of shortening integrated management of childhood illness guidelines training. Final report*. Geneva: World Health Organization.

Zinanga, A., Bouzidi, M., & Korte, R. (1990). Community-based distribution programme in Zimbabwe. In *Family planning for life: Experiences and challenges for the 1990s. Papers presented at the Conference on Management of Family Planning Programmes, Harare, Zimbabwe, 1–7 October 1989* (pp. 37–44). London: International Planned Parenthood Federation. Retrieved June 14, 2013, from, http://www.cabdirect.org/abstracts/19901884586.html;jsessionid=624368FA4B81168991A7123BA3973D12

Chapter 5
Social Class and Sexual Stigma: Local Interpretations of Emergency Contraception in Egypt

L.L. Wynn, Hosam Moustafa Abdel Hafez, and Ahmed Ragab

5.1 Introduction

In 2008, American anthropologist Lisa Wynn and Egyptian physician Hosam Moustafa Abdel Hafez embarked upon a research project to examine local interpretations of several reproductive health technologies in Egypt, including emergency contraception (EC).[1] Emergency contraception is broadly defined as any form of contraception that is used after sexual intercourse and includes both the post-coital insertion of the copper intrauterine device (IUD) as well as high doses of the same hormones found in many regular oral contraceptive pills.

Egyptian women have long used traditional folk methods for post-coital contraception, including vaginal douches and herbal infusions, some of which are in fact abortifacients and may post considerable health risks (Ragab 1997). For decades, Egyptian women have also had widespread access to hormonal contraceptive pills through Egypt's long-standing and state-subsidized family planning program, so the ingredients for do-it-yourself dosing have long been available for emergency contraceptive purposes. Yet it is only since 2007 that Egypt has had its own dedicated emergency contraception pill (ECP).[2] In that year, Contraplan II™ appeared in

---

[1] Funding for this research was provided by Macquarie University.

[2] The term "dedicated product" is used to describe pills that are packaged and marketed specifically for emergency contraceptive use, to distinguish from the common practice of cutting up packages of regular oral contraceptive pills for emergency – i.e. postcoital – use.

L.L. Wynn, Ph.D. (✉)
Department of Anthropology, Macquarie University, North Ryde, NSW, Australia
e-mail: lisa.wynn@mq.edu.au

H.M. Abdel Hafez, MBBCh.
Klinikum Luedenscheid akademisches Lehrkrankenhaus der Universitaet Bonn,
Luedenscheid, Germany

A. Ragab, M.D., Ph.D.
International Islamic Center for Population Studies and Research,
Reproductive Medicine Unit, Al-Azhar University, Cairo, Egypt

A. Kulczycki (ed.), *Critical Issues in Reproductive Health*, The Springer Series on
Demographic Methods and Population Analysis 33, DOI 10.1007/978-94-007-6722-5_5,
© Springer Science+Business Media Dordrecht 2014

Egyptian pharmacies, sold and marketed by DKT-Egypt, an affiliate of an international non-profit organization that operates in 16 countries to promote family planning and HIV/AIDS prevention.[3]

We had been searching for coverage of EC in the Egyptian press, but we had found next to nothing written about it other than the advertisements placed in several newspapers and radio programs by DKT-Egypt. This in itself piqued our interest. In many countries, the introduction of EC and attempts to make it available without prescription have been accompanied by considerable public debate and controversy (Foster and Wynn 2012). Debates have generally centered on one or more of the following issues: the drug's mechanism of action (i.e. how it works in the body to prevent pregnancy), concern that availability of post-coital contraceptive options will lead to reduced condom use and thus increased exposure to sexually transmitted infections, speculation about hypothetical health risks entailed in repeat use of high doses of contraceptive hormones,[4] and concerns about the consequences of decreasing reliance on biomedical authorities if women can purchase EC without prescription. In the U.S., for example, all of these issues were raised in public debates and media coverage, with EC opponents mobilizing a complex mixture of religious-moral and public health arguments to try to prevent the government from allowing ECPs to be sold without prescription (Wynn and Trussell 2006a, b).

Egypt is no less socially conservative than the United States. Surveys have shown that whether they are part of the Muslim majority or the small Christian minority, Egyptians are deeply religious, with 98 % of Egyptians declaring that religion is an important part of their daily life (Mogahed 2006).[5] Induced abortion is illegal in Egypt unless two physicians attest that it is necessary to save the life of the pregnant woman (Ragab 1997). By these indicators, at least, Egypt would certainly appear to be *more* socially conservative than the United States. Yet we could not find a whiff of public controversy associated with the introduction of EC in Egypt. Why?

To ask this very question, Dr Abdel Hafez decided to visit the offices of DKT-Egypt. The DKT-Egypt offices are located in Maadi, a leafy Cairo suburb where many expatriates reside, on the 31st floor of a posh apartment building with windows overlooking the Nile and views of some dozen ancient pyramids scattered throughout the bordering desert. Abdel Hafez made an appointment and showed up on time. When he arrived, he was told that no one had time to meet with him, despite his appointment. He offered to wait. They left him sitting in the reception area for some three hours. He concluded that the DKT-Egypt management was signaling his lack of importance, hoping that he would leave without insisting on a meeting.

---

[3]For more information about this non-profit group which is based in Washington, D.C. and operates in countries of Africa, Asia and Latin America, see its website and annual report (DKT International 2011), http://www.dktinternational.org/. DKT International's programs are known especially for social marketing of low-cost contraceptives.

[4]According to the World Health Organization (WHO), even repeated use of emergency contraceptive pills poses no known health risks (WHO 2004).

[5]In the same poll, only 68 % of Americans surveyed said that religion was an important part of their daily life. Egyptians ranked higher even than Saudis in personal religiosity, and only Indonesians ranked higher than Egyptians.

After three hours of waiting, Abdel Hafez was finally ushered into the office of one of the associates of DKT-Egypt, where he was coolly received. He introduced the research project and explained that he was working with an American anthropologist who was based in Australia. They told him very little, answering his questions curtly and rather evasively. They insisted that they had not a single copy of any of their marketing or promotional materials to show him. When he asked for information about what dates they had placed advertisements for Contraplan II™ in local newspapers and magazines so that he could find examples in the archives, they gave him the wrong dates. He left empty-handed and frustrated, only to spend more frustrating hours searching through archives for advertisements that were not there. Yet the veiled insult and elaborate runaround only served to further pique his curiosity: why were the employees of DKT-Egypt so reluctant to talk to him and reveal their EC marketing strategies?

A couple of months later, Wynn visited Egypt and, together with Abdel Hafez, made an appointment to meet with the management of DKT-Egypt. This time, we were kept waiting only a couple of minutes before being ushered into the director's office. Wynn introduced herself and established her connection to several individuals who are well known in the international community of EC researchers and activists. Two of the DKT-Egypt managers then spoke with Wynn and Abdel Hafez at length about the history of EC in Egypt, the contraceptive needs of the population, their print and media campaigns as well as the social marketing strategies they were piloting in rural communities. After answering all of Wynn's and Abdel Hafez's questions, they provided each with a bag full of glossy, colorful prints of the ads and physician information sheets – in short, copies of all of the Contraplan II ™ marketing materials that they had previously claimed were not available.

We were both amused and perplexed. What could explain the radical about-face between the cold reception Abdel Hafez encountered during his first solo visit and the cheerful openness with which Abdel Hafez and Wynn were received during our joint visit? When we recounted the story to colleagues in Egypt, Australia, and the U.S., two primary interpretations emerged. The first explained the encounters in terms of class snobbishness. Abdel Hafez is a young Egyptian physician from a middle-class village background who was trained from the age of 5 in al-Azhar Islamic educational institutions. His mannerisms are marked by deferential but self-assured politeness, his accent reveals his village origins, and an aura of religiosity permeates his speech patterns. In contrast, Wynn is an older American woman who speaks Egyptian Arabic rather clumsily. American and European foreigners in Egypt are often treated with enthusiasm and deference. The employees of DKT-Egypt are Westernized, upper-middle class urbanites. Some of our colleagues thought it unsurprising, therefore, that they would snub a local villager but welcome an American.

Other colleagues framed an explanation in terms of the politics of reproductive health activism in Egypt. Abdel Hafez had, at that time, little connection with the reproductive health research and activism community in Egypt. In contrast, Wynn's credentials within the global EC movement (which she flaunted deliberately in the hope that this would make the DKT-Egypt representatives more welcoming) were easily established. Some colleagues speculated that DKT-Egypt's wariness when talking with Dr. Abdel Hafez during his solo visit might be explained by the somewhat tenuous position of EC in Egypt. Perhaps, they suggested, the DKT-Egypt employees feared that someone with a religious background might try to infiltrate their organization or stir up religious opposition to the technology. This explanation hints at the social stigma lurking around ECPs, despite the lack of public controversy around the drug.

This encounter is revealing for what it tells us about EC in Egypt. We can never know for sure why the employees of DKT-Egypt received Abdel Hafez and Wynn the way they did. Yet reporting their actions and the speculative interpretations of reproductive health activists as social phenomena can help us to understand the economy of silences that attend reproductive health activism. The introduction of new reproductive health technologies is quite often attended by intense debate about who will use them and how they will transform sexual behavior in society. For example, in the U.S., religious opposition to EC contended not only that EC was an abortifacient (despite the fact that ECPs contain the same ingredients and work in the same way as oral contraceptive pills) but also that it would lead to an "epidemic" of sexual promiscuity amongst teenagers, with one government official going so far as to speculate that it would lead to teenagers forming urban "sex-based cults" centered around use of the drug (Wynn and Trussell 2006a, b; Davidoff and Trussell 2006). Egyptian reproductive health activists, well aware of the international context of EC debates, were probably eager to avoid similar controversies, and as we shall show in this paper, their marketing strategies are specifically designed to portray the likely user of EC as a respectable married woman, preempting controversy over adolescent (and premarital) use. Yet their marketing strategies, which target a young, unmarried, English-speaking and elite audience, belie the portrait they publicly draw of the most likely users.

In short, this little vignette suggests the importance of understanding reproductive health activism in terms of the politics of what can and cannot be said about sexuality in a particular society, as we examine how activists construct a health problem (and its solution) for public consumption. This chapter, therefore, examines the strategies used to market EC and define its users in Egypt, and situates the status of EC in Egypt within the context of Islamic jurisprudence and social concerns about the sexuality of young Egyptians.

5.2   EC in Egypt

5.2.1   Marketing a Drug and a Concept

Egypt has a long history of government-sponsored and subsidized family planning programs (El Shakry 2005), and both oral contraceptive pills and IUDs have for decades been widely available and inexpensive. The ECP brand Postinor™ tablets (manufactured by Gedeon Richter) were part of the National Family Planning

Program for several years, donated by several countries including Australia and Japan. However, introduction of Postinor™ was never accompanied by marketing or awareness-raising efforts, and most of the stock of these donated tablets was expired and never replaced, so this EC product did not have much impact on the Family Planning Program (Ministry of Health Official, June 2011, personal communication). It was not until 2007, when Contraplan II™ (2 tablets of 750 mg levonorgestrel) was approved for marketing, that an ECP was advertised to the public. While imported Postinor™ tablets can still be purchased in some pharmacies, Contraplan II™ (which is mainly distributed by two large drug distribution companies, Al Muttaheda and Ibn Sina) is the dominant pill brand on the market.

The company behind Contraplan II™, DKT-Egypt, started operations in 2004 with the mission of encouraging private-sector provision of low-cost contraceptive products. It operates in an environment where the government is increasingly cutting its subsidies of pharmaceutical products, and the company's representatives told us that DKT-Egypt receives no support from the Egyptian government, community service providers, pharmaceutical companies, or from any other organization, whether Egyptian or foreign. DKT-Egypt is responsible for two inexpensive IUDs, two brands of condoms, vaginal spermicide suppositories, and a 3-month injectable contraceptive, in addition to the ECP Contraplan II™, and in 2009 they sold over one million condoms, 138,000 IUDs, and 114,000 packages of ECPs. In 2008, DKT-Egypt had a sales team consisting of a national distributor and 15 medical representatives who covered the entire country, reaching 3,200 gynecologists and 18,000 pharmacies. By 2011, the sales force had 35 medical representatives (Hanna 2010). Medical representatives visit physicians both to market products and assess patient needs and attitudes to inform their advertising and educational outreach campaigns. In interviews, they described their agenda as "creating a need in the market." Like many pharmaceutical companies, they not only sell drugs, they sell the idea of a need for a drug.

In Egypt, this meant marketing the idea of post-coital contraception in a country where it is very little known. In 2005, the Egyptian Demographic Health Survey found that only 5.5 % of currently married women knew of EC, and only 0.1 % had ever used it (Hanna 2010). Further, there was a widespread misconception among healthcare professionals that ECPs were abortifacient (Hanna 2010). Initially, the drug was promoted mainly through DKT-Egypt's medical representatives who travelled the country visiting clinicians at their clinics to explain the medical benefits of the product and appropriate use. Drugs may be promoted to clinics and physicians without government permission, but no drug can be marketed to the public and advertised in the media without special approval from the Ministry of Health and Population. Similarly, Ministry approval is required before marketing research (e.g. focus groups and interviews) can be conducted for any drug.

DKT-Egypt promoted Contraplan II™ in obstetrics and gynecology clinics, family planning clinics, and hospitals. The drug was presented to clinicians both through personal visits by medical representatives and brochures. These brochures framed the need for EC in terms of public health, with statistics describing global rates of unintended pregnancy as well as the mortality associated with it. (The headline above the graphic representation of unintended pregnancies read, "A major, sometimes fatal, problem affects the world.") These pamphlets also described the drug's mechanism of action, emphasizing its status as a contraceptive, not abortifacient. The mechanisms of action listed were interference with ovulation (by disrupting luteal function and LH surge) and changes to the reproductive tract (including alteration of the cervical mucus) that would interfere with the movement and function of sperm. The possibility that EC might work by preventing the implantation of a fertilized egg was described as "unlikely to be the primary mechanism of action," and the pamphlet emphasized that ECPs would not be effective once implantation occurs. The pamphlet concluded by urging doctors to provide women with an advance supply of the drug not only to reduce unintended pregnancy but also to "[assure] comfort and satisfaction."

Once the company received government approval to market the drug to the public, they launched a series of advertisements in radio and print media. Print advertisements and commercial articles were run in Al-Ahram newspaper (the most widely distributed newspaper in Egypt) in March and May 2008, in the English-language Al-Ahram Weekly in April 2008, and in Broadcast and Television Magazine and a magazine called Layla (Night) in June 2008. In total, more than 21 ads were placed in 7 newspapers and magazines (Hanna 2010). A 50-second radio ad also ran for several months in late 2007 and early 2008.

In contrast with the ads targeting clinicians, these ads mixed colloquial Egyptian Arabic with Modern Standard Arabic, and rather than focusing on mechanism of action and the public health dangers of unintended pregnancy, they focused on the situations in which someone might need emergency contraception. They described four typical scenarios where people might need EC: married women who regularly use contraceptives but miss a dose, experience a condom tear, or have a problem with their IUD; situations where a husband and wife who do not want to get pregnant have unprotected intercourse; situations where the husband suddenly returns from travel or work abroad and so the couple fails to use contraception; and cases of rape. The majority of these scenarios, thus, framed EC need and use in terms of a marital relationship. However, the venue where the radio commercials appeared belies this framing of the typical EC user. The radio advertisements for Contraplan II™ appeared on Nogoom FM, which is the most popular FM radio station in Greater Cairo (comprising Cairo and its sister city across the Nile, Giza), and self-described by the radio station as having a largely young adult (unmarried) audience.

By 2010, demand for Contraplan II™ had increased, but sales dropped dramatically (to 66,500 ECP packs) because the Egyptian Ministry of Health had halted production of the drug at the pharmaceutical factory that produced it because of what the company described as "technical difficulties." A small pharmacy survey conducted by Professor Ahmed Ragab found that some pharmacies that had previously struggled to sell the drug were now experiencing shortages. Production of Contraplan II™ resumed in 2011, and it is currently available for 4 Egyptian pounds per one-use package (the 2011 official exchange rate is 6 Egyptian pounds to 1 US dollar).

5.2.2 Egyptian Attitudes Towards EC

In 2008–2010, Wynn, Abdel Hafez, and Ragab conducted small-scale ethnographic research on Egyptian attitudes towards EC. Using purposive sampling, we conducted semi-structured and informal interviews with approximately 50 women and men from a range of age groups, marital status, and educational and class backgrounds in Cairo. In addition to these lay opinions, we also conducted interviews with physicians and pharmacists to assess professional attitudes towards this contraceptive method.

Physician attitudes were mixed. Some felt that the drug would disrupt the morals of the community by facilitating illicit sexual relationships between unmarried men and women. Others had a more neutral attitude toward the drug, pointing out that there was another ECP previously available (Postinor™) that was distributed by the Ministry of Health and Population in family planning clinics. According to interviews with two pharmaceutical representatives, the main reason that Egyptian physicians were leery of EC was because it was not taught in the curricula of medical schools, so it was an unfamiliar concept. By and large, physicians did not refuse to prescribe the drug on ethical grounds, even if they suspected that its availability would lead to increased illicit sexual activity. According to a DKT-Egypt area manager, out of 1,500 physicians he had targeted for EC education, only eight refused the drug for ethical reasons.

Pharmacist attitudes tended less to the moral and more to the economic. In 2008, many regarded Contraplan II as a "burned drug," a colloquial expression that refers to a drug that does not sell. While the drug was available in most pharmacies in middle-class suburbs of Cairo, including Wast el-Balad, Dokki, Mohandiseen, Heliopolis, Nasr City and Maadi, it was rarely stocked in the lower-class suburbs on the outskirts of Cairo, suggesting that the drug is perceived by pharmacists to be used only by the wealthier classes and/or that the DKT-Egypt representatives were not pushing the drug in lower-class markets.[6] Yet only one pharmacy in all of Egypt that DKT-Egypt had approached refused to sell the drug on ethical grounds.[7]

In our informal interviews with laypeople, we encountered a range of opinions about the drug. Wealthier informants tended to have more tolerant attitudes towards

---

[6]A DKT-Egypt official told Dr Abdel Hafez that most sales of Contraplan II were to Nasr City, Heliopolis and Mohandiseen, three of Cairo's most elite suburbs. After those, sales of the drug were highest in Red Sea resort towns Sharm el-Sheikh and Hurghada, a fact which DKT-Egypt attributed to the familiarity of the concept of EC amongst tourists. A small-scale pharmacy survey of several districts of Cairo, Kafr el-Sheikh, and Menoufiyya conducted in 2009 by Dr Abdel Hafez found that the drug was rarely stocked by pharmacists in other areas of Cairo and its neighboring villages. Of the pharmacies that Dr Abdel Hafez visited in lower – to middle-class districts of Cairo (Hadayek al-Kobba, Abbasiyya, Ein Shams, Al-Obour City, Al-Darassa, Al-Azhar, Ataba, Kafr El-Sheikh, and Shebin al-Koum), the only ones that stocked Contraplan II at that time were large chain pharmacies on the main streets of Abbasiyya.

[7]The pharmacy that refused to stock the drug on ethical grounds was in Tanta, a large city in the north of Egypt.

EC users, but the predominant stereotype we encountered was that it was mostly young people, teens, and sex workers who would use EC. We did not encounter any woman who admitted to having ever used EC – unsurprising given the low overall use rates (0.1 % of women had ever used ECPs in 2005, and on average less than 100,000 units were sold over the past three years in a country with a population of over 80 million).

Clearly there exists in Egypt a generally negative stereotype about EC use. DKT-Egypt was at pains to counteract this with the portraits it drew of the typical users being married couples. While this negative stereotype never coalesced into opposition to the product, it may have been fear of such opposition that prompted the cautious attitude towards an unknown Egyptian researcher which we described at the start of this chapter.

In all these murmurs and silences about the drug – murmurs that prophesy its potential to corrupt the morals of Egyptian youth, and silences that hint at fears that these cultural stereotypes will develop into organized religious opposition – it is worth noticing what is *not* controversial about EC in Egypt: its mechanism of action. In many countries where new ECPs have been introduced or old ones made available over the counter, the Catholic Church and evangelical Christian organizations have claimed that EC is abortifacient, because of the theoretical (but unproven) possibility that it might work by preventing the implantation of a fertilized egg (Wynn and Trussell 2006a). Indeed, during the U.S. government hearings about making an ECP available without prescription, the drug's manufacturer anticipated such arguments and went to lengths to argue that the pill mainly worked by preventing ovulation and not by preventing the implantation of a fertilized egg (ibid). In contrast, none of our interviews or ethnographic research suggested that Egyptians are concerned with EC's mechanism of action, and while the DKT-Egypt brochures for clinicians explained the mechanism of action, this seems to be intended to establish the fact that ECPs are different than the so-called French abortion pill.[8] According to an area manager of DKT-Egypt, no Christian physician had refused to prescribe or recommend the drug on ethical grounds.

5.3   Emergency Contraception in Islamic Jurisprudence

So what is the Islamic position on EC and its mechanism of action? Unlike the Roman Catholic Church, there is no central hierarchy within Islam that is vested with the authority to interpret Islamic law for the entire community of Muslims. When the Qur'an and *sunnah* (recorded traditions of the Prophet) are silent on a contemporary social issue (as is the case with hormonal contraception), Islamic

---

[8]Mifepristone is not available in Egypt but is widely known as the "French abortion pill." Misoprostol (a drug which can be used to treat ulcers, start labor, or induce abortion) is readily available from Egyptian pharmacies (and an inexpensive product is produced by DKT-Egypt for treating post-labor bleeding), but few lay Egyptians know that it can be used as an abortion drug.

positions are derived through a process of interpretation, reasoning and analogy. Many countries have official state-sanctioned bodies responsible for issuing interpretations of Islamic law, i.e. *fatāwa* (sing. *fatwa*). These interpretations of Islamic law vary from country to country, depending on sect and school of Islamic jurisprudence.[9] Even where such state-sanctioned (and often state-controlled) bodies of religious leadership exist, there may be variation of opinion within that organization. There may also be clerics or experts of Islamic jurisprudence in that country who are not state-sanctioned but who have considerable popular influence (in Egypt, the most prominent example would be the Muslim Brotherhood which in 2011 was still officially banned by the government but had considerable popular influence). In short, there is a diversity of interpretation on most social issues in Islam and so while we can point to majority views, to speak of a singular Islamic position is nonsensical (Wynn et al. 2005).

That said, most Islamic scholars permit modern forms of contraception within a marital relationship (though many scholars only condone reversible contraceptive methods), and according to the United Nations, no Muslim-majority country actively limits family planning access (Hassan 2000; United Nations 2009). In Egypt, the official state-sanctioned body tasked with interpreting Islamic law is Dar el-Ifta ("House of Islamic Jurisprudence"), which is connected with Al-Azhar University, an ancient and venerable institution of Islamic learning. Egypt's Al-Azhar scholars have a long history of supporting family planning and modern contraception (Dardir and Ahmed 1981), but when we first began this research project, we did not know if Al-Azhar had taken an official position on EC, so we searched the Dar el-Ifta archives for rulings. We found not a single *fatwa* devoted to EC. Traditionally *fatāwa* are issued in response to a particular request for a ruling, and these requests may come from the state or from individuals. At Dar el-Ifta, trained experts in Islamic jurisprudence hold daily open houses where any individual can request an official *fatwa* in response to a personal dilemma or question. All these personalized *fatāwa* issued by Dar al-Ifta are then archived in their enormous online *fatwa* database. The fact that no *fatwa* existed on EC until we solicited one is thus a telling indicator of the lack of controversy and publicity surrounding the technology.

Professor Ahmed Ragab interviewed two Islamic scholars to seek their position on EC. One was Professor Rafaat Osman, a former Dean of the Faculty of Shari'ah at al-Azhar University, Professor of Jurisprudence and member of the High Islamic Research Academy, who is well-known for his scholarship on the religious aspects of medical discoveries. The second was Dr. Salem Abdel Galeel, who in early 2011 was Egypt's Deputy Minister of Religious Endowments (*awqāf*). Both prefaced their comments on EC by describing Islam as a code of life which not only deals with questions of faith and worship but also regulates moral behaviour, social interaction, and marital relationships, including

---

[9]There are four schools of Islamic jurisprudence within Sunni Islam, and many other sects including Shi'a, Sufi, and Ismaili.

sexuality, family formation, family planning, and abortion. Both religious leaders prefaced their interpretation by noting that the key question in developing a ruling on EC would be whether it affected human life. Ragab explained the drug's mechanism of action, including the possibility that it could prevent the implantation of a fertilized egg, and noted that EC therefore does not interrupt an established pregnancy.[10]

Both scholars reviewed the Islamic position on when life begins. The Qur'an describes the fetus as undergoing a series of transformations before becoming human. Sura 22:4, for example, describes fetal growth thus:

> O mankind: If you are in doubt as to resurrection,
> Consider that we have created you of earth
> then of a blood like clot then of a lump of flesh (which is)
> formed and not formed so that we may demonstrate to you [our
> power], and we establish in the wombs what we will till a
> stated term; then we bring you out as infant.

Sura 23:12–14 reads,

> We created man of a quintessence of clay. Then we
> placed him as semen in a firm receptacle, then we formed the
> semen into a blood-like clot; then we formed the clot into a
> lump of flesh; then we formed out of that lump bones and
> clotted the bones with flesh. Then we made him another
> creation. So blessed be God the best creator.

These verses describe fetal development metaphorically, but they do not establish the time at which "ensoulment" occurs. This is described in two significant <u>hadiths</u>, or sayings of the Prophet Muhammad as recorded by his peers, that describe fetal development:

> Each of you is constituted in your mother's womb for
> forty days as a 'nutfa', then it becomes an 'alaqa' for
> an equal period, then a 'mudgha', then an angel is sent,
> and he breaths the soul into it.

> When forty-two nights have passed over the [semen] drops,
> Allah sends an angel to it, who shapes it and makes its
> ears, eyes, skin, flesh and bones. Then he says, "Lord!
> Is it male or female?" And your Lord decides what He wishes
> and the angel records it.[11]

---

[10] Theories about EC's mechanism of action are evolving. A decade ago, most EC researchers and activists accepted a 3-part mechanism of action. Yet in recent years, the post-fertilization mechanism of action has been increasingly disputed, and in April 2011, the International Federation of Gynecology and Obstetrics (FIGO) and the International Consortium for Emergency Contraception (ICEC) issued a joint statement claiming that "Review of the evidence suggests that LNG ECPs cannot prevent implantation of a fertilized egg" and "Language on implantation should not be included in LNG ECP product labeling" (FIGO/ICEC 2011).

[11] It is difficult to fully understand the above translations without elaborating on the meanings of the Arabic terms used to describe stages of fetal development. <u>Nutfa</u> literally means "a drop of fluid," which refers to semen. `<u>Alaqa</u> literally means "something that clings or adheres (to the

In short, these Qur'anic verses and <u>hadith</u> describe ensoulment (or the moment at which a fetus becomes a human being) as occurring at either 40 or 120 days, and have been the basis for most Islamic rulings on abortion. Dr. Abdel Galeel declared that Muslims believe that point to be at the end of the fourth month of pregnancy, while Professor Osman declared that point to occur at the end of 42 days, when organ differentiation begins. While these Egyptian scholars disagreed about the time of ensoulment (with implications for the stage of pregnancy at which abortion would be permitted in Islam), both of these scholars agreed that there is nothing in either the Qur'an or the <u>hadith</u> to indicate that it would make any difference to Islamic jurisprudence whether emergency contraception worked before or after fertilization, since that is not the moment at which life begins in Islamic theology.

Thus while EC's mechanism of action is a central aspect of debate in Latin America and other Catholic-dominated countries (Foster and Wynn 2012), Egypt's Islamic scholars are not particularly concerned with questions of whether EC works before or after fertilization. A far more likely area of concern to religious Egyptians is the influence that a reproductive health technology like EC might have on the sexuality of unmarried users. Most Islamic scholars are firm in their opinion that sexuality must only be expressed within the context of marriage, and contraception, therefore, is only permissible for married people. As we will see, while Islamic scholars have ruled EC to be acceptable, there is considerable social anxiety about whether new reproductive health technologies will encourage sex amongst unmarried people. It is this cultural anxiety which DKT-Egypt worked so hard to avoid triggering in their advertising campaigns for Contraplan II™. This social anxiety must be understood within the context of changing sexual norms in Egypt, particularly amongst young, unmarried people.

5.4 Sexuality of Young Egyptians

There is an Egyptian proverb that says, "She has the desire [for sex] but she is afraid of getting pregnant" (<u>'Ayza wa khaifa min el-habal'</u>). Many Egyptians believe that if women are provided with means of preventing pregnancy, they will be more likely to give in to desire. In recent years, there has been considerable social concern about the introduction of new technologies that disguise (and therefore facilitate) lack of

---

uterus/womb)," and elsewhere is translated as "clot." It is usually interpreted as referring to what contemporary science understands to be the fertilized egg at implantation (blastocyst). Finally, <u>mudghah</u> means "a piece of flesh that has been chewed," sometimes translated as "a lump," and is interpreted as referring to the embryo. In the first hadith cited above, direct reference is made to the ensoulment of the fetus after 120 days from the time of fertilization. At the same time, some of the commentators of the Qur'anic texts hold that the words "khalqan akher" (i.e. another act of creation) at the end of the first Qur'anic verses above signify the ensoulment of the fetus, and that the stage of "mudghah ghayer" (i.e., the lump not yet completely created) in the second Qur'anic verse denotes the stages when no soul had yet been breathed into it. It is noteworthy that the second hadith states that organ differentiation occurs 42 nights after fertilization.

virginity. For example, lawmakers have called for a ban on imports of a popular Chinese-produced artificial "hymen" (a gelatin-encased vaginal suppository containing fake blood), and while hymenoplasty has been approved by several of Egypt's highest ranking Islamic scholars, many physicians believe the procedure to be immoral and responsible for a rise in premarital sexual activity. Similarly, a post-coital contraceptive method is thought to be a temptation to young, unmarried people, who are unlikely to plan contraceptive use before sexual activity, unlike married people who are thought to be both better informed about contraception and better prepared to use it.

Sexual health services for adolescents are very limited in Egypt. As Egyptian boys or girls reach puberty, they are given little if any information about sexual and reproductive health, and no comprehensive sexuality education (Ragab and Mohamoud 2006). Sex education for youths is strongly opposed by many of Egypt's religious leaders, even though at the time of the Prophet Muhammad, comprehensive sex education was provided side by side with other teachings of Islam (Ragab 2009). Medical and educational services for youth are often scarce, under-funded, and of poor quality. Teachers and health professionals are not prepared to address sexuality and understandably bring their own biases, fears and misinformation to the subject. In terms of proper sexuality education, there is no local research that can serve as the basis for evidence-based public policy. For example, the school curriculum in the 9th grade provides a small chapter that focuses mainly on the biological aspects of sexuality. Though this chapter is small, it is neglected by many teachers and students alike, and even on the few occasions when teachers approach these topics, students are discouraged from discussing it in detail or at length.

Premarital sexual relations do exist despite the taboo. Egyptian sociologists El-Zanaty and El-Daw found that in a survey of university students, approximately 26 % of the males and 3 % of the females reported having had sexual intercourse at least once. The number of females reported as having premarital sex in this survey is also misleading because most female counterparts of the men interviewed were younger and less educated (they were not university students), and so were not part of the survey (El-Zanaty and El-Daw 1996).

In a more recent study, El Tawila and Khadr (2004) studied patterns of marriage and family formation in Egypt. Young men and women were asked if they knew someone close to them who had been involved in a sexual relationship. Approximately 13 % of single young males responded affirmatively, compared to only 3.4 % of single females. The number increased to 22 % when the question was posed to engaged young males, but remained the same for engaged young females. Married males reported the lowest number among the men at just 9 %, while married females at 3 % were on par with single females (El Tawila and Khadr 2004, p. 64). The study also revealed that sexual activity was far more prevalent in urban areas than in rural areas — single, engaged or married men and single and engaged women all reported that the majority of cases they knew were in urban governorates or in urban areas of lower and upper Egypt; the only discrepancy was with married women who reported slightly higher incidences in rural lower Egypt. When the same respondents were asked to give their own experiences, the numbers decreased considerably; only 1.4 % of males reported such an experience compared to less than 1 % of females.

In the same study, 70 % of single male respondents and 59 % of single female respondents reported that dating relationships among youth are very common. From these respondents, 27 % of males and 24 % of females admitted they had been involved in a relationship, and these percentages increased slightly for engaged or ever-married respondents (El Tawila and Khadr 2004).

In addition to premarital dating, there is another type of quasi-marital relationship that is becoming increasingly common in Egypt as a way for young people to express sexual intimacy without the expense and formal arrangements of an orthodox marriage: the 'urfi marriage. The practice of 'urfi (Arabic for "customary") marriage is a contemporary practice with roots in Sunni Islam. Such marriages are usually clandestine and involve a man and a woman drafting their own marriage contract and opting not to register it with public authorities. While far from illegal, 'urfi marriages grant no rights to the wife except to file for divorce – if she is able to prove that there was a marriage in the first place. 'Urfi marriages are increasingly popular among Egyptian youth. The high cost of marriage forces many young couples to wait several years before they marry. Since sex before marriage is forbidden by religion, law, and cultural tradition, consequently many young people consider 'urfi marriage a solution. 'Urfi marriage is a simple procedure that a couple with only two witnesses can perform.

While premarital sexuality is theoretically prohibited for both men and women, in practice it is women whose virginity is most scrutinized and women, not men, who pay the social price for premarital and extramarital sex (Foster 2002). The religious penalties imposed by shari`a (Islamic) law are severe (Zuhur 2006), but rarely applied, as the required burden of proof is nearly impossible to achieve. Yet if evidence of a woman's premarital sexual activity comes to light – through pregnancy or if the hymen is found to be torn – the social consequences can still be severe. She may be socially ostracized and at risk of violence by family members; her child would be legally considered illegitimate and face lifetime stigmatisation, and she might find it difficult or impossible to ever marry.

Young Egyptians are well aware of the social dangers of premarital sexual activity for women, and they employ several methods to mitigate the consequences. Several young people interviewed suggested that non-penetrative sex is widely practiced, both to keep the hymen intact and to avoid pregnancy. One young man from Sharqia Governorate said that his girlfriend gave him leave to "enjoy and play" with her sexually, so long as he kept her hymen intact. Withdrawal is also widely practiced both within and outside of marriage to prevent pregnancy.

Yet increasingly Egyptian women are making use of new reproductive health technologies, including medication abortion, hymenoplasty, and EC, to control their reproduction and hide the fact that they have had premarital sex. Interviews with gynecologists working in different parts of Egypt (Cairo, Mansoura, Alexandria and Sharqia) affirmed both the existence of premarital sexual relations and the increasing use of medical technologies to cover it up. They claimed that young women are increasingly coming in to request hymen reconstruction surgery. One female doctor who is also a feminist activist carried out an unpublished study on abortion which found that many doctors specialize in providing illegal abortions for unmarried women (El-Damanhoury 2009). It is in this context – one in which Egyptians are uneasy about changing social norms surrounding sex at the same time that they are increasingly aware of the availability of new medical technologies that can disguise the evidence of sexual activity – that we must situate both the cultural stereotypes about EC users and DKT-Egypt's careful strategies to promote Contraplan II™ in a way that would avoid triggering a social or religious backlash against the drug.

5.5   Conclusions: Placing the Egyptian Experience in a Global Context

New medical technologies offer a unique vantage point for studying cultural attitudes towards religion and the body (Wynn and Trussell 2006a). In particular, debates about new reproductive health technologies reveal a society's attitudes towards ideal and proscribed sexuality, gender role expectations, beliefs about families, cosmologies about when life begins and how an individual relates to God, and expectations about the role of government and medical experts in individuals' sexual and reproductive lives. Reproductive health technologies often become associated with certain stereotypes about typical users. These imaginations are built on cultural ideas about normal and abnormal sexuality, popular understandings of the workings of the body and the technology's mechanism of action.

The stereotype about EC users in Egypt (as largely young, unmarried women) is not atypical. In the US, for example, EC opponents claimed that nonprescription availability of EC would lead to an epidemic of sexually transmitted diseases amongst teens. And the U.S. Food and Drug Administration originally rejected the application to make an ECP available without prescription on the grounds that there was insufficient data on how teens would use it (Wood 2005; Wood et al. 2005).

Yet clearly there are differences between the cultural imaginations of this reproductive health technology in US and Egypt. In Egypt, while there is considerable public debate about the increasing availability of hymenoplasty and fake hymen products facilitating premarital sexuality, Egyptians are not nearly as concerned about EC. Even more notably, concern over mechanism of action, which has been the center of EC debates in many countries, is almost completely absent in Egypt. In Latin America, the United States, and some countries in Europe, there has been intense debate over whether EC works before or after implantation to prevent pregnancy, and these public debates over EC's mechanism of action have led Latin American researchers to undertake several scientific studies to investigate this (Croxatto et al. 2001, 2004; Ortiz et al. 2004). In contrast, no debate about the permissibility of EC in Islam has attended the introduction of this reproductive health technology in Egypt. While the brochures and leaflets distributed by DKT-Egypt were quick to point out that Contraplan II™ was not an abortifacient, there was little discussion of its mechanism of action beyond declaring it to be a contraceptive. In contrast, the careful profiling of EC users as primarily married couples suggests that reproductive health activists' main concern is that any opposition to EC will revolve not around the drug itself and its mechanism of action, but rather around its social use outside of marriage.

International reproductive health activists have often assumed that the promotion of EC in the Arab world would inevitably be a politically charged enterprise, perhaps assuming that attitudes towards the drug by social conservatives in one part of the world would naturally be reflected in similar attitudes elsewhere (Wynn et al. 2005). Yet EC is widely available in the Arab world, where the introduction of dedicated products has not met nearly the same level of opposition that it has in, for example, Latin America (Foster and Wynn 2012).[12] The apparently uncontroversial introduction of EC in Egypt compared to other (non-Muslim) socially conservative countries illustrates that social conservativism is far from monolithic when it comes to reproductive health technologies (Bowen 1997). It suggests the importance of fine-tuned ethnographic understanding of the local cultural and religious norms that shape local interpretations of global technologies.

5.6 Looking to the Future, Post-revolution

In recent years Egypt has witnessed a striking increase in Salafism and other fundamentalist forms of Islam. In the wake of the 2011 revolution that overthrew the Mubarak regime, these groups have become more visible and have actively sought to transform the social terrain of gender and sexuality in Egypt through proposed changes to legislation and even through violent demonstrations. For example, in March 2011 several people who were suspected of running a brothel or working in it were attacked and beaten by Salafist activists. There have also been calls to repeal the quota of women in parliament (under the Mubarak regime, 60 women were selected in separate elections) and to cancel some of the family laws protecting the rights of women and children (such as the minimum age of 16 for marriage). In May 2012, Al-Watan newspaper reported that a Salafist Member of Parliament, Nasser Shaker, had applied to change Act 242 of the Penal Code to no longer make it a

---

[12] In the Arab world, oral contraceptive pills that can be used for EC are available in every country. Dedicated ECPs are registered and sold in Algeria, Israel, Kuwait, Lebanon, Morocco, Tunisia, and Yemen. The pills available in most of these countries are NorLevo (manufactured by HRA Pharma, a French pharmaceutical company) and Postinor-2 (manufactured by Gedeon Richter, a Hungarian pharmaceutical company), which are the two most widely available pill brands internationally (the exceptions are Pregnon in Algeria and Duet in Yemen; both of these dedicated ECPs are produced by an Indian pharmaceutical company, FamyCare International). Saudi Arabia has a dedicated ECP registered but it is not sold in the country. Egypt is the only Middle Eastern country to have a locally manufactured ECP. While dedicated ECPs are not registered in Bahrain, Iraq, Libya, Oman, Qatar, Syria, and the United Arab Emirates, travelers have reported that imported boxes of NorLevo and Postinor-2 can sometimes be found in the pharmacies of the small Arab Gulf states, even though there is no officially registered product. No Arab country bans ECPs, unlike some countries in Latin America which have made the use of EC illegal. While there was some controversy over the registration of EC in Morocco, there was none in Tunisia or Lebanon (Foster and Wynn 2012).

criminal offense to circumcise girls as long as the procedure was carried out under the supervision of a medical doctor, and this attempted legislative reform (still under consideration at the time this book went to press) was supported by several other members of Parliament from the Muslim Brotherhood. As of June 2012, many Egyptian reproductive health activists were afraid that the Salafists or the Muslim Brotherhood will take power and institute changes that will be detrimental to reproductive and sexual health, in spite of the fact that the majority of Egyptians seemed to be mostly optimistic about the political changes afoot in Egypt.

It is difficult to disaggregate the principled calls for radical social change from backlash against the overthrown regime and its corruption. For example, the campaign to end female genital cutting (alternatively known as female circumcision or female genital mutilation) was previously sponsored by Suzanne Mubarak, the wife of the former president. In the wake of the revolution, billboards with an anti-female circumcision message that had been up for years in Cairo had by April 2011 been removed and replaced with revolutionary slogans about rebuilding a democratic Egypt. Many reproductive health activists claim that, post-Mubarak, a popular surge in demand for female circumcision has occurred. Is this a burgeoning of demand for a cultural institution that was previously suppressed by anti-female circumcision legislation, or is it a symbolic challenge to the priorities of the *ancien régime*? It is impossible to separate the two, and the challenge faced by reproductive health activists who previously sought partnerships with the government will be to distance themselves from the old regime without delegitimizing their agendas.

In the case of EC, it is difficult to predict how government policy will change. Before the January 2011 revolution, DKT-Egypt had offered the Ministry of Health free samples of Contraplan II in the hopes that it would be included in the National Family Planning Program. Post-revolution, a number of inquiries were being undertaken into drugs that were adopted onto the government's list of essential drugs or into various government programs (like the National Family Planning Program) because of claims that pharmaceutical companies had bribed government officials to have their products included in these lists and programs. Some reproductive health experts in Egypt have wondered whether Contraplan II™ will be challenged.

Yet it is notable that potential challenges to EC in the post-revolutionary period are being framed in the language of corruption and the practices of pharmaceutical companies, not in terms of the morality of the drug or its use. In 2011, Contraplan II™ was introduced into 20 % of the health units in Menoufia Governorate, with a supply donated by DKT-Egypt. In 2012, the Egyptian Ministry of Health in collaboration with the United Nations Family Planning Agency (UNFPA) bought the equivalent of LE two million in Contraplan II™ supplies to be introduced into the family planning programs of five governorates (Menoufia, Sharqiyya, Fayoum, Beni Suif, and Assiut).[13] These appear to be positive steps toward the eventual widespread

---

[13]Personal communication with a senior program officer in the Ministry of Health (Dr. Amal Zaki, head of outreach workers division (Raedat Rifiat) in the family planning sector), 14 May, 2012.

adoption of emergency contraception in Egypt's National Family Planning Program. The continuation of such policies that expand women's reproductive health choices will, in part, depend on whether DKT-Egypt (or another international ECP manufacturer) can build new alliances with emerging social and political actors in postrevolutionary Egypt.

References

Bowen, D. L. (1997). Abortion, Islam, and the 1994 Cairo population conference. *International Journal of Middle East Studies, 29*, 161–184.

Croxatto, H. B., Devoto, L., Durand, M., Ezcurra, E., Larrea, F., Nagle, C., Ortiz, M. E., Vantman, D., Vega, M., & von Hertzen, H. (2001). Mechanism of action of hormonal preparations used for emergency contraception: A review of the literature. *Contraception, 63*, 111–121.

Croxatto, H. B., Ortiz, M. E., & Müller, A. L. (2004). Mechanisms of action of emergency contraception. *Steroids, 68*, 1095–1098.

Dardir, A. M., & Ahmed, W. (1981). Islam and birth planning: An interview with the Grand Mufti of Egypt. *Popular Science, 2*, 1–5.

Davidoff, F., & Trussell, J. (2006). Plan B and the politics of doubt. *Journal of the American Medical Association, 296*, 1775–1778.

DKT International. (2011). *Annual report 2010*. Washington, DC: DKT International. Available at: http://www.dktinternational.org/index.php?section=10

El Shakry, O. (2005). Barren land and fecund bodies: The emergence of population discourse in Interwar Egypt. *International Journal of Middle East Studies, 37*, 351–372.

El Tawila, S., & Khadr, Z. (2004). *Patterns of marriage and family formation among youth in Egypt*. Cairo: National Population Council.

El-Damanhoury, H. (2009). *Determinants of induced abortion in Cairo*. Cairo: New Woman Foundation.

El-Zanaty, F., & El-Daw, A. (1996). *Behavior research among Egyptian university students*. Cairo: International Medical Technology Egypt (MEDTRIC) and Family Health International. Unpublished Report.

FIGO/ICEC. (2011). *Emergency contraception statement: Mechanism of action*. Available at: http://www.cecinfo.org/UserFiles/File/MOA_FINAL_2011_ENG.pdf

Foster, A. M. (2002). Young women's sexuality in Tunisia: The health consequences of misinformation among university students. In D. L. Bowen & E. A. Early (Eds.), *Everyday life in the Muslim Middle East* (pp. 98–110). Bloomington: Indiana University Press.

Foster, A. M., & Wynn, L. L. (Eds.). (2012). *Emergency contraception: The story of a global reproductive health technology*. New York: Palgrave Macmillan.

Hanna, S. (2010). *ECPs in Egypt: A challenging experience*. Cairo: DKT-Egypt.

Hassan, R. (2000). Is family planning permitted by Islam? The issue of a woman's right to contraception. In G. Webb (Ed.), *Windows of faith: Muslim women scholar-activists in North America* (pp. 226–237). Syracuse: Syracuse University Press.

Mogahed, D. (2006). *Ordinary Muslims (Gallup World Poll special report: Muslim world)*. Princeton: Gallup, Inc.

Ortiz, M. E., Ortiz, R. E., Fuentes, M. A., Parraguez, V. H., & Croxatto, H. B. (2004). Postcoital administration of levonorgestrel does not interfere with post-fertilization events in the new-world monkey *Cebus apella*. *Human Reproduction, 19*, 1352–1356.

Ragab, A. R. (1997). Abortion decision-making in an illegal context: A case study from rural Egypt. In E. Ketting & J. Smith (Eds.), *Abortion matters: International conference on reducing the need and improving the quality of abortion services: Proceedings*. Utrecht: Stimezo.

Ragab, A. R. (2009). Sexuality education and HIV/AIDS: Perspectives from North Africa and Middle East. *Egypt Journal of Fertility and Sterility 13*, 55–60. http://www.arsrc.org/resources/publications/sia/aug05/issue.htm

Ragab, A. R., & Mohamoud, M. (2006). Sex education for young people in Egypt: A community based study. In *Proceedings of the Cairo Demographic Center Conference* (pp. 559–569). Cairo: Cairo Demographic Center.

United Nations. (2009). *World population policies 2007*. New York: United Nations.

WHO. (2004). *Medical eligibility criteria for contraceptive use* (3rd ed.). Geneva: WHO.

Wood, S. F. (2005). Women's health and the FDA. *New England Journal of Medicine, 353*, 1650–1651.

Wood, A. J. J., Drazen, J. M., & Green, M. F. (2005). A sad day for science at the FDA. *New England Journal of Medicine, 353*, 1197–1199.

Wynn, L. L., & Trussell, J. (2006a). The social life of emergency contraception in the United States: Disciplining pharmaceutical use, disciplining women's sexuality, and constructing zygotic bodies. *Medical Anthropology Quarterly, 20*, 297–320.

Wynn, L. L., & Trussell, J. (2006b). Images of American sexuality in debates over nonprescription access to emergency contraceptive pills. *Obstetrics and Gynecology, 108*, 1272–1276.

Wynn, L. L., Foster, A. M., Rouhana, A., & Trussell, J. (2005). The politics of emergency contraception in the Arab world: Reflections on Western assumptions and the potential influence of religious and social factors. *Harvard Health Policy Review, 6*, 38–47.

Zuhur, S. (2006). Women's crimes and the criminalization of sex. *Al-Raida, 23*, 28–37.

Chapter 6
Using New Data and Improved Study Designs to Examine Infertility-Service Seeking and Adverse Maternal and Perinatal Outcomes in the South-Central United States

Suzanne Dhall and Andrzej Kulczycki

6.1 Introduction

The inability to produce a biological child can profoundly disturb mental and social wellbeing, although it does not in itself threaten physical health. Infertility is also a problem of global proportions, affecting about 4–14 % of couples worldwide (Nachtigall 2006), with estimates of couples experiencing involuntary childlessness for at least 1 year ranging from 10 to 30 %. After a long period of neglect, infertility is finally receiving increased public and research attention. Infertility treatments can assist those desperate to become parents, but they have also fallen under scrutiny for their potential adverse maternal and infant outcomes. In this chapter, we use a new data source and novel comparison group to consider the use of such services and their salient outcomes. Our application is to Texas, the second most populous and extensive state in the U.S., and which has some of its most glaring reproductive health disparities.

6.2 The Growth of the Infertility Field and Industry

Reproductive medicine has undergone relentless growth since the birth in 1978 of the first child by in vitro fertilization (IVF) (Carr et al. 2005; Fritz and Speroff 2011). Subsequent advances in the understanding, diagnosis and treatment of many

S. Dhall, DrPH (✉)
Department of Health Care Organization and Policy,
University of Alabama at Birmingham, Birmingham, AL, USA
e-mail: suzanne.roseman@gmail.com

A. Kulczycki, Ph.D.
Associate Professor, Department of Health Care Organization and Policy,
University of Alabama at Birmingham, Birmingham, AL, USA
e-mail: andrzej@uab.edu

A. Kulczycki (ed.), *Critical Issues in Reproductive Health*, The Springer Series on Demographic Methods and Population Analysis 33, DOI 10.1007/978-94-007-6722-5_6, © Springer Science+Business Media Dordrecht 2014

causes of infertility have led to a steady improvement in the pregnancy rates associated with assisted reproductive technology (ART), as well as the introduction of intracytoplasmic sperm injection (ICSI) to treat male infertility (see Table 6.1 for a glossary of commonly-used terms in infertility studies). There are now a wide variety of treatment options for couples experiencing infertility, ranging from the low-tech use of fertility drugs or surgery to the use of costly, high tech ARTs like IVF and ICSI. Ovulatory induction, or the use of powerful fertility drugs to stimulate egg production, has enabled thousands of couples to produce babies and, as with ARTs, has led to increases in the twin birth rate and in higher-order births (Wilcox et al. 1996; Martin et al. 2011).

These medical advances have also spurred a lucrative infertility industry whose value reached $4.04 billion by 2008 in the U.S. alone (Marketdata Enterprises 2009), adding to the ethical controversies surrounding the field. Many European nations have sought to regulate its practices more closely by, for example, restricting the number of children a sperm donor can father to well below the 25 that the American Medical Association recommends. Also, they more tightly regulate the number of embryos that can be transferred to enhance the implantation rate; the Nordic countries have moved toward elective single-embryo transfer whereas the American Society for Reproductive Medicine (ASRM) guideline allows five embryos for women over 40 years old (Pandian et al. 2009; Jones et al. 2011). This reflects concerns about the number of risky multiple births which may lead to increased maternal, newborn and pediatric complications (Bronson 1997; Hansen et al. 2005; Templeton and Morris 1998), as well as ethical, financial and other potential violations of a reproductive marketplace. The increased awareness of potential adverse maternal and perinatal outcomes associated with various infertility services has also led to a considerable expansion of the field of reproductive epidemiology (Macaluso et al. 2010). However, controversy about the health risks of multiple-embryo transfer for mothers and babies has not led to a global standardization of its regulation.

Childless women and men seeking to have their own baby view infertility treatment as very important. This is especially true if they live in countries where infertility is much stigmatized and children are highly prized for personal, economic, social and cultural reasons (Hollos et al. 2009; Inhorn and Balen 2002; Inhorn 2003); but unless wealthy and well connected, they have poor coverage of services and their needs are accorded low priority by governments challenged with addressing primary health care and other health services. In more affluent countries, infertility treatments are more widely available and although access to services may also be limited by income and other constraints, the number of births from such treatments will rise further with the development of new technologies.

Also, surveys show an increase in reported levels of infertility, in part because this issue was not measured until recently and in part due to increased public, media and research scrutiny. There is now much greater awareness of the risk of infertility from sexually transmitted infections (STIs) and pelvic inflammatory disease (PID), and much concern about environmental hazards possibly harming sperm and egg quality. With increased warnings from the media and medical community, women

Table 6.1 Glossary of key terms regarding infertility and its treatments

Term	Definition
Artificial insemination	Includes intrauterine insemination (see below) and its relatives.
Assisted reproductive technology (ART)	A group of different methods or technical procedures used to help infertile couples. ART works by removing eggs from a woman's body and mixing them with sperm to make embryos, which are then put back in the woman's body. Common methods of ART include GIFT, ICSI, and IVF (see below).
Embryo donation	Transfer of an embryo that did not originate from the recipient and her partner.
Gamete intrafallopian transfer (GIFT)	A procedure where eggs and sperm are transferred into the woman's fallopian tubes, so that fertilization occurs in the woman's body. Few practices offer GIFT as an option.
Impaired fecundity	This is a broader measure than 12-month infertility because it includes pregnancy loss as well as conception problems. It includes those subfecund, nonsurgically sterile, and a long interval without conception (36-month infertility).
Infertility	The inability to conceive after 12 months of regular unprotected sexual intercourse.
Intracytoplasmic sperm injection (ICSI)	A form of IVF often used for couples in which there are serious problems with the sperm, and sometimes also used for older couples or for those with failed IVF attempts. ICSI goes one step further than IVF by injecting a single sperm directly into a mature egg and then transferring the embryo to the uterus or fallopian tube.
Intrauterine insemination (IUI)	In this procedure, the woman's uterus is injected with specially prepared (washed and concentrated) sperm. The woman is sometimes also treated earlier with medicines that first stimulate ovulation. Not all countries classify this procedure under ART (e.g. the USA excludes it).
In vitro fertilization (IVF)	A laboratory procedure often used when a woman's fallopian tubes are blocked or when a man produces too few sperm, and used when other ARTs have failed. Male sperm are placed in a special dish with unfertilized mature eggs, and when fertilization occurs, the resulting healthy embryo(s) is implanted (transferred) into the woman's uterus (with the aim being to establish a successful pregnancy and the birth of a baby) or cryopreserved (frozen) for future use.
Non-ART infertility treatment	Any fertility enhancing drugs (e.g., Clomid, Pergonal), artificial insemination or intrauterine insemination used to initiate the pregnancy.
Ovulation induction	This is one of the simplest and least invasive fertility treatments available. It involves a series of hormone injections or drug treatments that are designed to stimulate ovaries to produce more than one egg per menstrual cycle, thus increasing the likelihood of becoming pregnant. Nearly 90 % of infertility cases may be treated through drug or advanced non-ART infertility treatments like ovulation induction.

and couples may be seeking medical help more quickly than in the past and earlier than the 12 month threshold commonly used to define as infertile those couples remaining childless after actively seeking to become pregnant. Compositional changes also play a role due to higher age at marriage and delayed childbearing, which may lead to ovarian aging and associated infertility. However, the expanding literature on ARTs and infertility more generally largely overlooks that women and couples more often seek less expensive fertility drugs and other treatments.

This chapter proceeds with a brief comparative overview of infertility treatment use and results in the U.S. and in the UK, as well as in Europe more generally. It then describes infertility and infertility-service seeking in the U.S. and some of the databases used to collect such information. These population-based datasources do not, however, report information from non-assisted reproductive technology (non-ART) infertility treatments, although their use and potential associated adverse outcomes may be equally significant. To explore this situation further, we exploit a newly available source of information, the 2003 revision of the U.S. live birth certificate, which is slowly being implemented across U.S. states and which carries information on infertility treatments. This permits the effects of both ART and non-ART infertility treatments on maternal and perinatal outcomes to be studied while controlling for the effects of infertility itself.

We use Texas live birth files for 2005–2006 to assess maternal characteristics, co-morbidities and complications of pregnancy, as well as adverse infant outcomes, among live births from non-ART and ART treatments. Texas accounts for almost one in ten of the nation's births (Martin et al. 2011), though it has its lowest level of health care coverage. As outlined further below, the state's overall reproductive health profile is poor and is the source of a bitter political dispute, making Texas of special interest. Also, despite higher rates of infertility among low-income and non-White women (Chandra et al. 2005), there has been comparatively less focus on variation in structural aspects of infertility such as income, race, and ethnicity, and on the unbalanced rates and outcomes of non-ART use by low-income or non-White patients (Inhorn et al. 2009; Shanley and Asch 2009). This chapter pays attention to these important issues, but its key objective is to examine the information available from the revised birth certificate and to examine if this new data source can shed light on whether non-ART treatments are, like ARTs, equally associated with an increased risk of adverse outcomes.

6.3 Comparative Overview of Infertility Treatment Use and Success Rates in the United States, the United Kingdom, and Other European Countries

Data on infertility treatment use are not entirely statistically comparable across countries due to the lack of standardized data collection and reporting of results. Since the ultimate goal of ART is to have a pregnancy and deliver a child, success rates are typically presented in terms of pregnancy and delivery rates. However, some of the key differences between reported European and U.S. data consist of those published by the European Society for Human Reproduction and Embryology (ESHRE) including intrauterine insemination (IUI), while U.S. data collected and published by the Centers for Disease Control and Prevention (CDC) and the Society for Assisted Reproductive Technology (SART) only report on ARTs. Further, the causes of infertility are not available for ESHRE data, and age of the recipients is not available from each ESHRE reporting country. European data also reflect tighter regulatory laws that limit the number of embryos that can be cultured and transferred and thereby reduce the likelihood of having multiple births (Gleicher et al. 2006; Myers et al. 2008; Sutcliffe and Ludwig 2007). Nevertheless, it is still possible and instructive to briefly review experiences across countries where these procedures are more common and better recorded, along with some of their results.

Both the UK and the U.S. report their clinic success rates annually but differently, and neither is required to report their patient selection criteria that also influence success rates. The ensuing difficulties in interpreting the clinic success rates may mislead both physicians and the lay public in estimating the likelihood of a successful ART outcome and in making decisions about whether to attend a particular clinic or to receive services at all (Abusief et al. 2007). The availability, access, and utilization of infertility-related services also differ within and between the U.S. and UK, as do ethical perspectives and legislative policies. The U.S. situation is clearly less regulated and leads to great differentials, but even with its national health care system and national regulatory system for reproductive technologies, the UK also experiences problems related to access, availability, and affordability of ART and other infertility-related services for couples that meet the criteria for services.

For the UK, the Human Fertilisation and Embryology Authority (HFEA) regulates and determines access to infertility-related clinics and protects human infertility-related research. It also gathers data from all licensed fertility centers and publishes annual ART clinic outcome statistics. The most detailed assessment of long-term data available in 2012 was for 1992–2006, during which time 122,043 babies were born following IVF and ICSI treatment (Kurinczuk and Hockley 2010). The number of live births increased steadily to 10,250 in 2006, by when 29 women in every 100 treated gave birth (29 %). In 2006, 37,531 women started fertility treatment at 84 clinics licensed by HFEA and 49,391 cycles were carried out. Of the 35,452 women who had one or more cycles of IVF or ICSI, 98 % tried to conceive a baby during that treatment cycle, with others involved in egg sharing, egg or embryo storage for later use (with such fertility preservation typically done in advance of receiving cancer treatment), and others sought to produce embryos for donation for use by other couples or as part of a surrogacy arrangement.

As a result of the IVF and ICSI fertility treatments received in 2006, 13,052 babies were born. Of these live births, 61 % were singleton births, 38 % were twins, and 1 % were triplets or higher order multiples. Also, 58 % of triplet (or more) pregnancies following IVF or ICSI resulted in the birth of all the babies, whereas 84 % of twin pregnancies resulted in the birth of both the babies and 88 % of singleton pregnancies resulted in the birth of a baby. Over time, fertility treatment success rates and multiple birth rates have fallen, and in 2009, HFEA set a maximum multiple birth rate which clinics should not exceed in an attempt to bring down over time the overall rate to 10 % (Kurinczuk and Hockley 2010).

The European IVF Monitoring program (EIM) is a joint IVF data collection program for Europe associated with the European Society for Human Reproduction and Embryology (ESHRE), which also collects data on other ART treatments from national registers in Europe. The most recent results of ART treatments initiated in 36 European countries show that 1,051 clinics reported 532,260 treatment cycles in 2008 (Ferraretti et al. 2012). In 19 countries where all clinics reported to the ART register, IVF and ICSI clinical pregnancy rates per aspiration and per transfer all averaged at about 30 %, although major differences exist between countries. In IVF and ICSI cycles, one, two, three, and four or more embryos were transferred in 22, 53, 22 and 2 %, respectively. The proportions of singleton, twin and triplet deliveries after IVF and ICSI (combined) were 78, 21 and 1 %, respectively, giving a total multiple delivery rate of 21.7 %. Compared with earlier years, the reported number of ART cycles has increased further, fewer multiple embryos (3+) are transferred per treatment, and there have been marginal increases in pregnancy rates and declines in multiple deliveries (Ferraretti et al. 2012; Nyboe Andersen et al. 2009).

A recent comparison of ART-involved pregnancy and delivery outcomes between the U.S. and 23 European countries showed that the latter utilized ART at approximately twice the rate of the U.S., but U.S. patients had significantly higher clinical pregnancy and delivery rates per started cycle, and they also received significantly more embryos per embryo transfer and experienced a significantly higher multiple pregnancy rate (Gleicher et al. 2006). For the U.S., the higher efficacy rate (measured in terms of better pregnancy and live birth outcomes) may be explained in part by the transfer of larger embryo numbers. However, there are also other factors not considered in such analyses and which bias the results. These include differences in patient selection (other than age), aggressiveness of stimulation, reduction policies, cancellation rates, and other factors that may affect the practice of ART (and other infertility treatments) and outcomes. Additionally, the benefit may be higher for individuals in Europe where the cost is lower and insurance coverage is higher, and the number of cycles per million population is higher. Most importantly, multiple pregnancy rates are lower in Europe, reducing neo- and post-natal care costs (Nygren et al. 2006). Also, it should be noted that Europe is far from homogenous and the situation varies between countries.

6.4 Infertility and Infertility-Service Seeking in the United States

As noted above, published data sources on infertility and its treatment provide limited information on the topic for the U.S. Data compiled on the type, number, and outcome of ART cycles performed annually in U.S. fertility clinics show that by 2009, such procedures had doubled since 1997; additionally, the number of infants conceived this way (60,190) was more than two times higher than in 1998 and represented well over 1 % of all live births (CDC/ASRM/SART 2011). However, these clinic success rates are limited to ART procedures, do not yield demographic information other than the age of the service users, and are not publicly available. Also, with the unit of analysis being the cycle rather than the individual patient, these data are very difficult to link to other data sources and document only if a cycle led to live birth, but they do not collect other infant or maternal outcomes. The Pregnancy Risk Assessment Monitoring System (PRAMS) is an annual follow-back survey of a stratified sample of postpartum women, which collects data on infertility treatment and pregnancy outcomes. Although PRAMS surveillance is conducted in 40 U.S. states, each state's questionnaire is unique and PRAMS data offer less information regarding infant outcomes than about maternal complications in pregnancy, labor and delivery. Also, PRAMS data are not representative of all pregnancies and the validity of its questions on infertility treatments has been challenged because mothers may self-report information about their use of infertility services during a previous pregnancy instead of in their current pregnancy (Schieve et al. 2006).

The National Survey of Family Growth (NSFG) collects information on factors affecting childbearing and family life, and is the primary source of nationally representative data on the prevalence of infertility and on the receipt of medical help for it. The 2006–2010 NSFG shows that 7.1 million women aged 15–44 (10.9 % of this population) had fertility problems, reflecting either 12-month infertility or impaired fecundity. Also, 11.9 % of women of childbearing age had ever used medical help for infertility, and 32.0 % of those with fertility problems had ever done so. In absolute numbers, 7.4 million women aged 15–44 overall had ever sought infertility services of any kind (NCHS 2012). However, this population-based survey does not allow estimates from individual states and only considers men and women ages 15–44 years, which may exclude some infertility treatment seekers. Also, these self-reported data do not provide outcomes data relevant to our study purpose.

Most women seeking medical help for infertility receive a consultation, advice or testing only. They may then proceed to use ovulation drugs or help to prevent miscarriage, but rarely do they resort to ARTs. Although the non-economic costs and consequences of ARTs are often discussed, they have arguably not always been given due consideration. It is perhaps even less widely appreciated that a growing share of infants are born after non-ART fertility treatments, such as ovulation induction or controlled ovarian stimulation, and that these may also carry increased risks of multiple birth and concomitant sequelae and adverse outcomes, even among singleton births. Even among women who reported fertility problems, NSFG data show that in 2006–2008, only 1.8 % had ever had ART whereas 13 % had ever had fertility drugs of some kind; an additional 5.8 % had ever had artificial insemination and 2.5 % had ever had tubal surgery. A recent estimate indicates that non-ART treatments account for 4.6 % of all U.S. births, or about four times more than the number conceived through ART use (Schieve et al. 2009).

U.S. data-sources recording non-ART infertility treatments are also very limited. This is despite the increasingly widespread use of such treatments and their established risks, which may include a higher incidence of multiple births and accompanying maternal and infant morbidity (Wang et al. 2002). A few studies have reported maternal, infant or other demographic characteristics among non-ART users in the U.S. using available sources of data such as the National Birth Defects Prevention Study and PRAMS (Duwe et al. 2010; Lu et al. 2008). These data sources introduce potential sampling bias and other biases due to maternal self-reporting of exposure (including non-ART infertility treatments). Studies have also used large fertility-related databases (notably the National ART Surveillance System) that have often linked the collected data to vital records so as to obtain information on selected maternal, and almost all infant, outcomes (Schieve et al. 2007).

Previous multivariate analyses have shown the strongest correlates of receipt of medical help for infertility as being ever-married, nulliparous, over 30 years of age, college-educated, and having higher income and private health insurance (Chandra and Stephen 2010). After controlling for these factors, there is no net effect of race or ethnicity on the use of such services, but socio-economic status (especially private insurance) and race are also important correlates of the more costly and medically intensive forms of help. Despite non-ART treatments being less expensive and probably more accessible, it is unclear if they differ in maternal and infant outcomes from ART and spontaneously conceived (SC) births. This study considers these issues by comparing non-ART births to both SC births and ART births. We first discuss the relevance of the new birth certificate data and provide relevant contextual information on the state of Texas.

6.5   New Information on Infertility in the Revised U.S. Birth Certificate

Notwithstanding the severe constraints to U.S. published data sources on infertility and its treatment, the gradual adoption of an improved birth certificate means that a new source of information may slowly become available to researchers.[1] Birth certificate data contain a wide range of reliable information for a very large number of live births on maternal socio-demographic (e.g. age, education, race/ethnicity, marital status) and infant characteristics (such as birthweight). The ability of birth certificate data to make available methodologically rigorous and reliably collected information on select exposures and outcomes on a large number of mother-infant pairs makes it appealing for multiple research purposes.

The 2003 revised birth certificate is especially helpful for our purpose because it modified the 1989 checkbox, "pregnancy resulted from infertility treatment," by asking those who responded affirmatively to report additionally whether they had used either:

---

[1]The U.S. standard certificate of live birth, first introduced in 1900, is the model for state birth certificates and provides reasonably accurate information for maternal demographic characteristics. It is revised every 10–15 years to improve data quality and the collection of comparable and relevant birth data (Kulczycki 2008).

- Fertility enhancing drugs, artificial insemination or intrauterine insemination; [or]
- Assisted reproductive technology (e.g.: in vitro infertilization (IVF), gamete intrafallopian transfer (GIFT)).

These revised questions on the birth certificate have been extensively pre-tested and the data have shown that non-ART infertility treatments (fertility enhancing drugs, artificial insemination or intrauterine insemination) and ARTs are mutually exclusive in the information collected by the birth certificates. Crucially, this allows us to separate ART and non-ART treatments. We analyze Texas data for reasons outlined below and because the state implemented the revision in January 2005, earlier than most states, and made these data on ART and non-ART treatments available to us. In 2005–2006, Texas had the largest number of births captured since the implementation of the revised birth certificate, when it accounted for 20 % of all U.S. annual births. By 2008, only 27 states had implemented the revised birth certificate, representing 65 % of all U.S. births (Osterman et al. 2011), and several of these states did not include the expanded question on infertility treatments in the implemented revision.

6.6   The Texas Context

Over 1970–2011, the population of Texas more than doubled in size to reach 25.8 million people. Texas has experienced more population growth in the last decennial decade (2000–2010) than any other U.S. state. In 2010, 46 % of the population comprised non-Hispanic White Americans, 12 % were African American (about the national average), 4 % were Asian Americans, and 38 % identified themselves as Hispanics (be they White or non-White).[2] Hispanics, or Latinos, account for two-thirds of the state's growth in the last decade, mostly from births to families already living in the state, with migration continuing to play a significant though declining role. Texas also has one of the most unequal income distributions of any state and spends less on each of its citizens than does any other state. It has the third-highest poverty rate, the second-highest imprisonment rate, the lowest proportion of high-school graduates, and the highest proportion of people (over 25 %) lacking health insurance of all 50 states.

---

[2]The U.S. Census Bureau collects and tabulates race and ethnicity data following the U.S. Office of Management and Budget's (OMB) standards, the most recent issued in 1997. These identify five race groups: white, black or African-American, American Indian or Alaska Native, Asian, and Native Hawaiian or Other Pacific Islander. The Census Bureau also utilized a sixth category ('some other race'). Hispanic-origin information is also collected to give data on ethnicity by two categories: "Hispanic or Latino" and "Not Hispanic or Latino."

Texas has a poor reproductive health profile relative to the rest of the country, with significant socio-economic and racial/ethnic differentials. It has the fourth highest pregnancy rate and the third highest birth rate for females aged 15–19, as well as the fourth lowest rate of condom use at last intercourse (56 %) among high school students, 39 % of whom report being currently sexually active (Bridges 2008). Sexually transmitted infection (STI) and HIV rates are disproportionately higher among African American and Hispanics. The high risk for negative sexual health outcomes makes comprehensive sexuality education and access to contraception more important than ever to the health of Texas' youth, but major deficiencies in these areas have become accentuated in recent years.[3]

Texas women's reproductive rights have been spotlighted by the neglect of evidence-based policy and political disregard for women's health. In 2011, the Republican-controlled legislature and governor curtailed the state budget for family planning services by two-thirds so as to cut off public money for Planned Parenthood (the largest reproductive health care provider in the state) and other clinics affiliated with abortion service providers.[4] Republican lawmakers also passed a law shutting out Planned Parenthood from funding through the state's Medicaid-supported Women's Health Program.[5] This serves hundreds of thousands of low-income women with free birth-control pills, cervical and breast cancer screenings and exams critical for the early detection of such cancers, and it provides grants to many clinics, including non-Planned Parenthood facilities. The Texas cuts are part of a nationwide effort by conservative lawmakers and their supporters to defund family planning services at the state level. In contrast, better-off women and couples find it relatively easy to secure reproductive health services, including for infertility treatment.

---

[3]U.S. teen pregnancy and birth rates declined by more than one-third over 1990–2008, but in 2008, their public costs (federal, state, and local) still amounted to $10.9 billion and in Texas, teen childbearing (with over 80 % of such births unintended) cost taxpayers at least $1,193 million, substantially more than for any other state (National Campaign to Prevent Teen and Unplanned Pregnancy 2011). Among other factors, the negative consequences for the children of teen mothers include increased costs for health care, child welfare and foster care, lost tax revenue due to decreased earnings and spending.

[4]Planned Parenthood uses private contributions and patient fees to provide abortions, but not federal or state funds as this is not permitted under U.S. law. The sharply curtailed funding has led to the closure of numerous clinics in the state.

[5]Medicaid is a joint federal-state program that finances health care for poor women. Under U.S. law, those who depend on Medicaid have to be able to access healthcare from clinics that accept Medicaid. The Medicaid-supported Women's Health Program generates $9 in federal funding for every $1 dollar spent by Texas. This match makes it a very good investment for the state and provides a safety net that is often the only health care many low-income women receive. In 2011, a lower court overruled the measure to bar Planned Parenthood (the program's largest provider, serving nearly half the women in the program with their primary health and family planning) and abortion affiliates from continuing as members of the Women's Health Program. This move was then appealed by the powerful Republican governor, whose presidential candidacy and coveting of social conservatives led his party to push more firmly against spending money on contraception and further limit access to reproductive health services.

6.7 Methods

6.7.1 Theoretical Model

Use of the new birth certificate data and of two different comparison groups (ART, as well as spontaneously conceiving (SC), mothers) allow us to establish the impact of non-ART infertility treatments on adverse maternal and infant outcomes. Such outcomes are determined by a complex array of factors, not all of which can be readily measured, so we restrict our analysis to factors that can be reasonably assessed using the birth certificate data. A cross-sectional design is used to describe the differences in the distribution of maternal characteristics and co-morbidities among ART and non-ART groups, and these are initially contrasted with the situation for women who had spontaneously conceived. A retrospective cohort design is then used to determine and compare adverse maternal and infant outcomes among the non-ART and SC groups, as well as among the two infertility treatment groups. In keeping with the exploratory nature of our study, the results of these comparisons are presented in the form of testing the following a-priori hypotheses:

For the SC vs. non-ART comparison, our three hypotheses are:

1. the mean maternal age for live-births resulting from non-ART infertility treatments is greater than or equal to the mean maternal age for SC live-births;
2. non-ART mothers are more likely to be married, and have higher educational and socio-economic attainments (more likely to be married, to have a college degree or higher, to be privately insured, and less likely to use WIC food);
3. when controlling for maternal demographic characteristics and plurality, the risk of adverse maternal and infant health outcomes is higher for the non-ART infertility treatment groups.

Similarly, results of the ART vs. non-ART comparison are presented in the form of tests for these three a-priori hypotheses:

4. the mean maternal age for live-births resulting from non-ART infertility treatments is less than or equal to the mean maternal age for live-births from ART;
5. there are no differences in marital status, educational attainment, insurance status, WIC food use, and self-reported race or ethnicity among the mothers of ART and non-ART live born infants;
6. when controlling for maternal demographic characteristics and plurality, there are no differences in the risk of adverse maternal and infant health outcomes between the ART and non-ART infertility treatment groups.

Several factors related both to the exposure (or type of infertility treatment) and to maternal and infant outcomes are treated as confounders. For example, older maternal age is directly associated with the need for infertility treatment as well as with pregnancy-induced hypertension and gestational diabetes mellitus (GDM). Maternal age, therefore, plays the role of a confounder between the effects of type of infertility treatment on GDM. Also, certain adverse maternal outcomes can in turn influence infant outcomes, for instance, infants born to mothers with pregnancy-induced hypertension may have higher risk of preterm birth. Birth plurality is treated as a confounder because it is related both to the exposure (non-ART and ART-births are each associated with higher risk of plural births) and to maternal and infant outcomes. Gestational age is measured as the best obstetric estimate of the infant's gestation in completed weeks based on the birth attendant's final estimate of gestation.

6.7.2 Study Variables

Our variables were derived from the 2003 revision of the birth certificate as implemented by Texas. The main predictor variable was the type of infertility treatment, defined as either: (1) ARTs: procedures that involve the handling of both sperm and (oocytes) eggs, e.g. IVF and GIFT; and (2) non-ART infertility treatments: use of fertility enhancing drugs, artificial insemination, and/or intrauterine insemination not meeting the ART definition. The dependent variables comprised both infant and maternal outcomes. The maternal outcomes considered include dichotomous responses for:

1. preeclampsia/eclampsia,[6] which are hypertensive disorders of pregnancy that enhance risk of maternal mortality, placental abruption, and adverse fetal outcomes including fetal growth restriction;
2. non-vertex presentation, defined as any nonvertex fetal presentation including breech, shoulder, brow, face, transverse or compound lie;[7] and
3. gestational diabetes (GDM), defined as glucose intolerance during pregnancy which requires treatment and is associated with increased risk of birth trauma for the mother and for several adverse fetal outcomes.

Infant outcomes included the following abnormal conditions of the newborn:

- low birthweight (<2,500 g);
- preterm birth (<37 weeks gestation, based on the 'best obstetric estimate');

---

[6]Pre-eclampsia can be a dangerous pregnancy complication in which hypertension is diagnosed during the pregnancy along with significant amounts of protein in the urine (proteinuria). There is no known cure for this set of symptoms, whose most visible sign is elevated blood pressure (above normal for age, gender, and physiologic condition) but which may also involve more generalized damaged to the kidneys and liver. It is more common among women who are pregnant for the first time and in women with a multiple gestation (twins or multiple birth), and it may occur in the immediate post-partum period when it can be more dangerous. Some women develop pregnancy-induced hypertension (high blood pressure without proteinuria), which also requires careful monitoring of mother and fetus. Eclampsia can occur after the onset of pre-eclampsia and is an acute and life-threatening complication of pregnancy. This form of hypertension includes seizures or coma.

[7]In keeping with prior literature (Nuojoa-Huttunen et al. 1999), non-vertex presentation is considered here as a maternal outcome, although it can also be viewed as a predictor for other adverse infant outcomes. In this dataset, the most significant predictors of non-vertex presentation were twin and triplet or higher order births, type of infertility treatment, preterm birth, and low birthweight.

- Five minutes Apgar score (with a low score, defined as ≤ 3 based on previous research, used to triage infants needing immediate medical attention);[8]
- need for assisted ventilation following delivery;
- admission to a neonatal intensive care unit (NICU);
- infant living at time of the report. (For the latter dichotomized variable, in most cases, 'no' meant that the infant was reported as not alive, but it also included cases where the infant had required transfer to another facility, or its status was unknown).

Confounding factors included both maternal socio-demographic characteristics (age, marital status, education, race/ethnicity) and health status variables (smoking, pre-existing illness, and plurality). Specifically:

- maternal age, with advanced maternal age defined as >35 years of age;
- marital status (with the reference category being married, the expected lower risk group);
- education (the reference group, women with at least college education, is expected to have lower risk);
- race (with the reference group being White race);
- ethnicity, dichotomized into Hispanic and non-Hispanic (the latter being the reference);
- smoking (both pre-pregnancy and during pregnancy) and pre-existing illness (existing diabetes and hypertension); for these dichotomous variables, the reference groups were non-smokers, non-diabetics and normotensives;
- plurality (or multiple birth), examined as singletons (the reference group), twins and triplets and higher order births.

We also considered two surrogate maternal socio-economic indicators collected in the birth certificate. These included the source of payment for delivery and WIC food use,[9] a federal healthcare and nutrition assistance program for low-income pregnant and breastfeeding women, non-breastfeeding postpartum women, and infants and children under the age of 5.

---

[8] The Apgar score, the very first test given to a newborn, is a systematic measure used for evaluating the physical condition of the infant at specific intervals following birth. Apgar scores range from 0 to 10, with scores 3 and below generally regarded as critically low and requiring immediate medical care (ACOG/AAP 2006). However, the Apgar score has its limitations and is neither a good indicator of long-term complications, nor of the etiology of a problem.

[9] The Special Supplemental Nutrition Program for Women, Infants and Children (abbreviated as WIC) is a Federal grant program whose target population are those at low-income and nutritionally at risk (for more information, see http://www.fns.usda.gov/wic/aboutwic/wicataglance.htm). To be eligible for WIC and for Medicaid during the time period evaluated, households had to have an income that was at or less than 185 % of the federal poverty level (i.e. an eligible family of four could earn up to $37,000 in 2006); and needed to have had a child younger than age 5 years, or a woman who was pregnant, breastfeeding, or up to 6 months postpartum (Texas Department of State Health Services 2012). Those with private health insurance can still apply for WIC and U.S. citizenship is not a requirement for eligibility.

6.7.3   Statistical Analysis

The analysis involved both descriptive and multivariate logistic regression analyses. We first reviewed the distribution of maternal demographic characteristics, co-morbidities and complications of pregnancy, as well as adverse infant outcomes among the non-ART and ART groups, and for SC mothers. Relevant hypotheses were tested by computing two commonly used techniques: the Students t-test for continuous variables (such as maternal age and birthweight) and chi-square for discrete variables (such as maternal education, race, ethnicity, GDM and low birthweight). Separate multiple logistic regression models were computed using backward elimination for the maternal and infant outcomes of interest, until all included variables left in a model were significant ($p < 0.05$) and no further improvement was possible. All statistical analyses were completed using STATA 10.0. This study involved publicly available data and did not use any protected health information, making it exempt from requiring further ethical review board approval.

6.8   Results

6.8.1   Descriptive Statistics

We first compared maternal characteristics among the three groups before proceeding to compare outcomes for the two treatment groups. Compared to SC mothers, women who used any type of infertility-related services were significantly older, more educated, more often White and without Hispanic-origin ethnicity, as well as more likely to be married (not shown) and to rely on private insurance (Table 6.2).

Table 6.2 Percent distribution of maternal socio-demographic and health status characteristics, co-morbidities and risk factors, among women who spontaneously conceived and those who used ART and non-ART infertility treatments, Texas, 2005–2006

Characteristic	Spontaneously conceived (n = 795,599)	Non-ART (n = 3,491)	ART (n = 767)
Bachelor's degree or higher	19	63.4	70.6
Hispanic origin ethnicity	50.2	14.1	12.2
White race	75.8	85.7	87.2
Privately insured	35.4	89.6	87.1
WIC food use	52.4	8.0	5.2
Chronic hypertension	1.0	3.0	2.3
Chronic diabetes	0.6	0.9	1.4
Smoking during pregnancy	5.9	1.2	0.1
Mean maternal age, y (SD)	26.4 (6.1)	33.0 (5.0)	34.5 (6.5)

Notes: *y* years, *SD* standard deviation

A smaller proportion of ART mothers reported smoking during (and prior to) their pregnancy. Otherwise, there were no significant differences found in maternal co-morbidities and risk factors during pregnancy (pre-existing diabetes, hypertension, previous preterm births, and previous poor pregnancy outcomes) across the infertility treatment groups (Table 6.2). On the other hand, there were major differences in plural births, and for maternal and infant outcomes unadjusted for confounders among non-ART and ART live births. In particular, there was a higher incidence of singleton births[10] and lower incidence of twin births, non-vertex presentation, and poor 5 min Apgar scores among non-ART births, without adjusting for confounders.

Compared to the SC group, mothers in the non-ART group were significantly older (36.1 % were older than age 35 compared to 11.2 % among the SC mothers) and were over three times as likely to have a bachelor's or graduate degree. They were also significantly more likely to be married (96.2 % vs. 61.3 %), White (85.7 % vs. 75.8 %) or Asian (6.5 % vs. 3.5 %), and to be privately insured (89.6 % vs. 35.4 %). They were also significantly less likely to be Hispanic (14.1 % vs. 50.2 %), or to use WIC food during pregnancy (8.0 % vs. 52.4 %). Hence, we accept the null hypotheses 1 and 2. The non-ART mothers had a higher prevalence of chronic hypertension (3.0 % vs. 1.0 %) and chronic diabetes (0.9 % vs. 0.6 %), and previous pre-term births. In addition, they had a lower prevalence of smoking prior to (2.2 % vs. 6.5 %) or during pregnancy (1.2 % vs. 5.9 %).

Overall, the non-ART and ART groups appear closer to each other than to SC women, but some significant differences are evident among the two infertility treatment groups. In particular, the mean maternal age was significantly lower among non-ART mothers. Although higher proportions of ART mothers were married and had a bachelor's or graduate degree, and fewer had Hispanic-origin ethnicity, these findings did not reach statistical significance. We therefore fail to reject both the fourth and fifth null hypothesis (that there are no differences in mean maternal age, marital status, higher educational attainment, or self-reported ethnicity among the treatment groups). On the other hand, non-ART mothers were more likely to use WIC food during pregnancy and to be privately insured. They were also less likely to be of White race. Consequently, we reject the null hypothesis that there are no differences in insurance status, WIC food use, or self-reported race, among the mothers of ART and non-ART live born infants. Mothers who conceived with the help of infertility treatments (non-ART or ART) tended to have higher incidence of pre-pregnancy diabetes, chronic hypertension, previous preterm birth, and lower prevalence of smoking before and during the pregnancy.

We used multiple logistic regression to evaluate the effects of non-ART infertility treatments on several maternal and infant outcomes. A number of sociodemographic correlates were explored. The final set of models included controls for the following confounders: older maternal age (defined as >35 years), marital status

---

[10]Results for plurality are calculated incidence rates, whereas other demographic characteristics and co-morbidities are prevalence rates because they were computed with cross-sectional data.

Table 6.3 Adjusted maternal and infant outcomes, no infertility treatment versus non-ART treatments (N=799,090), Texas, 2005–2006

Characteristic	All live births (n=795,599) No. (%)	Non-ART births (n=3,491) No. (%)	p-value[a]
Non-vertex presentation	7,395 (1.0)	193 (6.0)	<0.001
Gestational diabetes	27,344 (3.4)	270 (7.7)	<0.001
Preeclampsia	36,667 (5)	388 (11.1)	<0.001
Eclampsia	1,143 (0.1)	14 (0.4)	0.29
Maternal ICU admission	2,304 (0.3)	22 (1.0)	0.41
Birthweight, g:			<0.001
Normal (≥2,500)	730,123 (91.7)	2,316 (66.3)	
LBW/VLBW (<2,500)	65,476 (8.3)	1175 (33.7)	
Gestational age:			<0.001
Term	707,289 (88.9)	2,097 (60.0)	
Preterm (<36 weeks)	88,310 (11.1)	1,394(40)	
Plurality:			<0.001
Singleton	773,651 (97.2)	2,097 (60.0)	
Twin or higher order	21,909 (2.8)	1,394 (40)	
Assisted ventilation required for >6 h	9,505 (1.1)	255 (7.3)	<0.001
NICU admission	49,309 (6.2)	1,031 (29.5)	<0.001
Infant alive at discharge[b]:			<0.001
Yes	790,448 (99.3)	3,423 (98.05)	
No	5,023 (0.63)	67 (1.9)	
5 min Apgar score:			<0.001
≥4	777,516 (99.5)	3,408 (98.5)	
≤3	3,745 (0.5)	52 (1.5)	

Note: *g* grams
[a]Chi-square test was used to compare the categorical variables
[b]Infant status unknown at discharge for 128 SC infants and 1 non-ART infant

(being not married), less than college educated status, non-White race, Hispanic ethnicity, smoking prior to and during the pregnancy, chronic hypertension and chronic diabetes, twin and triplet or higher order birth, non-privately insured status, and use of WIC food during pregnancy.

6.8.2 Logistic Regression Model Results

The effects of type of infertility treatment and various confounders on individual maternal and infant outcomes were evaluated using logistic regression analysis. We first note that maternal and infant outcomes are worse in the non-ART group when compared to SC mothers (see Table 6.3). Non-ART infertility treatment was found to be an independent predictor of worse outcome for each maternal and infant outcome examined except eclampsia, maternal ICU admission and the need for assisted ventilation immediately after delivery. Also relative to the SC group, ART-mothers fared worse for each maternal outcome examined except eclampsia and for each adverse infant outcome (data not shown). Mothers who conceived with the help of infertility treatments had higher incidence of GDM, pre-eclampsia and non-vertex presentation during pregnancy than did mothers who conceived naturally. The mean birthweight and gestational age were lower for infants born from infertility treatments, and other infant outcomes also tended to be poorer. Hence we accept null hypothesis 3, except for eclampsia and maternal ICU admission, where there were no statically significant differences observed.

Table 6.4 presents results for the more direct comparisons drawn for ART- and non-ART live births after controlling for confounders. The predictors are shown in the left hand column, with positive signs indicating an increase in odds and negative signs denoting a decrease in odds. When controlling for plurality and other confounders, there were no differences in the ART vs. non-ART groups among maternal and infant outcomes except for non-vertex presentation, low 5 min Apgar score, and NICU admission; with ART mothers having higher odds of non-vertex presentation and low 5-min Apgar. The odds of NICU admission were lower for infants born from ART treatments, but this may be artifactual with a greater proportion of these infants requiring transfer to a higher acuity facility, and consequently lost to follow up at the time of registration of the birth certificate. Based on these observed differences, we fail to reject the null hypothesis that there are no differences in the risk of adverse maternal and infant health outcomes between the ART and non-ART infertility treatment groups, after controlling for maternal demographic characteristics and plurality. However, we reject the null in the case of non-vertex presentation, poor 5-min Apgar score and NICU admission. It was not possible to detect any other increased risk of other adverse infant health outcomes stemming from the infertility treatment itself.

We also observe that twin and triplet/higher order births increased the odds of all outcomes examined, with the exception of eclampsia and GDM. Plausibly, the odds ratios may be higher for plurality because outcomes may be rare in singleton (non-plural) births. Smoking during pregnancy (which is a known risk behavior) was not found to alter the odds of any outcome, a finding that may be due to the small number of mothers in our two treatment groups who acknowledged smoking during pregnancy.

6.9   Discussion

Previous studies have shown that compared to SC infants, ART live-born infants are at higher risk of various adverse outcomes. However, such research often ignores that mothers who require ARTs are biologically different from women who conceive spontaneously. Also, studies have overlooked that non-ART use tends to be far more widespread than resort to ARTs. This chapter has attempted to help answer

Table 6.4 Odds of adverse maternal and infant outcomes by maternal/birth characteristics and type of infertility treatment (non-ART vs ART; N=4,258), Texas, 2005–2006

Predictors	Outcomes										
	Pre-eclampsia	Eclampsia	Non-vertex presentation	GDM	Maternal ICU admission	LBW	Preterm birth	Poor 5-min Apgar score	Assisted vent >6 h	NICU admission	Infant not living
Non-ART treatment	+		−					−		+	
Age > 35		+							+		
Marital status (unmarried)							−				
< college education			+	+		+	+	+	+		
Non-White race			+	+		+					+
Hispanic ethnicity								−	+		+
Smoke pre-pregnancy				−							
Smoke during pregnancy		+									
Chronic diabetes			+							+	
Chronic hypertension			+	+	+	+	+			+	
Twin birth	+		+			+	+	+	+	+	+
Triplet or higher order birth	+		+	+	+	+	+	+	+	+	+
Non-privately insured								+			
WIC food use	+							−			

Notes: *GDM* gestational diabetes mellitus, *LBW* low birthweight, *ICU* intensive care unit, *NICU* neonatal intensive care unit, *WIC* Women, Infants and Children program (a U.S. federal government-funded, special supplemental health and nutrition program to support low-income women and children up to age 5 who are at nutritional risk; see also footnote 9)

A blank box indicates there was no statistically significant association between the maternal or infant outcome and the infertility treatment type or maternal/birth characteristic considered whether the non-ART infertility treatment increases the risk to the mother and infant for that pregnancy, and whether outcomes vary by the type of treatment. To do so, we considered mothers who conceived spontaneously or by utilizing ART as two control groups for non-ART use. We found almost no differences in outcomes among the ART and non-ART groups. This is in contrast to the striking differences found in outcomes in either the ART or non-ART group women when compared to those who spontaneously conceived, even after controlling for confounders. These results bring into sharp relief several clear policy messages considered further below. Their significance is given added weight by the higher incidence of non-ART compared to ART-assisted births and, consequently, the greater public health impact of adverse outcomes associated with such procedures.

In the U.S., the ASRM has recommended minimum standards for infertility specialists and certified facilities to provide ART treatments and monitors clinic success rates using certain key metrics nationally. On the other hand, non-ART treatments are probably being delivered not just by infertility specialists, but also by general obstetricians and gynecologists and possibly even general practitioners, in a much less controlled and monitored environment. Presently, there exists no mandate for reporting of non-ART treatments, which are less expensive and may be perceived as safer. The heterogeneity of settings delivering these non-ART infertility treatments may also make it more difficult to counsel couples considering these treatments about their potential adverse maternal and infant outcomes. The 2003 birth certificate revision has still not been implemented by several states, while others have decided not to implement the modified question that asks about the type of infertility treatment that led to the index live birth.

In this chapter, we explored the Texas vital statistics data from 2005 to 2006 to establish that women requiring infertility treatments as a group differ from those who conceive spontaneously, and that non-ART treatment births differ significantly from SC births, and resemble ART births in terms of maternal and infant outcomes when controlling for factors like maternal age and co-morbidities as well as plurality. There is an urgent need to record not only the contribution of non-ARTs to the birth cohort, but also to educate couples considering these treatments about the risks of adverse maternal and infant outcomes from these births. Since the contribution of infertility treatments to the birth cohort is growing in many developed countries, these inferences apply also to other nations that lack systems to monitor these births and to counsel recipients of these non-ART infertility treatments.

Several other noteworthy messages emerge. Compared to non-ART mothers, those who underwent ART treatment tend to be older, more educated, more likely to be White and to self-pay, as well as less likely to use WIC or smoke. Using multiple logistic regression to control for a number of confounders, ART treatment remained an independent predictor for increased odds of non-vertex presentation and poor 5 min Apgar score, as well as for decreasing the odds of NICU admission. The higher risk of non-vertex presentation is biologically plausible for several reasons that could not be examined here. These include preferential attempts to facilitate lower implantation of an embryo in ART users, as well as their higher plurality and lower gestational age (Romundstad et al. 2006).[11] Although it is unclear why ART use was found to be more associated with lower 5-min Apgar outcomes and a lower risk of NICU admission, ART-mothers could have poorer 5-min Apgar scores relative to non-ART users due to their lower gestational age. The lower risk of NICU admission is hard to explain but may be an artifact of the data, with a higher proportion of ART infants possibly being transferred due to their higher frequency of poor Apgar scores.

To the best of our knowledge, previous U.S.–based studies have not looked at outcomes for non-ART mothers by race/ethnicity, although they have examined such differences for prevalence of infertility and infertility risk factors (Wellons et al. 2008). For mothers requiring infertility treatments (ART and non-ART), non-White race was independently associated with: higher odds of GDM, LBW, and infant not alive or requiring transfer at time of report. It is possible, if not probable, that the reported race-ethnic differences in infertility outcomes may really be a surrogate for other socioeconomic factors such as income that could also not be measured adequately here. Instead, birth certificate data collect information on source of payment and WIC food use.

This study found that non-privately insured status increased the odds of poor 5 min Apgar score. The authors are not aware of previous U.S. studies that may have explored the effects of insurance on maternal or infant outcomes among women who have used infertility-related services, although they have evaluated such factors as access to insurance and barriers to coverage, which we were unable to study here. Further, the impact of insurance status on outcomes is difficult to interpret because mothers who are not privately insured could be self-paying or on Medicaid (our birth-certificate data were categorized as private pay vs. everything else). A more thorough discussion regarding insurance coverage at both the individual and state levels is beyond the scope of this study, but future research could investigate this issue further, including its relationship to other variables not considered here, such as decisions regarding the number of embryos transferred.

Similarly, it is difficult to interpret the significance of WIC food use during pregnancy. WIC food use was found to be associated with increased odds of pre-eclampsia, as well as decreased odds of poor Apgar and need for assisted ventilation. However, birth certificate data do not indicate how mothers qualified for Medicaid or WIC, nor the timing and duration of WIC participation, so it is not possible to hypothesize a causal association between pre-eclampsia and WIC use. On the other hand, infant outcomes come after WIC use in this study, so the decreased odds of adverse infant outcomes appear to be biologically plausible.

Another caveat concerns our findings with regard to smoking, because small numbers of mothers in both the ART and non-ART groups acknowledged smoking. Pregnancy is cited as the most common reason among women to quit smoking and

---

[11] This was evident when gestational age was studied as a continuous variable, although the preterm birth difference was not shown to be significantly different among the two infertility treatment groups when it was looked at as a categorical variable.

women undergoing ART treatments may have more frequent encounters with medical professionals regarding the harmful effects of smoking. The ASRM has issued strongly worded practice guidelines encouraging smoking cessation prior to ART. Moreover, the prevalence of smoking during pregnancy has been shown to decline with age (in the examined cohort, women undergoing ARTs were older than non-ARTs).

This study has several methodological strengths with respect to both the data source and the methods used. A major strength concerns our ability to use birth certificate data which are publicly available (although special permission was needed to use information on the infertility treatments), inexpensive, and include all births that occurred in Texas. Unlike SART data, birth certificates collect information on a wide range of socio-demographic variables. The facility worksheet is abstracted from medical records, so the data are not self-reported for many of these variables (e.g. birthweight, gestational age, co-morbidities) and are more likely to be accurate. The birth certificate data collection process has numerous built-in error checks, which help improve data quality. Additionally, we have analyzed recently released 2005–2006 data, making our results timely and relevant.

In addition, the new birth certificate data from Texas has information available from non-ART and ART mothers which has allowed us to use a novel and more appropriate comparison group. It should be noted, though, that not all states which have adopted the revised 2003 U.S. birth certificate have information available from both non-ART and ART mothers. Our first two sets of study hypotheses were explored using cross-sectional analyses, as birth certificate data on exposure (ART/non-ART) and on the variables are collected simultaneously. Also, there is no biological reason for these variables to have a certain temporal relationship with exposure, in contrast to the situation for birth outcomes. The retrospective cohort analysis used to explore our final study hypothesis allowed us to evaluate multiple maternal and infant outcomes using the birth certificate data. This approach is preferable to a case control study design which permits analysis of only one outcome and multiple exposures.

Although this study represents a first, several limitations to our data should also be stated. In other ongoing work not shown here, we have detected some evidence that infertility treatment-related live births may be somewhat underreported in the Texas revised BC data; it is unclear if this may have had any impact on our findings. We did not examine paternal characteristics due to a large number of missing information items regarding many demographic and other factors. The data neither offer information on the duration of infertility nor on the specific type of treatment procedure followed. Although our comparative analyses allow us to "partially" control for the independent effects of infertility, we can neither explain the effects of the underlying cause of infertility on outcome, nor determine how the specific procedure related variables (e.g. freezing, site of implantation) may have affected an outcome. However, this situation is still preferable to using the SC group as a comparison group (Romundstad et al. 2008). Lastly, the results may not generalize fully to other geographic areas with different demographic, institutional, and socio-political backgrounds.

Further research is needed to definitively ascertain the validity of the new data item examined here on ART/non-ART treatment in the birth certificate. However, this question was extensively pre-tested prior to its adoption, and with the novelty of the 2003 birth certificate gradually 'wearing off' and as more recent current data become available, it will be possible to explore this issue further and to see if data quality has improved over time. It should also prove possible to validate these study findings in comparison to other data sources.

Our study findings suggest several policy implications. There is need to strengthen secondary and tertiary prevention efforts focused on reducing poor maternal and infant outcomes for infertility treatments. Continued public health surveillance of these pregnancies should include those resulting from non-ART treatments. There is also continued need to design accurate educational materials – which should be up-to-date, culturally, and linguistically competent, as well as widely accessible in alternative format – for both ART and non-ART treatments, and for women and their partners. Additionally, practitioners taking care of infants conceived following infertility treatments (ART and non-ART) need to be made aware of these results and of the policy implications.

Acknowledgments The authors would like to thank the Texas Department of State Health Services for granting access to data used in this study.

References

Abusief, M. E., Hornstein, M. D., & Jain, T. (2007). Assessment of United States fertility clinic websites according to the American Society for Reproductive Medicine (ASRM)/Society for Assisted Reproductive Technology (SART) guidelines. *Fertility and Sterility, 87*(1), 88–92.

ACOG/AAP [American College of Obstetricians and Gynecologists; American Academy of Pediatrics]. (2006). The Apgar score. ACOG Committee Opinion no. 333. *Obstetrics and Gynecology, 107*(5), 1209–1212.

Bridges, E. (2008). *Texas' youth: Focus on sexual and reproductive health.* Washington, DC: Advocates for Youth. Available at: http://www.advocatesforyouth.org/publications/publications-a-z/641-texas-youth-focus-on-sexual-and-reproductive-health. Accessed 15 Apr 2012.

Bronson, R. (1997). How should the number of embryos transferred to the uterus following in-vitro fertilization be determined to avoid the risk of multiple gestation? *Human Reproduction, 12*(8), 1605–1618.

Carr, B. R., Blackwell, R. E., & Azziz, R. (2005). *Essential reproductive medicine.* New York: McGraw-Hill.

Centers for Disease Control and Prevention (CDC), American Society for Reproductive Medicine (ASRM), Society for Assisted Reproductive Technology (SART). (2011). *2009 assisted reproductive technology success rates: National summary and fertility clinic reports.* Atlanta: U.S. Department of Health and Human Services (especially Section 5: ART Trends 2000–2009). Available at: http://www.cdc.gov/art/ART2009/section5.htm. Accessed 21 June 2012.

Chandra, A., & Stephen, E. H. (2010). Infertility service use among U.S. women: 1995 and 2002. *Fertility and Sterility, 93*(3), 725–736.

Chandra, A., Martinez, G. M., Mosher, W. D., Abma, J. C. & Jones, J. (2005). Fertility, family planning, and reproductive health of U.S. women: Data from the 2002 National Survey of Family Growth. *Vital Health Statistics, 23*(25), 1–160. Atlanta: National Center for Health Statistics. Available at: http://www.cdc.gov/nchs/data/series/sr_23/sr23_025.pdf. Accessed 21 June 2012.

Duwe, K. N., Reefhuis, J., Honein, M. A., Schieve, L. A., & Rasmussen, S. A. (2010). Epidemiology of fertility treatment use among U.S. women with liveborn infants, 1997–2004. *Journal of Women's Health, 19*(3), 407–416.

Ferraretti, A. P., Goossens, V., de Mouzon, J., Bhattacharya, S., Castilla, J. A., Korsak, V., Kupka, M., Nygren, K. G., Nyboe Andersen, A., & The European IVF-monitoring (EIM) Consortium. (2012). Assisted reproductive technology in Europe, 2008: Results generated from European registers by ESHRE. *Human Reproduction, 27*(9), 2571–2584.

Fritz, M. A., & Speroff, L. (2011). *Clinical gynecologic endocrinology and infertility* (8th ed.). Philadelphia: Lippincott Williams & Wilkins.

Gleicher, N., Weghofer, A., & Barad, D. (2006). A formal comparison of the practice of assisted reproductive technologies between Europe and the USA. *Human Reproduction, 21*(8), 1945–1950.

Hansen, M., Bower, C., Milne, E., de Klerk, N., & Kurinczuk, J. J. (2005). Assisted reproductive technologies and the risk of birth defects – A systematic review. *Human Reproduction, 20*(2), 328–338.

Hollos, M., Larsen, U., Obono, O., & Whitehouse, B. (2009). The problem of infertility in high fertility populations: Meanings, consequences and coping mechanisms in two Nigerian communities. *Social Science and Medicine, 68*(11), 2061–2068.

Inhorn, M. C. (2003). *Local babies, global science: Gender, religion, and in-vitro fertilization in Egypt*. New York: Routledge.

Inhorn, M., & van Balen, F. (Eds.). (2002). *Infertility around the globe: New thinking on childlessness, gender and reproductive technologies*. Berkeley: University of California Press.

Inhorn, M. C., Ceballo, R., & Nachtigall, R. (2009). Marginalized, invisible, and unwanted: American minority struggles with infertility and assisted conception. In L. Culley, N. Hudson, & F. Van Rooij (Eds.), *Marginalized reproduction: Ethnicity, infertility and reproductive technologies* (pp. 181–197). London: Earthscan.

Jones, H. W., Cohen, J., Cooke, I., Kempers, R., Brinsden, P., & Saunders, D. (2011). International federation of fertility societies surveillance 2010. *Fertility and Sterility, 95*(2), 491.

Kulczycki, A. (2008). Birth certificates. In S. E. Boslaugh (Ed.), *Encyclopedia of epidemiology* (pp. 96–97). Thousand Oaks: Sage.

Kurinczuk, J. J., & Hockley, C. (2010). *Fertility treatment in 2006 – A statistical analysis*. London: Human Fertilisation and Embryology Authority, HFEA. Available at: http://www.hfea.gov.uk/docs/Fertility-treatments-2006.pdf. Accessed 20 July 2012.

Lu, E., Barfield, W. D., Wilber, N., Diop, H., Manning, S. E., & Fogerty, S. (2008). Surveillance of births conceived with various infertility therapies in Massachusetts, January–March 2005. *Public Health Reports, 123*(2), 173–177.

Macaluso, M., Wright-Schnapp, T. J., Chandra, A., Johnson, R., Satterwhite, C. L., Pulver, A., Berman, S. M., Wang, R. Y., Farr, S. L., & Pollack, L. A. (2010). A public health focus on infertility prevention, detection, and management. *Fertility and Sterility, 93*(1), 16.e1–10.

Marketdata Enterprises. (2009). *U.S. Fertility clinics & infertility services: An industry analysis*. Tampa: Marketdata Enterprises, Inc.

Martin, J. A., Hamilton, B. E., Ventura, S. J., Michelle, J. K., Osterman, M. J. K., Kirmeyer, S., Mathews, T. J., & Wilson, E. C. (2011). Births: Final data for 2009. *National Vital Statistics Reports, 60*(1), 1–102. Hyattsville: National Center for Health Statistics.

Myers, E. R., McCrory, D. C., Mills, A. A., Price, T. M., Swamy, G. K., Tantibhedhyangkul, J., Wu, J. M., & Matchar, D. B. (2008). Effectiveness of assisted reproductive technology (ART). *Evidence Reports/Technology Assessments, 167*, 1–195 (AHRQ Publication No. 08-E012). Rockville: Agency for Healthcare Research and Quality.

Nachtigall, R. (2006). International disparities in access to infertility services. *Fertility and Sterility, 85*(4), 871–875.

National Campaign to Prevent Teen and Unplanned Pregnancy. (2011). *Counting it up: The public costs of teen childbearing*. Washington, DC: National Campaign to Prevent Teen and Unplanned Pregnancy. Available at: http://www.thenationalcampaign.org/costs/. Accessed 15 Apr 2012.

NCHS [National Center for Health Statistics]. (2012). *Key statistics from the National Survey of Family Growth*. Special tabulations by NCHS. Available at: http://www.cdc.gov/nchs/nsfg/abc_list_i.htm#infertility. Accessed 9 July 2012.

Nuojua-Huttunen, S., Gissler, M., Martikainen, H., & Tuomivaara, L. (1999). Obstetric and perinatal outcome of pregnancies after intrauterine insemination. *Human Reproduction, 14*(8), 2110–2115.

Nyboe Andersen, A., Goosens, V., Bhattacharya, S., Ferraretti, A. P., Kupka, M. S., de Mouzon, J., Nygren, K. G., & The European IVF-monitoring (EIM) Consortium, for the European Society of Human Reproduction and Embryology (ESHRE). (2009). Assisted reproductive technology and intrauterine inseminations in Europe, 2005: Results generated from European registers by ESHRE. *Human Reproduction, 24*(6), 1267–1287.

Nygren, K. G., Nyboe Andersen, A., Felberbaum, R., Gianoroli, L., de Mouzon, J., & Members of ESHRE's European IVF-monitoring (EIM). (2006). On the benefit of assisted reproduction techniques, a comparison of the USA and Europe. *Human Reproduction, 21*(8), 2194.

Osterman, M. J. K., Martin, J. A., Mathews, T. J., & Hamilton, B. E. (2011) Expanded data from the new birth certificate, 2008. *National Vital Statistics Reports, 59*(7), 1–28. Hyattsville: National Center for Health Statistics. Available at: http://www.cdc.gov/nchs/data/nvsr/nvsr59/nvsr59_07.pdf. Accessed 9 July 2012.

Pandian, Z., Bhattacharya, S., Ozturk, O., Serour, G., & Templeton, A. (2009). Number of embryos for transfer following in-vitro fertilization or intra-cytoplasmic sperm injection. *Cochrane Database of Systematic Reviews, 2*, CD003416.

Romundstad, L. B., Romundstad, P. R., Sunde, A., von During, V., Skjaerven, R., & Vatten, L. J. (2006). Increased risk of placenta previa in pregnancies following IVF/ICSI; A comparison of ART and non-ART pregnancies in the same mother. *Human Reproduction, 21*(9), 2353–2358.

Romundstad, L. B., Romundstad, P. R., Sunde, A., von During, V., Skjaerven, R., Gunnell, D., & Vatten, L. J. (2008). Effects of technology or maternal factors on perinatal outcome after assisted fertilization: A population-based cohort study. *Lancet, 372*(9640), 737–743.

Schieve, L. A., Rosenberg, D., Handler, A., Rankin, K., & Reynolds, M. A. (2006). Validity of self-reported use of assisted reproductive technology treatment among women participating in the pregnancy risk assessment monitoring system in five states, 2000. *Maternal and Child Health Journal, 10*(5), 427–431.

Schieve, L. A., Cohen, B., Nannini, A., et al. (2007). A population-based study of maternal and perinatal outcomes associated with assisted reproductive technology in Massachusetts. *Maternal and Child Health Journal, 11*(6), 517–525.

Schieve, L. A., Devine, O., Boyle, C. A., Petrini, J. R., & Warner, L. (2009). Estimation of the contribution of non-assisted reproductive technology ovulation stimulation fertility treatments to US singleton and multiple births. *American Journal of Epidemiology, 170*(11), 1396–1407.

Shanley, M. L., & Asch, A. (2009). Involuntary childlessness, reproductive technology, and social justice: The medical mask on social illness. *Signs, 34*(4), 851–874.

Sutcliffe, A. G., & Ludwig, M. (2007). Outcome of assisted reproduction. *Lancet, 370*(9584), 351–359.

Templeton, A., & Morris, J. K. (1998). Reducing the risk of multiple births by transfer of two embryos after in vitro fertilization. *The New England Journal of Medicine, 339*(9), 573–577.

Texas Department of State Health Services. (2012). *Texas Department of State Health Services, Women, Infants and Children Program (WIC)*. Available at: http://www.dshs.state.tx.us/wichd/. Accessed 15 June 2012.

Wang, J. X., Norman, R. J., & Kristiansson, P. (2002). The effect of various infertility treatments on the risk of preterm birth. *Human Reproduction, 17*(4), 945–949.

Wellons, M. F., Lewis, C. E., Schwartz, S. M., Gunderson, E. P., Schreiner, P. J., Sternfeld, B., Richman, J., Sites, C. K., & Siscovik, D. S. (2008). Racial differences in self-reported infertility and risk factors for infertility in a cohort of black and white women-The CARDIA Women's Study. *Fertility and Sterility, 90*(5), 1640–1648.

Wilcox, L. S., Kiely, J. L., Melvin, C. L., & Martin, M. C. (1996). Assisted reproductive technologies: estimates of their contribution to multiple births and newborn hospital days in the United States. *Fertility and Sterility, 65*(2), 361–366.

Part II
Advancing Policy

Chapter 7
The Evolution of Consensus on Population and Development: Prospects for Resurgent Policy and Program Action

Andrew B. Kantner

7.1 Introduction

The world's total population increased from 2.5 billion in 1950 to 7.0 billion in 2011. This nearly three-fold increase constitutes the most rapid gain in human numbers in recorded history. Much of this increase has been concentrated in the world's poorer regions. Between 1950 and 2011, the total population of the developed world rose from 0.8 to 1.2 billion while developing countries grew from 1.7 to 5.8 billion over the same period (United Nations 2010a).

Population growth rates rose substantially in many less developed countries as fertility remained high (or only gradually declined) while mortality rates, principally among infants and children, began reductions that were to accelerate over coming decades. The average annual rate of population growth in less developed countries peaked at 2.5 % between 1965 and 1970 with countries such as Brazil, China, Egypt, India, Indonesia, Nigeria, and Pakistan growing at rates between 2.2 and 2.6 % at this time (United Nations 2010a).

During the first decades following the Second World War there was a widely-held consensus that rapid gains in human numbers posed a serious impediment to prospects for development. Beginning in the late 1950s, more affluent countries began to explore the feasibility of establishing family planning programs in developing countries to reduce high rates of fertility. Sweden was an early pioneer in this effort along with several private American foundations; namely, the Ford and Rockefeller Foundations and the Population Council. In the 1960s, these early exploratory efforts gave way to far larger bilateral and multilateral efforts to promote family planning services. Over the 50 year period that followed, it can be reasonably argued that the three most successful development initiatives were gains

A.B. Kantner, Ph.D. (✉)
Independent Consultant
e-mail: abkantner@gmail.com

A. Kulczycki (ed.), *Critical Issues in Reproductive Health*, The Springer Series on Demographic Methods and Population Analysis 33, DOI 10.1007/978-94-007-6722-5_7, © Springer Science+Business Media Dordrecht 2014

in agricultural productivity and food consumption associated with the introduction of Green Revolution technologies; enhanced child survival stemming from declines in the number of high risk births, improvements in nutrition, and the prevention and treatment of childhood diseases; and the reduction of high fertility through the widespread adoption and use of modern family planning methods.

Between 1960–1965 and 2005–2010, population growth rates fell substantially as fertility rates responded to the growing use of modern contraception and gradual gains in the age at marriage and first birth. Over this period, the average population growth rate in the world's less developed countries fell from 2.3 % per annum to 1.5 %. However, these reductions were not achieved in all regions. In the world's least developed countries (primarily in Eastern, Central, and Western Africa), the population growth rate was still 2.3 % as of 2005–2010, a figure little changed from 1960 to 1965 (United Nations 2010a). Many countries in these regions are growing by at least 2.5 % per year (or doubling times of 28 years or more when rates are held constant) and have made little progress in reducing fertility rates that are often as high as 6–8 births per woman.

Owing partly to falls in population growth in the world's most populous developing countries since 1960–1965, population dynamics (the size, growth, and distribution of population) now tend to be accorded less importance as factors influencing development outcomes. At best, population is now viewed by many development economists as a secondary factor influencing prospects for economic growth. However, while population growth rates have slowed substantially in recent decades, it should be noted that they have not fallen as rapidly as implied by reductions in fertility owing to considerable success in reducing infant and child mortality. Population momentum stemming from the young age distributions of most developing countries has also propelled population totals beyond what one might anticipate from the fertility declines that have typified most developing countries.[1]

Attention to demographic issues in the developing world has also waned over the past two decades. Concerns surrounding rapid population growth, high fertility, and the strengthening of family planning programs were deemphasized in favor of sexual and reproductive health (SRH) services, women's empowerment, and reproductive and human rights. The *1994 International Conference on Population and Development (ICPD)* held in Cairo, Egypt, and the *1995 Fourth Conference on Women* in Beijing were the seminal events that signaled this change in focus. The Cairo paradigm affirmed the ability of women to freely choose the number and spacing of their children and (where legal) whether to carry their pregnancies to term. It promotes efforts to strengthen the availability, accessibility, and quality of SRH services (including family planning), but within a larger human rights framework.

---

[1] A case in point is India where the 2011 Population Census recently reported that the country's total population rose from 1.020 billion in 2001 to 1.210 billion in 2011 (Government of India 2011). The 2001–2011 annual intercensal population growth rate of 1.7 % (while lower than in previous decades) will, if unaltered, double India's population in approximately 40 years. The enormity of this projected increase is difficult to ignore.

The SRH and human rights sensibilities that guide the ICPD Plan of Action (PoA) have not gone unchallenged despite their affirmation by the UN's member states at Cairo (United Nations 1995). Most notably, there has been a growing effort in recent decades to limit women's right to an abortion. The "pro-life movement" in the United States and elsewhere received political support from a resurgent conservative politics that dominated the United States during much of the first decade of the twenty-first century. Pro-life advocates often embraced a broad definition of abortion that views modern family planning methods as little more than additional forms of pregnancy termination. The growing cultural and political divides between pro-choice and pro-life advocates have greatly polarized what remains of the population field and has undermined the bi-partisan political support for domestic and international family planning programs that typified much of the post-war period.

It is unclear whether a broad international consensus currently exists on population and development. Some observers argue that population dynamics still matter and are important factors influencing educational attainment, health outcomes, food availability, prospects for employment and income growth, the depletion of natural resources, and the potential for civil disorder. Others now maintain that demographic conditions have lost their saliency since fertility rates have fallen substantially throughout much of the developing world (outside sub-Saharan Africa) over the past half century. Still others believe that population was decoupled from development at Cairo (Cleland 1996). They maintain that the ICPD largely succeeded in casting women's decisions pertaining to the number and spacing of their children as immaterial to societal as opposed to individual well-being.

The attention currently given to population dynamics as factors influencing development outcomes can be seen in the effort mounted by the United Nations to craft Millennium Development Goals (MDGs) for the twenty-first century. The original MDGs adopted by the United Nations in 2000 did not include any objectives directly pertaining to population growth, fertility reduction, and universal access to family planning and other SRH services. Only later was the importance of family planning and other SRH elements acknowledged to be important in reducing maternal mortality. MDG 5 that calls for a 75 % reduction in maternal mortality by 2015 eventually incorporated a sub-objective for achieving universal access to SRH services. However, this somewhat belated achievement, while of note as a bureaucratic triumph, has not coincided with significantly greater global funding support for family planning and other SRH services.

It has been 20 years since the 1994 ICPD dramatically reshaped thinking on population and development and altered the post-war landscape for international population assistance. But how well has this new paradigm fared? Have women's health outcomes demonstrably improved since ICPD? Has the broader SRH paradigm agreed to at Cairo been successfully incorporated in service delivery programs? To what extent has the HIV/AIDS epidemic, only faintly glimpsed in 1994, influenced the provision of SRH services. And looking forward, what are the prospects for more effectively addressing women's health needs in future years?

7.2 The Shifting Post-War Consensus on Population and Development

Unprecedented post-war population growth rates led to growing calls to reduce high fertility rates as a means of accelerating the pace of social and economic advance in less developed countries. However, there was little agreement on how to do this. The debate tended to divide between those who argued that small family norms, lower fertility preferences, and the demand for contraception had to be generated before family planning programs could become effective in reducing fertility rates. Only by increasing educational attainment, improving child survival and health conditions, and raising incomes and labor force participation would it be possible to convince families to have fewer children. This demand-side approach, as it became known, essentially maintained that development was the best contraceptive. Many also argued that family planning programs, if effectively managed, could rapidly reduce high rates of fertility, improve women's health, and make important contributions to improving living standards. This supply-side position saw the establishment of family planning services as a pressing priority for foreign assistance.

The 1974 World Conference on Population in Bucharest, Romania, while not bereft of rancorous debate, essentially came to a meeting-of-the-ways between these opposite positions. Development was still acknowledged to be an important precursor for transitioning to low regimes of fertility and mortality, but it was also agreed that development could be achieved more rapidly in settings that had attained lower fertility rates. The phrase "whatever your cause, it's a lost cause without contraception" became a commonly heard mantra at Bucharest.[2]

The 1970s and 1980s saw a major commitment of new resources for family planning programs. In terms of total resources expended for family planning services, the effort was led by the United States, but many European countries (e.g., Norway, Sweden, the Netherlands, and the United Kingdom) and Japan were also major contributors. The United Nations Fund for Population Activities (UNFPA), later renamed the United Nations Population Fund, was founded in 1969 and became the principal multilateral agency providing support for family planning.

Taiwan, South Korea, and Hong Kong were among the initial family planning success stories during the 1960s. These programs received support from international donors (principally private foundations based in the US) and gave encouragement to the view that fertility rates could fall rapidly when women had ready access to modern forms of contraception and could freely determine the number and

---

[2]The Bucharest Conference was also notable for being the venue at which John D. Rockefeller III, an early proponent and funder of international family planning programs, deserted the ranks of the neo-Malthusians. He became convinced by the arguments of a Rockefeller Foundation employee that family planning programs, as constituted at the time, were not serving the best interests of women. This was the first major crack in the ranks of neo-Malthusians who maintained that controlling rapid population growth in less developed countries was an imperative for achieving more rapid and sustainable development. A more extensive review of this historical record can be found in Kantner and Kantner (2009).

spacing of their children. In the 1970s and 1980s, family planning programs achieved considerable success in such countries as Bangladesh, Brazil, Egypt, Indonesia, and Thailand. And the two most populous countries in the world, China and India, made considerable headway in lowering fertility rates, at times through coercive measures that did much harm to the cause of international family planning.

The consensus that gradually emerged on population and development following the Bucharest Population Conference in 1974 did not survive for more than a decade. With the coming of the Reagan Administration in 1980, a concerted effort was made to deny the importance of population growth and begin de-funding international population programs. A new form of economic revisionism, which maintained that larger populations produced more technical innovation, faster economic growth, and greater poverty alleviation, gained prominence during this time. In addition, pro-life advocacy became more vocal and better funded during the Reagan years. At the 1984 Mexico City Conference on Population, the official US position was that population growth had been overstated as the root cause of poverty in less developed countries and that unfettered market mechanisms rather than investments in family planning offered the best hope for development.

The United States Government also announced its Mexico City Policy at this time (also known as the Global Gag Rule) which put severe restrictions on the ability of family planning programs receiving US assistance to offer information on pregnancy termination or any form of safe abortion service.[3] Funding for international family planning programs was also curtailed during the Reagan years, a setback that caused lasting damage to the momentum that family planning programs had attained in many developing countries by the mid-eighties, especially in countries such as Bangladesh, Egypt, Indonesia, and Kenya that had been receiving significant assistance from the United States Government.

While contraceptive prevalence rates were rising and fertility rates falling by the mid-1980s in many less developed countries, there was also growing concern that the quality of family planning services often fell short in meeting the reproductive health needs of many women. Concerns initially focused on problems associated with contraceptive side-effects and high rates of discontinuation for modern methods, especially reversible hormonal methods. There were also calls to make family planning service delivery more responsive to women's health needs and institute more client-centered approaches in providing care. Numerous facility-based guidelines for improving client-provider relations and service quality (e.g., COPE, REDI, and GATHER) were developed with support from USAID and became effective operational tools in many facilities (EngenderHealth 2010).

During the 1980s, serious efforts were also undertaken to eliminate demographic and contraceptive acceptance and user targets as management tools for measuring

---

[3]The Mexico City Policy was initially in force from 1984 until 1993, then rescinded during the Clinton years, reinstituted during the second Bush Administration, and then canceled yet again by President Barack Obama. Given the wide pendulum swings in American politics that seem to typify recent decades, it would not be safe to assume that the Mexico City Policy has been permanently banished from the stage.

program performance. Targets were increasingly seen as implicitly coercive and a threat to women's ability to freely make reproductive choices. In 1998, the United States Congress passed the Tiahrt Amendment that required family planning programs supported through organizations funded by the United States Government to ensure voluntarism, informed consent, and the abolition of incentive payments and performance targets.[4]

The growing attention given to improving the quality of family planning programs during the 1980s proved to be an important precursor to the crafting of a more holistic conception of women's reproductive health at the 1994 ICPD. Women's health advocates successfully adopted a SRH agenda that emphasized the provision of a broadened array of services including antenatal, delivery, and postnatal care; the diagnosis and treatment of sexually transmitted infections; HIV/AIDS prevention and care/support; safe abortion services (where legal) and post-abortion care; emergency obstetric care; specialized information and clinical services for adolescents, and the diagnosis and treatment of reproductive cancers in women. Family planning was consigned to being just one element in a broad constellation of interventions needed to ensure improved health outcomes for women.

The SRH agenda embraced at the 1994 ICPD, combined with the emphasis given to women's human rights at the *1995 Beijing Fourth World Conference on Women*, came together to form a new sexual and reproductive health and rights (SRHR) paradigm for addressing women's health issues and designing programs of assistance. Women's empowerment was increasingly viewed as a necessary precondition for achieving improvements in reproductive health and welfare, despite evidence that rapid fertility declines could occur without the transformations in gender power relations and women's status that were often seen as necessary preconditions for change. Bangladesh has often been cited as a case in point (Cleland et al. 2004). During the 1980s and 1990s, Bangladeshi women rapidly adopted modern contraception and achieved their stated preferences for smaller families without first making significant gains in education, economic participation, and social status.

The extent to which SRHR now constitutes a new international consensus can be debated. Certainly many members of the pro-life movement would hotly contest this supposition. But there is little question that the Plan of Action (PoA) agreed to at Cairo laid the ground-work for what became the SRHR agenda that now guides much international donor assistance on women's health. However, there continue to be concerns that the SRHR approach, with its broadly defined objectives pertaining to gender, empowerment, and human rights may have diluted the more focused emphasis given to family planning and maternal and child health (MCH) services that received priority attention in the pre-Cairo era. This is a challenging supposition to either defend or reject with the evidence at hand, but it warrants a closer examination.

---

[4]Even though target systems were implemented with varying levels of efficiency and zeal in many countries and at times may have been unfairly castigated as a source of coercion and human rights abuse, they were increasingly falling out of favor in many less developed countries by the early 1990s.

7.3   Recent Levels and Trends in Fertility

Fertility has continued to fall throughout much of the developing world since the population field was recast by the ICPD in 1994. However, the pace of fertility decline has slowed over the past 20 years. Between 1970 and 1990, fertility rates in less developed countries fell from 5.2 births per woman to 3.9 (an annual decline of .064 births), while from 1990 to 2010, fertility fell from 3.4 births to 2.7 (a decline of .035 births per annum) (United Nations 2010a).

It is of course not surprising that the rate of fertility decline should slow as lower fertility levels are attained and women become more successful in achieving their fertility goals. However, there is evidence that fertility declines have faltered over the past 20 years in the least developed countries of the world that often continue to have high fertility – countries largely concentrated in the regions of sub-Saharan Africa (other than Southern Africa) and South Asia. It is not uncommon to find fertility rates ranging from 6 and 8 births per woman in such countries as Burkino Faso, Chad, Mali, and Niger and exceptionally low levels of family planning use. Recent results from Demographic and Health Surveys (DHS) show that adolescent fertility rates have actually risen in some sub-Saharan countries since 2000 (e.g., in Benin, Liberia, Mozambique, and Tanzania), which suggests that younger women in these and other sub-Saharan African countries are increasingly underserved by existing SRH services (Demographic and Health Surveys 2010).

There is growing concern that some developing countries in which fertility declines have been achieved may be stalling. Bongaarts has examined this issue extensively using DHS data. His most recent analysis of 40 developing countries found that the pace of fertility decline has stalled in half of the sub-Saharan African countries examined, and had not begun at all (CPR < 10 %) in Chad, Guinea, and Mali (Bongaarts 2008). Only one Asian country (Turkey) and one country in Latin America (Guatemala) had stalled. Recent evidence suggests that Bangladesh may have joined Tanzania in resuming its fertility transition after initially appearing to stall between two successive DHS surveys during the 1990s. It is not clear why much of sub-Saharan Africa has paused in its transition to lower fertility, but Bongaarts suggests that falling rates of economic growth and living standards, the HIV/AIDS epidemic, and declining support for family planning programs may be part of the story.

An analysis of trends in unwanted births using DHS information shows that many women are still having more children than they would like to have. This is even the case in countries that have experienced sizeable falls in fertility rates. The highest percentage of births that were reported as unwanted occurred in Bolivia and Swaziland (45 %), Haiti (38 %), Nepal and Peru (35 %), and Bangladesh, Honduras and India (all at 30 %) (Westoff 2010:19–20). Considerable potential remains for fertility to decline further in these and other developing countries once women are better able to determine the number and timing of their offspring.

There is a growing divide between countries that are transitioning to lower fertility and those that continue to have high fertility. Many countries with high fertility are continuing to face challenges in educating and feeding their populations, providing adequate water/sanitation facilities and housing, and generating ample economic opportunity. These pressures tend to moderate in countries that have achieved lower levels of fertility. Dependency ratios (typically defined as the population aged 0–14 and 65+ in relation to the economically active population between the ages of 15–64) have fallen substantially in countries with rapid declines in fertility. As the relative size of the economically active population increases, a favorable population balance, commonly referred to as the demographic dividend, is created that can help accelerate economic growth over several decades. However, once this dividend is used up, countries can enter periods of high old age dependency and slower economic growth. China, which currently has the world's most rapidly growing large economy, will enter the ranks of countries with high elderly dependency by 2030.[5]

7.4   The Implementation of Family Planning and Other Reproductive Health Services

7.4.1   Family Planning

Gains in the use of contraception have largely accounted for the declines in fertility recorded since 1960 in less developed countries. According to figures compiled by the United Nations, the percentage of currently married women aged 15–49 using any contraceptive method reached 61.2 % by 2009 in the developing world (United Nations 2010b).[6] However, in the world's least developed countries, all method prevalence was still only 31.4 % in 2009. Most least developed countries continue to have prevalence rates below 20 % and typically report little change in levels of use. Bangladesh, Nepal and Zambia were the only least developed countries with prevalence rates well above the group average.

The rate at which women in developing countries have been adopting contraception has slowed over the past 15–20 years. Clearly, some diminution in the rate at which prevalence rises can be expected in countries that have attained moderate to

---

[5]Demographic factors are contributing, but not necessarily decisive factors in securing economic growth. Long-term shifts in age-related dependency burdens have little to say about what caused the Asian economic crisis in 1997–1998, the global great recession in 2008–2009, or arguably even the current commodity price inflation for food, energy, and precious metals, etc. Good economic policy, effective governance, the efficiency of capital markets, and educational and human resource capacities may matter even more – factors that tend to be overlooked in writings on the demographic dividend.

[6]An analysis of global family planning programs in 2008 concluded that the use of contraception avoided 188 million unintended pregnancies, 1.2 million neonatal deaths among infants, and 230,000 maternal deaths (with approximately one-third of these averted maternal deaths resulting from reduced reliance on unsafe abortion) (Singh et al. 2009).

high levels of use (e.g., among countries in Eastern and Southeastern Asia and much of Latin America), but there is also evidence that women in low prevalence countries are becoming less inclined to adopt and use contraception. For example, among developing countries with fertility rates greater than 4.0, Burundi, the Central African Republic, Chad, Cote d'Ivoire, the Democratic Republic of the Congo, Ghana, Ivory Coast, Mozambique, Niger, Nigeria, Sudan, and Togo reported reductions in the rate at which contraceptive use increased when contrasting the periods from 1980 to 1995 with 1995–2010 (United Nations 2010b). Some sub-Saharan African countries continue to have contraceptive prevalence rates below 10 %; namely, Angola, Burundi, Chad, Guinea, Mali, Mauritania, Sierra Leone, and Sudan (United Nations 2010b).

Family planning programs in developing countries generally provide better service quality than a generation earlier. However, they also tend to emphasize a limited range of methods, have high contraceptive discontinuation rates, and weak counseling and follow-up services. Some country programs are heavily reliant on a limited range of methods, (e.g., oral contraceptives in Bangladesh, injectables in Indonesia and IUDs in Egypt and Jordan). Countries such as India and Nepal still rely on female sterilization and continue to have weak provision of reversible methods more suitable for women wishing to space births.

The extent to which women are able to access family planning services is often assessed by levels and trends in unmet need. This concept is usually defined as the percentage of women who are not using any method of contraception and say they want to delay their next birth or want to stop childbearing completely. Non-users who want to delay their next birth are said to have an unmet need for spacing methods while non-users who want no additional children are said to have limiting need. While the concept of unmet need has not gone unchallenged by women's health advocates (e.g., see Dixon-Mueller and Germain 1992), it has tended to serve as a common-ground concept for family planners and SRHR advocates promoting broader transformative agendas.

Recent estimates for developing countries indicate that global unmet need for family planning among currently married women aged 15–49 in the developing world has fallen slightly from 13.6 % in 1990 to 11.4 % by 2009 (United Nations 2010b). The world's least developed countries report the highest unmet need as of 2009 (24.2 %) compared to all developing countries (9.3 %). Unmet need has not fallen appreciably in the world's poorest countries, declining from 25.2 % in 1990 to just 24.2 % in 2009. Women in the sub-regions of Eastern Africa (27.6 %), Central Africa (22.6 %) and Western Africa (24.2 %) have the highest unmet need in the world.

7.4.2 Other Reproductive Health Services

The SRH framework adopted at Cairo argued for a more holistic approach to the provision of women's health services. While family planning remained an important element, program priorities could no longer be strictly established around the goal of reducing fertility through contraceptive use. Greater attention needed to be given to other SRH services, some of which had been long neglected.

The strengthening of maternal health services (antenatal, delivery, post-natal and emergency obstetric care) came to be seen as priorities for reducing high maternal mortality rates in many less developed countries. High levels of morbidity and mortality stemming from unsafe abortions and the lack of comprehensive post-abortion care also had not been receiving adequate attention. The adverse health consequences of female circumcision and morbidities associated with fistula had long remained underground as women's health issues. Reproductive cancers in women (primarily breast, cervical, and ovarian) still go largely undiagnosed and treated in many less developed countries, especially among poorer women.

The diagnosis and treatment of sexually transmitted diseases (STDs) has remained an underdeveloped service in many settings. And the most serious STD the world has ever encountered, HIV/AIDS, grew rapidly in sub-Saharan Africa, Eastern Europe, and parts of Asia and the Caribbean over the past three decades. Funding for the prevention of HIV and treatment of AIDS came to dominate SRH budgets in less developed countries (an eventuality not foreseen at Cairo), which contributed to the marginalization of funding support for family planning and other SRH services. Violence against women, especially domestic violence and the welfare of women and girls in conflict settings are also priority concerns for the human rights framework that informs the SRHR approach.

The full SRHR agenda has become a very full plate that exceeds the ability of most countries to fully address and fund. In the post-Cairo years, many countries initiated pilot projects (often donor funded) that attempted to introduce a more complete constellation of services and integrate these initiatives with pre-existing family planning or primary health care. Considerable efforts were also made to field-test various approaches for integrating SRH program elements with HIV/AIDS prevention and treatment services. While outcomes from program research trials often produced beneficial outcomes for a limited number of clients, clinic settings, and local communities, they usually did not lead to extensive replication or scale-up. Funding constraints and inadequate health system capacity (stemming from human resource, managerial, and technical limitations) made many scale-up recommendations naive and difficult to implement.

Three SRH issues highlighted by the 1994 ICPD PoA in need of priority attention were maternal mortality, safe abortion (where legal) and post-abortion care, and the prevention and treatment of HIV/AIDS. As noted previously, reducing maternal mortality by 75 % between 1990 and 2015 was established as MDG 5 and has been assigned higher priority than family planning, unsafe abortion, and other SRH needs in the MDG framework. These women's health issues have not been given their own MDG, but instead are seen as supportive of MDG 5. HIV/AIDS has also been assigned MDG 6 which calls for halting and reversing the spread of HIV and achieving universal access to HIV/AIDS treatment by 2010 "for all of those who need it" (UNDP 2011).

7.4.3 *Maternal Mortality*

While progress has been made in reducing levels of maternal mortality over the past two decades, it is unlikely that most developing countries will achieve a 75 % reduction in maternal mortality by 2015. Many countries still lack valid estimates of levels and trends in maternal mortality. According to estimates released by WHO (WHO et al. 2010), there has been a 34 % fall in the maternal mortality ratio (MMR) between 1990 and 2008 (from 400 to 260 maternal deaths per 100,000 live births).[7] This analysis concluded that 355,000 maternal deaths occurred in developing countries and just 3,200 in developed countries in 2008. Sub-Saharan Africa accounted for 57 % of all maternal deaths in the world (204,000), 9.0 % of which were due to HIV/AIDS-related causes. For MDG 5 to be attained by 2015, countries will need to achieve an annual decline of 5.5 % in the number of maternal deaths from 1990 to 2015, yet the annual percentage decline in MMR over the 1990–2008 period was only 2.3 %, less than half of the required level (WHO et al. 2010).

A second study conducted by researchers at the University of Washington employing various indirect methods and interpolation procedures in analyzing census, survey, vital statistics registration, and verbal autopsy data from 181 countries concluded that the MMR had fallen by 21.5 % between 1990 and 2008 (from 320 to 251 maternal deaths per 100,000 live births) (Hogan et al. 2010). The study also noted that 50 % of all maternal deaths occur in just six countries; namely, India, Nigeria, Pakistan, Afghanistan, Ethiopia, and the Democratic Republic of the Congo. The WHO and University of Washington MMR estimates for 2008 are remarkably similar. However, the evidence-base for both sets of estimates is not reassuring given the extent to which modeling assumptions applied to data of unknown quality have been relied upon to derive MMR estimates for many countries.

Countries with the most rapid declines in maternal mortality also tend to be those that report the most pronounced reductions in fertility. This is not unanticipated since women who are more successful in reducing high risk pregnancies (pregnancies that are spaced too closely together, take place at too young an age, or occur among older high parity women) are less likely to experience delivery complications. The availability and use of antenatal services for pregnant women has also improved in many less developed countries since 1990. Service providers are therefore better able to identify problem pregnancies and treat anemia and hypertension (pre-eclampsia and eclampsia). However, the majority of women in less developed countries still deliver at home and often lack ready access to safe delivery services and emergency obstetric care. In fact, in some sub-Saharan countries such as Tanzania there is evidence that the percentage of mothers delivering in clinic facilities has actually fallen in recent years (Riley 2008:96). Post-natal and post-abortion care services also tend to be inadequate and poorly attended in many countries with elevated maternal mortality.

---

[7]The range of uncertainty surrounding the 2008 MMR estimate falls between 200 and 370 maternal deaths per 100,000 live births (and between 220 and 410 in developing countries) which underscores the degree of imprecision underlying global MMR estimates.

7.4.4 *Abortion*

Unsafe abortions and the lack of post-abortion care are also major factors contributing to high levels of maternal mortality in many less developed countries. Obtaining valid estimates of spontaneous and induced abortions is a challenge in most settings.[8] The evidence available suggests that little change has occurred in the frequency and safety of the procedure in recent years. The number of induced abortions reportedly fell from 46 to 42 million between 1995 and 2003, which constitutes a decline in the induced abortion rate from 35 per 1000 women aged 15–44 in 1995 to 29 per 1000 in 2003 (Sedgh et al. 2007). Much of this decline occurred in Russia and other developed nations in Eastern Europe (where women increasingly substituted modern contraception for abortion) rather than in less developed countries with the highest levels of unsafe abortion.

Moreover, the number of unsafe abortions has actually increased slightly from 19.9 million in 1995 and 21.6 million in 2008 (Shah and Ahman 2010: 90–101). The WHO attributes much of this gain to the increase in the number of women of reproductive age over the period. The unsafe abortion rate actually fell from 15 unsafe abortions per 1,000 women aged 15–44 in 1995 to 14 in 2008. Unsafe abortions tend to be concentrated in less developed countries with poor health system capacity, underdeveloped post abortion care (PAC) services, and legal restrictions on the provision of safe abortion. Around 47,000 women were thought to have lost their lives to unsafe abortions in 2008. Most of these deaths could have been prevented if legal restrictions on providing safe abortions were removed, menstrual regulation and PAC made more widely available and accessible,[9] and unwanted pregnancies reduced through the greater use of contraception.

Soon after the 1994 ICPD, there was a major push to generate funding for PAC services. Pilot programs launched in such countries as Bangladesh, Bolivia, Kenya, Peru, Egypt, and Senegal found considerable demand for these services (Health Communication Partnership 2010:197–203). However, these early pilots were not widely replicated, with the result that PAC is still not a readily available service for most women in these countries. For example, one notable pilot program in

---

[8]Spontaneous abortions are essentially impossible to measure with any precision since the majority happen before women are even aware that they are pregnant. Induced abortions are often prone to underreporting, especially when abortions are illegal and performed surreptitiously. And the quality of abortion data is not clear in such countries as China and Vietnam where many legal abortions are performed.

[9]Menstrual regulation, which is provided in some countries as a back-up to contraception, is defined as the evacuation of the uterus for women up to 10 weeks since the start of their last menstrual cycle. Recent research from Bangladesh has shown that the provision of menstrual regulation services greatly reduces unsafe abortions occurring in the second and third trimesters of pregnancy and lessens demands on expensive post-abortion care. (Johnston et al. 2010:197–203).

Egypt was successful in improving the quality of PAC clinical practices, integrating PAC with pre-existing family planning services and enhancing client satisfaction (Nawar et al. 1997). But PAC services are still not widely available in Egypt. This has been an all-too-common result in many countries, and remains a major impediment to making more rapid gains in reducing maternal mortality.

7.4.5   HIV/AIDS

Efforts to prevent HIV transmission and treatment of AIDS patients has become the dominant global health initiative in terms of program commitment and resource allocation over the past 20 years. As of 2008, 33.4 million people were HIV positive, with most cases (22.4 million) occurring in sub-Saharan Africa (UNAIDS 2010). The rate at which new infections have been occurring has been gradually declining since 1996. In addition, antiretroviral treatments (ARVs) have risen substantially in recent years. They have improved survival times for people living with AIDS and reduced HIV transmission rates, especially if ARVs are started in the early stages of infection.[10] However, only one-third of all people with AIDS who are clinically indicated for care are currently receiving ARV treatment. Further, for every two people placed on ARV drugs, there are five newly infected people with HIV who will eventually require treatment. And new ARV treatment guidelines adopted by WHO in 2010 now recommend that ARV's be started sooner in the progression of the disease, which will entail having more people on treatment at any given time (WHO 2010). HIV/AIDS will likely be placing major demands on health systems and budgets for decades to come.

There has also been progress in making services that prevent HIV transmission from mothers to children (PMTCT) more widely accessible. By 2008, PMTCT services were available to 45 % of all pregnant women, although there were wide regional variations in PMTCT coverage levels (UNAIDS 2010). Potential programmatic linkages between PMTCT and SRH services have not been fully realized in many countries. The prevention of unintended pregnancies among women living with HIV should be an important component of efforts to limit mother to child transmission. Improved counseling on transmission risk factors and the protective benefits of condom use are other areas where there is clear overlap between HIV/AIDS and SRH services (WHO et al. 2010). However, family planning and other SRH interventions are conspicuously absent in many PMTCT service sites.

---

[10]Recent research findings indicate that HIV transmission can be reduced by 96 % if ARVs are started early in the onset of the disease. These encouraging results imply the widespread use of ARV's may be more effective in controlling the HIV pandemic than previously thought. See National Institute of Allergy and Infectious Diseases (NIAID 2011).

7.5   Prospects for Strengthening Family Planning and Other Sexual and Reproductive Health Services

Major gains have been made in reducing rapid population growth over the past 50 years. But the transition to low levels of fertility and mortality remains incomplete in some parts of the developing world. Much of sub-Saharan Africa continues to have exceptionally high fertility, and countries in other less developed regions, especially in South Asia, have only transitioned to moderately low fertility (TFR of between 3 and 4 births per woman) that may prove stubbornly resistant to reaching replacement levels. Birth dearth and population implosion theories of demographic change that have arisen to explain the historically low fertility rates of Europe and Eastern Asia do not apply to other regions of the world. It is generally the case that women in less developed countries are currently still having more children than they would prefer while women in developed countries are not having as many as they would like.

There is considerable evidence that the availability of SRH services and client outcomes is notably unequal in many developing countries. DHS findings show that less educated women residing in poorer households (often situated in more inaccessible urban slums or rural areas) are less likely to be using modern SRH services and experiencing better health outcomes. A review of family planning use by household wealth status found notable differences in the extent to which women from poorer circumstances were using contraception (USAID Health Policy Initiative 2007). However, there was considerable variation in the equity of contraceptive use within regions. In Asia, for example, Bangladesh, Indonesia, and Vietnam had more equitable patterns of family planning use, India and the Philippines were somewhat less equitable, while Cambodia, Nepal, and Pakistan appear to be significantly underserving their poorest women.

There is clearly considerable work ahead in ensuring that all women have access to the full-range of SRH services needed to improve women's health (and called for under MDG 5). But what are the future prospects for strengthening the accessibility, quality, and use of family planning and other SRH services? Can these services be given the priority they deserve in the rush to combat HIV/AIDS, TB, malaria, and a multitude of other infectious and chronic diseases? And what prospect is there for generating the global resources necessary to accelerate progress in meeting women's health needs?

7.5.1   The Status of Family Planning and Other SRHR Funding

Despite the commitment of new resources for women's health programs in recent decades, the more holistic SRHR paradigm that emanated from the 1994 ICPD and *1995 Beijing Conference on Women* has generally not received the attention and funding support to move much beyond local area pilots and models worthy of scale-up. Services for the diagnosis and treatment of sexually transmitted diseases, safe pregnancy termination and post-abortion care, emergency obstetric services, and reproductive surgical repair (e.g., for female circumcision and fistula treatment) remain poorly developed and underfunded in most less developed countries. While progress has been made in slowing the progression of the HIV/AIDS pandemic, it has come at considerable cost in terms of burdening underdeveloped health systems and compromising the flow of resources for other SRH services (including family planning).

While there have been substantial gains in funding for international population programs between 1995 and 2009, much of this increase resulted from the infusion of new funding for HIV/AIDS activities.[11] Funding for family planning has actually declined by roughly 30 % between 1995 and 2009 while funding for other reproductive health services (excluding HIV/AIDS) did not rise appreciably.[12]

In 2009 UNFPA revised the original cost estimates for achieving the objectives of the 1994 ICPD. These new funding requirements were much higher since they include new cost data for service delivery and commodities; greater outlays for HIV/AIDS prevention, care, and treatment; and reproductive surgical repair and cancer screenings/treatment that were not included in original ICPD cost estimates. Recent projections suggest that total population assistance (from both international and domestic resources) could be roughly $24 billion below required funding levels in 2010 (assuming that international donors contribute $10 billion and developing countries mobilize $31 billion in 2010). These levels of support are far from assured given the debt problems that are increasingly weighing on public-sector budgets in countries that have traditionally been the largest contributors to population activities.

Over the past decade, donor assistance from European nations has been increasingly allocated through sector-wide approaches that claim to provide countries with greater flexibility in setting program and budgetary priorities. Health program needs are also increasingly cast within larger poverty reduction strategies, often articulated in poverty reduction strategy papers that have been much favored by the

---

[11] It has become increasingly difficult to track funding allocations and expenditures for these four components since many donors no longer maintain budgets that correspond to these headings (e.g., family planning and reproductive health are often merged together). Donor expenditures that address poverty reduction strategies and health sector reform (increasing fashions among European donors and the World Bank) also do not track outlays in relation to original ICPD budget categories.

[12] In 2009, $10.4 billion was contributed by bilateral donors, multilateral organizations (mainly United Nations agencies such as UNFPA, UNAIDS, UNICEF, WHO and the World Bank), and private donors and foundations (United Nations 2011). Domestic resources generated in developing countries amounted to $28.9 billion in 2009 (this amount includes national government budgets, NGO resources and consumer expenditures for care). In 2009, this amount was nearly three times higher than the total international population assistance budget of $10.4 billion. The 1994 ICPD originally anticipated that developing countries should support two thirds of the total costs for implementing the Cairo Plan of Action. There has always been some concern about the validity of developing country expenditure data for population activities – results tend to be somewhat notional as they constitute best approximations that can be made from partial information.

World Bank, that juxtapose health spending against allocations for such sectors as education, food production, housing, transportation infrastructure, and employment generation. The sector-wide and poverty reduction strategy approaches have tended to marginalize family planning/reproductive health programs and budgets, with HIV/AIDS, malaria, TB, and child immunization services garnering ever-greater attention and financial resources.

The United States has been the largest provider of international population assistance over the past half-century. With the arrival of the Obama Administration, there were hopes that the newly announced Global Health Initiative (GHI) would bring new resolve and financial commitments to America's global health efforts, especially in sub-Saharan countries with high fertility and maternal mortality. During the first year of the GHI, impressive new leadership was recruited for the GHI and a greater emphasis on women's and girl's health was proposed, including additional funding for SRH programs. However, HIV/AIDS funding levels actually fell for the first time in the history of the pandemic, which prompted an outcry from the HIV/AIDS advocacy community.

Just as the GHI band wagon began to gather momentum, newly emergent funding uncertainties cast doubt on where this initiative will be heading. The American political pendulum swung yet again in 2010 and enabled conservative forces to propose major cuts in USAID's operational budgets, including sizable reductions in resources for family planning and other SRH program elements. This story remains to play out, but as in past decades, the United States may again prove to be an unsteady partner in providing international population assistance owing to the contentious nature of its domestic politics. This worry was partly confirmed when the GHI quietly disappeared from consideration in 2012.

Some major contributors to international population assistance in Europe (e.g., the Netherlands, and the United Kingdom) are facing large budget deficits stemming from the still-unfolding "great recession" and debt crisis of 2008–2009. Japan, another prominent contributor to bilateral and multilateral population assistance in past decades, faces major reconstruction challenges following the triple earthquake-tsunami-nuclear reactor disaster that struck in March, 2011. It will be understandable if Japan is forced to look inward to its own needs for a time. One awaits the arrival of China (and to a lesser extent India) as major contributors to international population programs. China is the one major world economy now positioned to make major contributions to the cause of family planning and SRH program support. China's international reputation would likely rise considerably if it were to redirect some of its US dollar surplus holdings (much of it American debt) to the cause of improving woman's health.

Some believe that private sources of assistance, if effectively mobilized and thoughtfully programmed, could fill some of the void in SRH funding created by budgetary and political confrontations in Washington. However, that promise has not been realized yet. With the possible exception of the Hewlett Foundation, most private foundation funding has been directed toward childhood immunization (most recently polio eradication), malaria and TB prevention and treatment, and HIV/AIDS. Fertility and family planning have somehow gotten lost in the mix, even though women with fewer high risk births have significantly better health outcomes and fitter children.

Nearly 20 years since the ICPD in Cairo, funding prospects for SRHR activities could be entering another difficult period. Many of the most important bilateral donors are facing economic challenges that could compromise their ability to sustain current foreign assistance budgets. And multilateral agencies may be facing growing resource constraints, compounded by having UNFPA committed to the implementation of overly diffused SRHR agendas within its country programs and the World Bank remaining essentially disinterested in family planning and SRH (other than HIV/AIDS).

The World Bank has never provided impressive funding support or intellectual leadership in family planning and reproductive health, despite the calls of Robert McNamara to take the issue of rapid population growth seriously during his presidential tenure from 1967 to 1983. Population issues were often treated as "externalities" by many economists working at the Bank during and after McNamara's time. The World Bank, along with other multilateral development banks and some bilateral donors, has instead given considerable attention to health system strengthening and reform over recent decades. Perhaps inadvertently, these efforts may have contributed to the marginalization of SRH service provision and funding.

7.5.2 Health Sector Reform and the Realignment of Health Priorities

In recent decades, the World Bank, along with other multilateral and bilateral donors, has made major efforts to alter the operational environment and capacity of health systems in less developed countries. These health sector reforms have varied in emphasis across countries, but they have generally included efforts to decentralize health services, more fully integrate essential service packages with primary health care, implement more cost recovery and fee-for service approaches to defray the cost of health services, encourage greater private sector participation in health care delivery, and strengthen human resource capacity.

The centralized command and control management structures that typified family planning programs until the early-1990s have been replaced in many countries by more decentralized systems in which local governments have greater control over the composition of health programs and budgets. Countries such as Bangladesh, Egypt, India, Indonesia, and the Philippines have attempted to decentralize the implementation of family planning and other SRH services to local governments and communities. To date, such initiatives have produced mixed results. There has been concern that service provision may have been frustrated when local health personnel or government representatives did not accord the same importance to SRH as central government health officials. In some settings, decentralization also appears to have led to greater problems in coordinating national policies and guidelines for implementing consistent administrative procedures, clinical practicums, and the reporting of program results.

The move to greater decentralization and the loosening of centralized administrative controls has led to less reliance on target setting for evaluating the performance of providers, health facilities, and program outcomes. At the 1994 ICPD, target systems for managing family planning programs were greatly vilified as the source of excessive zealotry for recruiting contraceptive acceptors and encouraging the use of coercion to achieve demographic targets. While there is little question that family planning targets were at times embraced with excessive managerial enthusiasm in such countries as India and Indonesia and likely triggered inflated reports of performance (e.g., see Warwick 1982), they were often not implemented effectively or used with much consistency.[13]

Health sector reform efforts have also focused on developing comprehensive monitoring and evaluation (M&E) procedures that provide clinic-based information on the full range of services being offered. These new M&E approaches, often referred to as integrated health management information systems, are designed to assess the effectiveness of service delivery and operational deficiencies (e.g., essential drug and equipment stock-outs) requiring remedial attention rather than a tool to monitor provider performance or client recruitment quotas. New surveillance systems are also being developed as part of integrated M&E approaches. For example, in Egypt, a national maternal mortality surveillance system is now in place to identify and evaluate every reported maternal death in the country. This system, which is unique in the developing world, is intended to enable health providers to better understand the circumstances and causes of maternal deaths in Egypt, and generate more accurate and timely information on Egypt's progress in attaining MDG-5.

Strengthening human resource capacity in the health systems of developing countries has been another important component of health sector reform. Many less developed countries continue to be plagued by shortages of well-trained doctors, nurses, trained midwives, and auxiliary health staff capable of providing good quality care. Long-term professional training in the medical and health sciences is often inadequate, salaries and working conditions are challenging, and staff turnover high and often depleted by permanent emigration. It's doubtful whether health system strengthening and health sector reforms will be successful without long-term human resource strategies in place.

The provision of family planning and other SRH services can be compromised in settings without staff trained to provide these services. For example, in Southern Sudan, current shortages of well-trained midwives pose major hurdles in providing safe delivery and emergency obstetric care in most regions of this newly emergent

---

[13] In India, the inability to meet prescribed targets for sterilization use led to reproductive and human rights abuses of the Emergency declared by Indira Ghandi from 1975 to 1977. This highly dysfunctional exercise in target setting eventually led to the scrapping of family planning provider and client targets in favor of a "community needs assessment" approach that has proven difficult to define and implement with any degree of uniformity across much of India (Narayana and Sangwan 2000). In addition, the additional number of indicators that needed to be tracked in the new approach added to administrative workloads. A case study of these issues in the State of Karnataka is provided in Murthy et al. (2002).

country. Family planning services are also not available in most areas, leading to a larger proportion of high risk births and one of the highest maternal mortality ratios in the world (over 1,000 maternal deaths per 100,000 live births in 2006) (Ministry of Health and Government of Southern Sudan 2008).

There have also been efforts to integrate family planning and other SRH services with primary health care (even in countries with weak primary care), child survival interventions, and HIV/AIDS programs. These initiatives often occurred before primary health care services were fully staffed and operational. While family planning and other SRH services are increasingly integrated in less developed countries, HIV/AIDS interventions still typically stand apart as vertical programs. In many sub-Saharan African regions (other than South Africa), HIV/AIDS services have actually displaced FP/RH services as HIV/AIDS funding swamped budgets for other activities. This appears to have happened in Kenya, a development that coincided with a stall in the country's fertility rate. In other Eastern, Central, and Western African countries, HIV/AIDS funding has dominated national health budgets, even when HIV prevalence was not particularly high, while family planning has been remarkably neglected, thereby precluding any serious attempt at integration.

Efforts to integrate essential services within primary health care facilities have sometimes added to the burdens of providers and reduced levels of attention previously given to a more limited array of services. In Egypt, the Family Health Model implemented by the Ministry of Health as the centerpiece of the country's health sector reform has introduced new screening, treatment and referral mechanisms for infectious and chronic diseases not previously incorporated as part of primary care. There have been concerns that the broadened set of responsibilities now given to primary care providers may take too much time away from family planning, antenatal care, and childhood immunization programs that were the core services provided at primary care facilities in earlier times.

Health sector reforms have been experimenting with cost recovery from clients able to pay more for services while subsidizing care for the poor. Different price scales have sometimes been established for different services and commodities based upon the income or poverty status of individual clients. This approach was attempted in Indonesia as part of the Keluarja Sejahtera (family welfare) campaign in the mid-1990s for attaining greater equity in the allocation of family planning services. In Egypt, Family Health Model clinics have experimented with separating subsidized services during morning service hours from "economic" fee-for-service care after 2 p.m. Revenues generated from both service tiers are placed in a Service Improvement Fund that is used to pay for clinic upgrades and operational costs not provided through regular budgets (Riggs-Perla et al. 2010:79).

There has also been growing attention given to developing insurance schemes for enabling more secure access to care, including obtaining essential drugs and supplies that many clients may not be able to afford. Such schemes have more typically been attempted in middle income developing countries, often through the auspices of private insurers. The extent to which health insurance schemes inspired by health sector reform have been able to reach lower income clients and households in less accessible urban slums and rural areas deserves further study. Of particular concern is the extent to which SRH services are typically covered by private rather than publicly-funded insurance systems.

Another aspect of health sector reform has been the growing reliance on private sector provision of SRH services. Some countries such as China and India continue to implement centralized (top-down) programs that are highly dependent upon public sector service provision. Other countries such as Bangladesh and Thailand have opted for more pluralistic service delivery systems that have greater civil society participation. However, in many countries with high private sector involvement, it is not always clear how private sector services compare with publically-provided care, especially with respect to quality of care. For example, in Egypt, private sector facilities are often not accredited and cannot be readily compared to public sector outlets in terms of quality and client satisfaction. Current health sector reforms being enacted through the country's Family Health Model are attempting to have private sector provision more fully accredited and discourage the use of doctors and facilities that may be providing sub-standard care.

Social marketing programs have played major roles in such countries as Bangladesh, India, Indonesia, and Thailand in making contraceptive commodities widely available and more readily used. The ability of women to purchase family planning commodities through local pharmacies and other commercial outlets has helped support the use of contraception in many countries. Research over recent decades has shown that women are willing to pay for their family planning supplies if commodities are priced at affordable levels. For example, in Bangladesh, women have increasingly relied on commercial outlets (primarily pharmacies) to meet their family planning needs. In 2007, pharmacies provided 45.0 % of all pills, 13.2 % of injectables, and 66.1 % of condoms in Bangladesh (NIPORT et al. 2009:67) – figures that now dwarf the provision of these methods by government fieldworkers, once the main source of supply for non-clinical contraceptive methods in Bangladesh.

7.6 Prospects for Resurgent Policy and Program Action in Family Planning and Reproductive Health

Family planning and other SRH programs have been neglected development priorities since the ICPD in 1994. Fertility declines in much of the developing world may have promoted complacency about addressing the full range of women's SRH needs. Donor resources for program services have also been defused across broad social and cultural agendas centered on gender and empowerment. These transformational initiatives, while often constructive and well-meaning in their own right, have tended to blur the earlier focus on program services that typified family planning and MCH efforts in the pre-Cairo period. In addition, there has also been a tendency to neglect family planning and other SRH services in favor of HIV/AIDS, malaria, and TB programs. The vertical program structures employed to implement these services are tightly delimited and fiercely advocated by well-entrenched constituencies that have not pushed for greater integration with SRH services.

The main challenge in providing women with access to effective and affordable family planning and other SRH services will be to ensure that comprehensive programs are available that offer internationally recognized standards of care. If SRH policies and programs are to become truly resurgent, efforts need to be centered on ensuring that comprehensive program services are accessible and of sufficient quality to instill women's confidence in their use. SRH services remain underdeveloped in many of the world's least developed countries (especially safe delivery services for mothers). The MDG 5 sub-objective of ensuring women access to SRH care can't be fulfilled if the services are not in place. Country programs should also not be overly beholden to prescriptive agendas and plans of action imported from abroad. Countries have different service requirements, health system characteristics, and sociocultural environments in which programs must function. These variable contexts need to be recognized if countries are to make lasting improvements in the provision and extensive utilization of women's health services.

It remains unclear whether future resource flows from developed countries will reach levels needed to provide universal access to family planning and other SRH services. Developed countries may find it increasingly difficult to maintain strong financial support for global health programs as their populations age, elderly dependency burdens rise, and economic growth slows in comparison to emerging market economies. Increasingly, many less developed countries will need to provide for their health services from domestic (national) resources rather than relying on the international foreign assistance that was so crucial during the latter half of the twentieth Century. However, in the world's least developed countries (situated primarily in East, Central and West Africa as well as South Asia), significant foreign assistance outlays will still be needed to provide women with the means to reduce unwanted fertility and obtain safe maternal health services (including access to emergency obstetric care and newly born care for infants).

New global challenges lie ahead, many of which will be driven by the very demographic dynamics that were effectively dismissed as salient concerns for development at the 1994 ICPD. While fertility and population growth have slowed in most regions of the developing world, the world's total population will almost certainly reach 9 billion by 2050, and may be considerably higher if the UN's current population estimates and projections prove overly optimistic with respect to current levels of fertility and the speed at which replacement fertility is reached in many developing countries.

The effect of climate change and global warming seem set to become more pressing concerns in the decades ahead. Growing inflationary pressures on air, water, energy, and other natural resource commodities will likely become greater constraints on economic growth in the twenty-first Century. The production of sufficient food stocks to feed the world's growing population may become even more problematic given the prospect of increasingly unsettled weather patterns stemming from global warming. Generating sufficient resources for education and employment generation will continue to be major hurdles in many regions of the developing world, especially in least developed countries that continue to have high rates of population growth. Rapidly growing rates of urbanization will also place large demands on such infrastructure investments as housing, sanitation and waste management, and transportation capacity.

Compared to the resource demands entailed in responding to these demographically-induced development challenges, investments needed to ensure that all women have access to modern family planning and other SRH services are extremely modest. An analysis conducted in 2008 concluded that an outlay of $6.7 billion would be required in that year to satisfy all unmet need for family planning services in the developing world (Singh et al. 2009). If the cost of maternal and newborn care needed to ensure a more comprehensive reproductive health service is included, the annual required budget would rise to $24.6 billion, a figure roughly double the actual outlay for SRH services in 2008. The world can ill-afford not to make the investments required if there are to be realistic prospects for improving the health, reproductive rights, and social welfare of women and achieving more equitable and sustainable social advance around the world.

References

Bongaarts, J. (2008). *Fertility transitions in developing countries: Progress or stagnation* (Poverty, Gender and Youth Working Paper Number 7). New York: Population Council.

Cleland, J. (1996). ICPD and the feminization of population and development issues. *Health Transition Review, 6*(1), 107–110.

Cleland, J., Philips, J., & Amin, S. (2004). *The determinants of reproductive health in Bangladesh.* Washington, DC: World Bank.

Demographic and Health Surveys. (2010). *STAT compiler.* Calverton: Measure 1 Project. Available at: www.statcompiler.com

Dixon-Mueller, R., & Germain, A. (1992). Stalking the elusive 'unmet need' for family planning. *Studies in Family Planning, 23*(5), 330–335.

EngenderHealth. (2010). *COPE: Client-oriented, provider efficient services.* New York: EngenderHealth. Available at: http://www.engenderhealth.org/our-work/improving-quality/cope.php

Government of India, Ministry of Home Affairs. (2011). *Census of India 2011.* New Delhi: Office of the Registrar General and Census Commission. Available at: http://censusindia.gov.in/

Health Communication Partnership. (2010). *Global/regional: Postabortion care (PAC).* USAID and the Center for Communication Program (CCP), Johns Hopkins Bloomberg School of Public Health and USAID, Washington, DC. Available at: www.jhuccp.org/hcp/countries/global_pac.html

Hogan, M., Foreman, K., Naghaui, M., Ahn, S., Wang, M., Makela, S., Lopez, A., Lozano, R., & Murray, C. (2010). Maternal mortality for 181 countries, 1980–2008: A systematic analysis of progress towards Millennium Development Goal 5. *The Lancet, 375*(9726), 1609–1623.

Johnston, H. B., Oliveras, E., Akhter, S., & Walker, D. G. (2010). Health system costs of menstrual regulation and care for abortion complications in Bangladesh. *International Perspectives on Sexual and Reproductive Health, 36*(4), 197–204.

Kantner, J., & Kantner, A. (2009). *International discord on population and development.* New York: Palgrave MacMillan.

Ministry of Health, Government of Southern Sudan. (2008, October). *Sudan Household Health Survey (SHHS), 2006.* Juba: Southern Sudan, MOH/GOSS.

Murthy, N., et al. (2002). Dismantling India's contraceptive target system: An overview of three case studies. In H. Nicole & M. Diane (Eds.), *Responding to Cairo: Case studies of changing practice in reproductive health and family planning* (pp. 25–57). New York: The Population Council.

Narayana, G., & Naveen, S. (2000). Implementation of the community needs assessment approach in India. In *Review of implementation of community needs assessment for family welfare in India* (pp. 1–18). Washington, DC: Policy Project II and the Futures Group International.

National Institute of Allergy and Infectious Diseases (NIAID). (2011, May 12). *Treating HIV-infected people with Antiretrovirals protects partners from infection.* Washington, DC: Press Release. www.niaid.nih.gov/news/newsreleases/2011/Pages/HPTN052.aspx

National Institute of Population Research and Training (NIPORT), Mitra and Associates, and Macro International. (2009). *Bangladesh demographic and health survey 2007.* Dhaka/Calverton: NIPORT.

Nawar, L. N., et al. (1997). *Scaling-up improved postabortion care in Egypt: Introduction to University and Ministry of Health and Population Hospitals: Final report.* Cairo: Egyptian Fertility Care Society and the Population Council.

Riggs-Perla, J., Carpenter-Yaman, C., Curtin, L., Kantner, A., Senlet, P., & Tanamly, M. (2010). *Egypt health and population legacy review.* Washington, DC: GH Tech Project and USAID.

Riley, L. A. (2008). *Population politics and development: From the policies to the clinics.* New York: Palgrave MacMillan.

Sedgh, G., Henshaw, S., Singh, S., Ahman, E., & Shah, I. H. (2007). Induced abortion: Estimated rates and trends worldwide. *The Lancet, 370*(9595), 1338–1345.

Shah, I., & Ahman, E. (2010). Unsafe abortion in 2008: Global and regional levels and trends. *Reproductive Health Matters, 18*(36), 90–101.

Singh, S., Darroch, J. E., Ashford, L., & Vlassoff, M. (2009). *Adding it up: The costs and benefits of investing in family planning and maternal and newborn Health.* New York: Guttmacher Institute and United Nations Population Fund.

UNAIDS. (2010). *AIDS epidemic update.* Geneva: UNAIDS.

United Nations. (1995). *Report of the international conference on population and development, Cairo, 5–13 September, 1994* (A/CONFF.171/13/Rev.1). New York: UN Publication.

United Nations. (2010a). *World population prospects: The 2008 revision.* New York: Population Division, Department of Economic and Social Affairs. Available online at: esa.un.org/unpp

United Nations. (2010b). *World contraceptive use 2010.* New York: Population Division, Department of Economic and Social Affairs. Available online at: un.org/esa/population/publications/wcu2010

United Nations Development Programme. (2011). *Millennium development goals.* MDG Homepage. New York: UNDP. undp.org/mdg/goal6.shtml

United Nations, Economic and Social Council. (2011, April 11–15). *Flow of financial resources for assisting in the implementation of the programme of action of the international conference on population and development* (44th session). New York: Commission on Population and Development.

USAID Health Policy Initiative. (2007, February). *Inequalities in the use of family planning and reproductive health services: Implications for policies and programs.* Washington, DC: The Policy Project.

Warwick, D. P. (1982). *Bitter pills: Population policies and their implementation in eight developing countries.* New York: Cambridge University Press.

Westoff, C. (2010). *Desired number of children: 2000–2008* (DHS Comparative Reports 25). Calverton: ICF Macro.

WHO. (2010). *New progress and guidance on HIV treatment* (*Fact Sheet*). Geneva: WHO. Available online at: www.data.unaids.org/pub.factsheet2010

WHO/UNICEF/UNFPA/World Bank. (2010). *Trends in maternal mortality: 1990 to 2008.* Geneva: WHO.

Chapter 8
How Problematic Will Liberal Abortion Policies Be for Pronatalist Countries?

Dennis Hodgson

8.1 Introduction

The twenty-first century begins with countries assessing induced abortion in widely divergent ways, from a murderous act that ends a human life to an individual woman's right that should be protected by the state. These varying state assessments of abortion take place in a world in which 210 million women become pregnant each year, over 84 million of whom did not intend to do so. These women give birth to approximately 135 million children, and experienced 22.2 million legal abortions, 21.6 million illegal abortions, and over 30 million spontaneous abortions and still births (WHO 2011; Sedgh et al. 2012).

Currently 112 countries, containing 60 % of the world's population, have policies in place aimed at altering their fertility levels: 71 countries, with 47 % of the world's population, have adopted antinatalist policies aimed at decreasing their fertility, and 41 countries, with 13 % of the world's population, have adopted pronatalist policies aimed at increasing their fertility. An additional 67 countries, containing 40 % of the world's population, either have a "no intervention" fertility policy or one aimed at "maintaining" their current fertility level. Policymakers in antinatalist countries fear that too high fertility is harming development efforts and policymakers in pronatalist countries fear that too low fertility is leading to the decline of their population and their economy. Induced abortion, ending more than half the world's unintended pregnancies, clearly affects whether countries attempting to lower or to increase their fertility will realize their population policy goals.

Those concerned with fostering both women's reproductive health and reproductive rights need to monitor closely the interplay between abortion and population policies. Currently the majority of countries with policies aimed at altering their fertility levels have abortion policies that are not in harmony with their fertility goals.

D. Hodgson, Ph.D. (✉)
Department of Sociology and Anthropology, Fairfield University, Fairfield, CT, USA
e-mail: hodgson@fairfield.edu

A. Kulczycki (ed.), *Critical Issues in Reproductive Health*, The Springer Series on Demographic Methods and Population Analysis 33, DOI 10.1007/978-94-007-6722-5_8, © Springer Science+Business Media Dordrecht 2014

Most antinatalist countries restrict women's access to abortion and most pronatalist countries permit women an easy access to abortion. This lack of harmony illustrates a significant way in which abortion differs from contraception. There is no longer much debate about the correctness of contraception or on the proposition that couples have the right to practice contraception to control their fertility. However, substantive debate remains about the correctness of induced abortion, and government leaders are far from a consensus about the proposition that all women should have uncomplicated access to abortion. Policymakers in a number of low-fertility European countries refuse to consider limiting a woman's access to abortion because they define access to abortion as a woman's right that must be protected by the state. Policymakers in a number of African and Latin American countries with still comparatively high fertility and active programs to distribute contraceptives refuse to liberalize their highly restrictive abortion policy because they define abortion as the taking of a human life. Cultural, religious, and political traditions clearly influence the make-up of abortion policies around the world in significant ways.

Yet countries attempting to alter their fertility levels do have clear demographic interests and the incidence of induced abortion helps shape every country's fertility level. A lack of harmony between a country's fertility policy and its abortion policy therefore makes policymakers susceptible to pressures to change their abortion policies. In antinatalist countries critics can blame restrictive abortion policies for worsening women's reproductive health and for keeping population growth rates high. In pronatalist countries critics can fault permissive abortion policies for exacerbating population decline and hastening a "demographic winter" of aging populations. The greater the felt urgency to alter a country's fertility level the greater this pressure will be. Clearly most countries' abortion policies are not solely determined by their fertility policies, but where fertility goals are a major priority a lack of harmony between these two policies will be a stress point for policymakers.

After discussing the sources of data used in this analysis, I will examine the two kinds of "stress points" being experienced by these policymakers. The stress point on policymakers in antinatalist countries will be seen to be working to further reproductive health goals. The stress point on policymakers in pronatalist countries will be seen to constitute a potential threat to reproductive rights. I will concentrate on examining the size and depth of this threat in light of UN projections that 69 % of the world's population by 2035 will be living in low fertility countries, defined as being countries with a total fertility rate (TFR) of 1.9 or less. I will identify the particular countries and regions most susceptible to this threat to reproductive rights, and will comment on how best to respond to this challenge.

8.2 Data

Information on abortion and population policies comes from the United Nation's database, *World Population Policies 2009* (UN 2010). I have excluded countries with populations of less than 100,000 from this analysis. The population projections are the UN medium estimates from the *World Population Prospects: The 2008 Revision* (UN 2009).[1]

The UN Population Division has maintained a country-specific database on abortion policies for over a decade, examining each country's criminal code as well as any public health or medical ethics codes that affect the application of abortion laws in particular situations. A three-volume work, *Abortion Policies: A Global Review* (UN 2002), contains treatments of the specific grounds on which each country permits abortion, duration-of-pregnancy limitations for specific grounds, a history of the country's abortion policies, and an assessment of its implementation of those policies. Seven standard grounds are used to categorize when countries permit abortion: to save the life of the woman, to preserve physical health, to preserve mental health, rape or incest, fetal impairment, for economic or social reasons, and on request. Every country places some duration-of-pregnancy limitations on when legal abortions are permitted, except for cases where the woman's life is in danger. In all cases where countries permit abortion on request or for economic or social reasons, the permission exists for a limited gestational period, in the range of 10–24 weeks. Either by limiting the allowable reasons for abortion or by offering greater protection of fetal rights as the gestation period increases, all states recognize that a difference exists between abortion and contraception. When abortions occur within the stipulated gestational period, contraception and abortion are most similar in terms of state regulation in those countries permitting abortion on request or for economic or social reasons since documentation of such a reason is rarely if ever required. Although some countries permitting abortion "to preserve mental health" liberally interpret its meaning, many countries permitting abortion for that reason are not so liberal in their interpretation. Therefore for this analysis I have defined "uncomplicated access to legal abortion" as living in a country that permits abortion on request or for economic or social reasons. In many "uncomplicated access" countries, however, a woman who discovers her pregnancy late, or who has difficulty finding an abortion facility, or who cannot afford a legal abortion still might find her access anything but "uncomplicated."

The World Population Policies 2009 database contains updated UN information on each country's 2009 abortion policies, its 1996 abortion policies, its population policies with respect to size and growth, age structure and spatial distribution, fertility levels, mortality levels, and migration levels for 1976, 1986, 1996, and 2009, as well as UN estimates of each country's relevant demographic and health measures for those 4 years. The database's primary source of policy information is official government responses to a UN requests for information on population policies. This is supplemented by an examination of government publications, documents and

---

[1]The manuscript for this chapter was finished before the release of the UN's *2010 Revision of World Population Prospects* in May of 2011. This most current set of projections covers the entire twenty-first century, not just the period to 2050. Since the projections relevant for this study end in 2035, the projections from the *2008 Revision of World Population Prospects* contained in this chapter do not significantly differ from those in the *2010 Revision of World Population Prospect* for the relevant time period.

statements, and by materials supplied by international organizations and NGOs (UN 2010: 2). I consider a country where "the government has policies in place to raise fertility levels" to be a pronatalist country, and a country where "the government has policies in place to lower fertility levels" to be an antinatalist country (UN 2010: 88). Although countries vary greatly in the effort that they invest in such policies, for this analysis I have used these simple UN groupings.

8.3   Abortion Policy and Population Policy

The great variation in population size among countries (from 100,000 to 1.35 billion in this case) means that the proportion of the world's population living under a particular abortion or population policy will be determined more by the population sizes of countries with that policy than by their number. Table 8.1 presents global abortion policies using both "countries" and "% of population" as units of analysis. In 2009, 32 % of countries with populations of 100,000 or more permitted abortion on request; they contained 41 % of the world's population. An additional 5 % of countries, containing 21 % of the world's population, permitted abortion "for economic or social reasons." Therefore in 2009, 37 % of countries granted women an uncomplicated access to legal abortion; they contained 62 % of the world's population. This is a conservative estimate since some additional countries permit abortion for liberally defined "health" reasons.

An uncomplicated access to legal abortion allows women experiencing unwanted pregnancies in antinatalist countries to terminate their pregnancies and thereby realize their own and their country's population goals. Table 8.2 indicates, however, that 86 % of antinatalist countries, containing 54 % of the population living in antinatalist countries, restrict women's access to abortion. Their abortion policy works against attaining their population policy goal. Conversely, women experiencing an unwanted pregnancy in pronatalist countries are very likely to be able to legally terminate that pregnancy: 81 % of pronatalist countries, containing 83 % of the population living in such countries, grant women an uncomplicated access to legal abortion.

Table 8.1 Grounds on which countries permit abortion, 2009

Reasons	% of countries (N = 179)	% of population (N = 6,808,352,000)
To save woman's life	97.2	99.4
To preserve physical health	69.3	78.9
To preserve mental health	65.4	76.3
Rape or incest	51.4	71.0
Fetal impairment	50.3	66.4
Economic or social reason	37.4	61.6
On request	31.8	41.0

Source: UN (2010) *World Population Policies 2009* (all countries 100,000 or more population)

Table 8.2 Countries' 2009 fertility policy by whether or not abortion is permitted on request or for economic or social reasons in 2009

Country's policy to modify fertility	Abortion permitted on request or for economic or social reasons		Total in fertility policy category	% of world's population in fertility policy category
	Yes	No		
Lower				
Number of countries	10	61	71	
Percent of countries	14.1	85.9	100	47.0
Percent of population	46.0	54.0	100	
Raise				
Number of countries	33	8	41	
Percent of countries	80.5	19.5	100	12.5
Percent of population	83.0	17.0	100	
Maintain				
Number of countries	11	14	25	
Percent of countries	44.0	56.0	100	24.9
Percent of population	89.7	10.3	100	
No intervention				
Number of countries	13	29	42	
Percent of countries	31.0	69.0	100	15.6
Percent of population	47.1	52.9	100	
Total				
Number of countries	67	112	179	
Percent of countries	37.4	62.6	100	100
Percent of population	61.6	38.4	100	

Source: UN (2010) *World Population Policies* 2009 (all countries 100,000 or more population)

These countries have abortion policies that make it easier for pregnant women to terminate unwanted pregnancies, even though such terminations reduce the country's birth rate. For policymakers in both sets of countries, the lack of integration of abortion and population policy produces a policy "stress point." These stress points are closely related to reproductive health issues in the case of antinatalist countries and reproductive rights issues in the case of pronatalist countries. The stress point works in the antinatalist context to sensitize policymakers to the health dilemmas faced by women with unintended pregnancies, while in the pronatalist context it works to desensitize policymakers to the reproductive rights of pregnant women.

8.4 The Antinatalist Stress Point

In the near term the most significant policy stress point is in the 61 antinatalist countries that restrict access to abortion. Most of these countries are African (34 of 61) and are categorized as "least developed" (32 of 61). Just 7.3 % of individuals in

Table 8.3 Where abortion is permitted on request or for economic or social reasons by development category and world region, 2009

	% of countries in category	% of population in category
Development category:		
More developed	88.9	92.5
Less developed	26.7	63.3
Least developed	8.3	6.9
World region:		
Northern America	100.0	100.0
Europe	89.7	88.0
Asia	40.4	72.7
Oceania	11.1	62.1
Latin America and Caribbean	20.0	21.2
Africa	7.7	7.3
Total:	37.4	61.6

Source: UN (2010) *World Population Policies 2009* (all countries 100,000 or more population)

Africa and 6.9 % in least developed countries have an uncomplicated access to legal abortion (Table 8.3). This policy stress point is a "natural" one in that success of the country's antinatalist fertility policy will lead to a rapid drop in desired family size. With desired family size declining rapidly, women have a new and urgent need for contraception but often must overcome cultural and service delivery barriers to its use, take time to find out where to obtain it, and learn how to use it correctly. During this period, unintended pregnancies are likely to increase in number even as contraceptive use is increasing (Hodgson 2009: 487). Significant problems will ensue as women with unwanted pregnancies confront the restrictive abortion policy, resort to illegal abortions, and suffer serious health consequences. Illegal abortions are many times more unsafe than legal abortions, especially in countries with poor health infrastructures. The World Health Organization (WHO) estimates that in Africa in 2008, where 97 % of its 6.2 million abortions were illegal ones, the case fatality rate (deaths per 100,000 abortion procedures) was 460 for women receiving illegal abortions, and in Latin America and the Caribbean, where 95 % of its 4.2 million abortions were illegal, it was 30. This compares with a case fatality rate of 0.6 for legal abortions done in the US (WHO 2011: 30; Sedgh et al. 2012: 628). An estimated 47,000 women die each year as a result of complications from unsafe abortions and five million need hospitalization (WHO 2011).

Abortion rates among countries vary little by the restrictiveness of their abortion laws (Singh et al. 2009: 17–18). Evidently women who are pregnant and who do not want to give birth strive to accomplish their goal regardless of legal barriers. The restrictive abortion policies of these 61 antinatalist countries, therefore, are not likely to result in markedly fewer abortions but only in high ratios of illegal to legal abortions, ratios that can significantly worsen women's health. Table 8.4 attempts to measure this impact by comparing the health and demographic measures of antinatalist countries with uncomplicated access to legal abortion to those of antinatalist

Table 8.4 Demographic and health measures of countries with a policy to lower fertility according to whether countries permit abortion on request or for economic or social reasons, 2009

Demographic/health measures	Abortion permitted on request or for economic or social reasons		Total
	Yes	No	
Count of countries	10	61	71
% of population in countries	46	54	100
Population growth rate (%)	1.37	1.97	1.70
Total fertility rate	2.74	3.71	3.27
Female life expectancy	66.7	64.7	65.6
Infant mortality rate	50.0	54.5	52.4
Under 5 mortality rate	72.7	81.5	77.5
Maternal mortality ratio	411	520[a]	470[a]
% Using modern contraception	51[a]	34[a]	42[a]
% Using any contraception	58[a]	42[a]	49[a]
GNI per capita, ppp 2006[b]	$3,136[a]	$2,810[a]	$2,960[a]

Source: UN (2010) *World Population Policies 2009* (all countries 100,000 or more population)
[a]Data missing for less than 1 % of the population
[b]GNI Source: GNI per capita, ppp (current international $) 2006 data is from the World Bank's World Development Indicators database; http://databank.worldbank.org/ddp/home.do

countries with a restricted access; all measures are "% of population" measures. The most telling difference is that the 46 % of the antinatalist population with an uncomplicated access to abortion has a 21 % lower maternal mortality ratio (411 vs. 520) than the restricted access population, a difference that suggests illegal abortions are leading to more maternal deaths in the restricted access population. The uncomplicated access population also experiences consistently better health and demographic conditions: an 8 % lower infant mortality rate (50.0 vs. 54.5), an 11 % lower under 5 mortality rate (72.7 vs. 81.5), a 30 % lower population growth rate (1.37 % vs. 1.97 %), a 26 % lower TFR (2.74 vs. 3.71), a 38 % higher use rate for all contraceptives (58 % vs. 42 %), and a 50 % higher use rate for modern contraceptives (51 % vs. 34 %). All evidence suggests that women in antinatalist countries that restrict access to abortion have more pregnancy-related deaths, poorer health conditions, higher fertility and population growth rates and lower contraceptive use rates. It is unlikely that their marginally lower GNI per capita ($2,810 vs. $3,136) can explain these inferior health and demographic conditions.

8.5 Exploiting the Antinatalist Stress Point

Advocates of enhancing the reproductive health of women in developing countries can effectively put pressure on policymakers in these 61 countries by exploiting this stress point. They need to publicize the above facts and focus on contrasting the health consequences of illegal vs. legal abortions. There is an obvious remedy for

Table 8.5 Total fertility rate (TFR) of populations living in each development category

Development category	1975[a]	1985[a]	1995[a]	2009[a]	2020–2025[b]	2030–2035[b]
More developed	2.12	1.85	1.67	1.63	1.67	1.73
Less developed	5.30	3.98	3.22	2.52	2.13	1.98
Least developed	6.64	6.31	5.76	4.56	3.52	2.95
World (total)	4.60	3.71	3.17	2.61	2.24	2.09

Sources: [a]UN (2010) *World Population Policy 2009*; [b]UN (2009) *2008 Revision of World Population Prospects*

higher population growth rates and poorer health conditions: permit abortion for economic or social reasons. Other remedies are difficult to identify. Improving hospital care for women suffering the consequences of illegal abortion is unlikely ever to eliminate the significant health disparities between illegal and legal abortion. Considering the weak state apparatus of most of these countries, enforcement of restrictive abortion laws offers no feasible solution. Additionally, strict enforcement only serves to highlight the policy contradictions of a state attempting to induce women to lower their fertility while simultaneously restricting pregnant women's access to abortion. Contraceptive failure is a frequent occurrence, happening to an estimated 33 million women annually (WHO 2011: 11). It is especially problematic when women attending government sponsored family planning clinics become pregnant and find that the state that desires them to use contraception offers no options when that contraception fails.

Over the last 50 years there has been a gradual extension of the legal grounds for abortion in developing countries, some of it stimulated by demographic concerns. Induced abortion has always been a significant factor affecting numbers of births and population growth rates (Himes 1932: 49; Davis and Blake 1956: 229–230; Frejka 1985: 230), and abortion policy has often been viewed as a potentially powerful means to accomplish a variety of population policy ends. It is not accidental that both India and China liberalized their abortion policies during the 1970s in the midst of strong government campaigns to lower national birth rates, nor that liberalization of abortion policies has been more prevalent among populous Asian countries with strong commitments to family planning programs than among Latin American and African countries with weak commitments to family planning programs. Historically, without the prod of a perceived significant population problem, policymakers have been less willing to confront religious and cultural traditions that view abortion as an immoral activity. Therefore exploiting the antinatalist stress point will not be easy since restrictive abortion policies now are so concentrated in African and Latin American countries.

Moreover, the world's annual rate of population growth peaked at 2.02 % in 1970 and now has fallen to 1.18 % (UN 2010). The TFR of the population of less developed countries, 70 % of the world's population, has declined from 5.3 children per woman in 1975 to 2.5 in 2009, just 0.4 of a child above the replacement level of 2.1 (Table 8.5). Even the population of the least developed countries, 12 % of the world's population, has seen its TFR fall by 1.2 children per woman over the last

14 years. With UN projections calling for continued significant fertility declines the demographic incentive for liberalizing abortion policies is rapidly dissipating.

Reproductive rights movements arose in many countries beginning in the late 1960s and put forward non-demographic rationales for liberalizing abortion policies. These movements have entered into alliances with antinatalist policymakers but have failed to convince all policymakers, especially those from Latin American and African countries, of the need to change abortion policies. Reproductive rights advocates assert that control of fertility is an individual woman's right, that every child should be a wanted child, and that women need access both to contraception and to legal abortion to accomplish that goal. However, there still is a general meshing of interests since antinatalist policymakers want to lower birth rates and reproductive rights advocates want to increase women's access to birth control. Progressively stronger alliances between the two were fashioned over the course of three UN sponsored international meetings on population and development: Bucharest in 1974, Mexico City in 1984, and finally Cairo in 1994. Antinatalist policymakers desired the legitimacy that reproductive rights movements can give to their efforts and the movements desired the additional resources that states can provide for fulfilling women's reproductive health needs. However, this has never been a perfect union. Two topics in particular have been sources of friction: population goals and abortion.

Excessive state enthusiasm for fertility control occasionally has led to women being coerced into having smaller families than they desired, but from a reproductive rights perspective, control of fertility is an individual woman's right that never should be constrained. The "common ground" position worked out at the Cairo conference did formally align both parties' population goals (Hodgson and Watkins 1997): redressing gender inequities is needed for lasting fertility control, and women have reproductive rights to freely determine their reproductive destinies. Abortion, though, has proved less amenable to a workable common ground solution. The population control movement historically has embraced a "contraception only" definition of family planning. Originally it did so to attract the many policymakers in less densely settled regions of the world, especially in Latin America and Africa, who were more interested in combating illegal abortion with their "family planning" programs than in solving population problems (Hodgson 2009). When reproductive health advocates attempted to include abortion in the Cairo conference's definition of the "reproductive health care" that all governments should provide, those past compromises and continuing religious opposition proved too strong an obstacle. The old abortion language of the Mexico City conference reappeared in Cairo's Program of Action (PoA): "In no case should abortion be promoted as a method of family planning."

Since Cairo the less developed world's population problem has receded from prominence and demographic arguments for liberalizing abortion policies have lost some of their potency. In international policy arenas the case for liberalization has focused more on reproductive health arguments largely because of successful efforts by conservatives to exclude any consideration of abortion as an effective and needed birth control method. Considering the nature of the twenty-first century's demographic trends, this exclusion may make defending women's reproductive rights more difficult.

8.6   The Twenty-First Century's Population Problem

Table 8.5 documents the departure of the twentieth century's "too high fertility problem" and the arrival of the twenty-first century's "too low fertility problem." By 2030–2035 the United Nations projects that the world will have replacement level fertility (2.09), the currently less developed population will have below replacement level fertility (1.98), and even the world's least developed population will have a TFR of less than 3. Over the next 25 years we can expect a significant decline in countries with antinatalist fertility policies and a simultaneous increase in countries with pronatalist policies. A general fear of rapid population growth may be being replaced by a fear of population decline.

This change in population agenda means that the past synchronization of the interests of state policymakers and reproductive rights advocates – both wanting to provide women with greater access to birth control – will likely end. The low fertility that states now find problematic is commonly accepted to be an expression of the actual fertility desires of women, given their social and economic circumstances. When states seek to increase the fertility of these women there is a much greater potential for the state to intrude on the right of the individual woman to determine her own fertility. While it might be possible for states to induce higher fertility while still respecting the reproductive rights of women, doing so without some element of coercion will require great care, an authentic state commitment to reproductive rights principles, and significant resources. The coming demographic regime is one in which women and states will have different fertility goals and an element of tension, not harmony, will affect the relationship between reproductive rights advocates and state policymakers.

8.7   The Pronatalist Stress Point

To the extent that abortion policy is a potentially powerful means to accomplish population policy ends, and that policymakers are willing to use it as such, abortion is likely to be one arena where these new tensions will play out. When policymakers experienced rapid population growth, and were truly concerned about resource shortages, unemployment, and economic stagnation, many came to see abortion as a health-promoting act for both society and the individual. When policymakers are faced with actual population decline and are truly concerned about a rapidly aging population and a faltering economy, many are likely to see abortion as a harmful act for both society and the individual. The more severe the population problem, the greater this inclination is likely to be. Policymakers will need an authentic commitment to reproductive rights principles not to succumb to such inclinations. As the significance of the pronatalist policy stress point increases, religious opponents of legal abortion and nationalists worried about the debilitating effects of population decline can be expected to exploit the mounting pressures felt by policymakers. They will be able to commandeer the demographic perspective and contend that liberal abortion policies are socially harmful and need to be changed. This changed policy environment constitutes a real threat not only to women's reproductive rights but to their reproductive health as well.

States worried about population decline can undertake, and have undertaken, unilateral changes in fertility and abortion policies that suddenly strip women of access to both contraception and abortion. The most notorious example of such a coercive pronatalist policy is Communist Romania's experiment in seeking to increase its birth rate (Baban 1999). Romania legalized abortion on request in 1957, before the development of many modern contraceptives, and abortion quickly became the main method of fertility control. In October of 1966 the Ceauşescu government, worried that fertility had fallen below replacement levels, abruptly restricted access to abortion as part of a package of coercive pronatalist policies that lasted for 23 years. This package grew to include banning the importation and sale of contraceptives, taxing childless couples, requiring monthly gynecological exams of working women aged 20–30, and the president proclaiming that "the fetus is the socialist property of the whole society" (David 1992: 13). In 1967 the crude birth rate spiked but then began a long term decline as women quickly resorted to illegal abortion. Maternal mortality rates more than doubled and thousands of unwanted infants were left at overcrowded "orphanages" (only 2 % of the residents were orphans) where they suffered high rates of psychological and neurological disorders (David 1992: 13). Tellingly, on December 26, 1989, the first day after the fall of the Ceauşescu regime, the restrictive abortion laws were repealed (Baban 1999: 200). The following year abortion related deaths declined 67 % (WHO 2004: 13). Romania's implementation of coercive pronatalism reveals the potential harm to reproductive health that can accompany such a policy shift.

Today the 33 pronatalist countries whose liberal abortion policies are not structured to further their pronatalist goals (Table 8.2) find themselves with a pronatalist policy stress point. It can be, and is being, exploited by opponents of women having an uncomplicated access to abortion. The population of these countries already has a stagnant annual growth rate (−0.02 %) and a TFR (1.46) well below replacement level. Twenty-four of these countries are European, of which 12 are now in their third decade of below-replacement fertility. Fourteen of these countries currently have declining populations and 11 have a median age over 40 (UN 2009). By 2025 the UN projects that 24 of these countries will be in population decline and 25 will have a median age over 40. Demographers and economists have extensively studied the problematic effects of low fertility on age structure, social security costs, health care costs, and labor force needs. Although not their intent, their findings have been taken up by opponents of liberal abortion policies who now lobby for a policy change with a demographic argument: liberal abortion policies are helping to bring about a socially harmful low fertility. Although most policymakers have not succumbed to such lobbying efforts, they are likely precursors of stronger future attempts to restrict access to abortion with demographic arguments and warrant examination.

8.8 Exploiting the Pronatalist Stress Point

Religious opponents of abortion, especially the Vatican, are focusing on low fertility European countries and fashioning demographic rationales for restricting abortion. They use current depopulation fears to portray new mothers as selfless and altruistic and women who end unwanted pregnancies as selfish and shallow. The number of abortions and the ratio of abortions to births are presented as measures of self-indulgence and of foregone beneficial population growth. Abortion is presented not simply as a moral problem, but as an activity that threatens the very existence of society. In 2002 Pope John Paul II (2002) told Italian legislators that Italy's future was threatened by:

the *crisis of the birthrate,* the demographic decline and the ageing of the population. Raw statistical evidence obliges us to take account of the human, social and economic problems which this crisis will inevitably impose on Italy in the decades to come. Above all, it encourages – indeed, I would dare to say, forces – citizens to make a broad and responsible commitment to favour a clear-cut reversal of this tendency.

In 2003 Cardinal Trujillo, then President of the Pontifical Council on the Family, identified abortion as the cause of Europe's "demographic winter" (Trujillo 2003):

Today, in almost every European nation, abortion is available up to the 12th week of pregnancy through a simple request by the mother… As a result, these countries often find themselves facing the grave consequences of a prolonged "demographic winter". They see their populations aging and diminishing numerically in a real and proper implosion that is draining the energies of their countries.

In his first year as pope, Benedict XVI echoed (2006) this theme: "Vast areas of the world are suffering from the so-called 'demographic winter', with the consequent gradual ageing of the population." In 2007 he identified (2007a) a selfish "individualism" behind this trend:

Unfortunately, from a demographic point of view, one must note that Europe seems to be following a path that could lead to its departure from history. This not only places economic growth at risk; it could also create enormous difficulties for social cohesion and, above all, favours a dangerous form of individualism inattentive to future consequences.

Pope Benedict XVI often explicitly related these population changes to abortion. He reviewed (2008) family change for Hungarian bishops and noted that it "has led to a drastic fall in the birth rate, made even more dramatic by the widespread practice of abortion." He appealed (2007b) to Austrian politicians "not to allow children to be considered as a form of illness, nor to abolish in practice your legal system's acknowledgment that abortion is wrong." He questioned (2007c) the validity of population and health arguments for liberalizing abortion policies in Latin America:

The pressures to legalize abortion are increasing in Latin American countries and in developing countries, also with recourse to the liberalization of new forms of chemical abortion under the pretext of safeguarding reproductive health: policies for demographic control are on the rise, notwithstanding that they are already recognized as dangerous also on the economic and social plane.

The Vatican that so adamantly decries population control efforts now offers a demographic rationale for banning abortion: the need to end the "demographic winter" brought on by below replacement fertility. In his 2009 encyclical, *Caritas in Veritate*, Pope Benedict XVI argued against "the tragic and widespread scourge of abortion" with sophisticated demographic analysis:

> In economically developed countries, legislation contrary to life is very widespread, and it has already shaped moral attitudes and praxis, contributing to the spread of an anti-birth mentality… formerly prosperous nations are presently passing through a phase of uncertainty and in some cases decline, precisely because of their falling birth rates; this has become a crucial problem for highly affluent societies. The decline in births, falling at times beneath the so-called "replacement level", also puts a strain on social welfare systems, increases their cost, eats into savings and hence the financial resources needed for investment, reduces the availability of qualified labourers, and narrows the "brain pool" upon which nations can draw for their needs.

8.8.1 National Case Studies of the Pronatalist Stress Point

So far these arguments have had some limited appeal, most notable in post socialist Eastern and Central European countries, several of whom have questioned the liberal abortion policies associated with their socialist past. The fall of communist regimes produced a new political environment that included both nationalist parties alarmed over population decline and an empowered Catholic Church desirous of aligning state policy with church doctrine. In Poland laws were changed in 1993 to permit abortions only to save a woman's life, preserve her health, in case of rape or incest, or if the fetus experienced irreversible damage (Kulczycki 1999). Abortions had to be performed in state hospitals and were not permitted for social or economic reasons, the grounds for 97 % of Polish abortions prior to this change in law (Titkow 1999). These restrictions, although contested several times since 1993, are still limiting Polish women's access to abortion, especially among the poor. There are consistently less than a thousand "official" abortions taking place in Poland each year. After Poland's entry into the European Union its strict enforcement of its restrictive abortion laws have produced clashes with the Council of Europe's human rights institutions. In March of 2007 the European Court of Human Rights awarded Alicja Tysiac €25,000 in damages after Polish doctors refused her request to abort a pregnancy that they knew posed serious risk to her sight (*BBC News* 2007).

Admittedly many Polish women with unwanted pregnancies travel to neighboring countries for legal abortions, but it is unclear the extent to which illegal "internal" abortions are available to women unable to afford a "tourist" abortion. It is clear, though, that these restrictions have done little to revive Polish fertility. Poland's TFR was 1.93 in 1992 and today it has declined to 1.27. Yet the debate over abortion continues, with the voices calling for even more stringent restrictions seemingly as strong as those calling for more liberal laws. In 2007 36 % of Polish parliamentarians voted for a constitutional amendment to end all abortion, a proposal put forward by the ultraconservative League of Polish Families party. This was short of the two thirds majority needed for passage, but several amendments then proposed by the late President Lech Kaczynski that would have enshrined Poland's current restrictive abortions laws in its Constitution, came much closer to passage with majorities of over 60 % (*New York Times* 2007).

Although up until now only Poland has traveled far down this path, other post socialist Eastern and Central European countries, including Russia, have nationalist parties worried about population decline, antiabortion religious traditions, and a history of the state imposing significant fertility initiatives. Some already have tightened certain abortion regulations, and so the possibility that they might end uncomplicated access to abortion cannot be dismissed. In 2003 a Russian nationalist lawmaker with support from the Russian Orthodox Church proposed legislation that would prohibit all abortions in Russia after the 12th week of pregnancy. The legislation never came up for a vote but it did trigger negotiations with the Ministry of Health and new regulations that severely limited the grounds for abortions after the 12th week of pregnancy. In this case religious antiabortion sentiment fueled by concerns over population decline worked to limit Russian women's access to abortion (Myers 2003).

In January 2010 Health Minister Tatyana Golikova stated (AFP 2010a) that Russia needed to cut its abortion rate still further in order to boost population growth: "The topic of reducing abortions is definitely on today's agenda. This won't solve the birthrate problem 100 %, but around 20–30%." The Russian "birth rate problem" is its current 1.37 total fertility rate. Russia's population has already lost eight million people from its 1995 level, and continued low fertility is accelerating this decline. Health Minister Golikova views "reducing abortions" as being a means of "solving the birthrate problem." She is clearly considering a coercive pronatalist abortion policy. The size of the birth rate, not the number of abortions, is her problem. At this stage in Russia's fertility transition abortions can be reduced by giving Russian women greater access to modern contraceptives, but such a policy shift would do very little to solve "Russia's birth rate problem." The fact that "Nashi," the Kremlin backed nationalist Russian youth group, links opposition to abortion and opposition to contraception in its policy positions hints that a more comprehensive solution to the "birth rate problem" might not be opposed in certain government circles (Arnold 2008).

Every country places some duration-of-pregnancy limitations on when legal abortions are permitted, and often there are limitations for specific grounds. The "incrementalist" regulatory changes that Russia has undertaken are examples of restriction occurring gradually in stages. Restriction also can happen through changes in the enforcement of abortion laws. This might be currently taking place in South Korea. It has had restrictive abortion laws on its books since the

1950s, but after South Korea initiated a very successful family planning campaign in 1962 abortion on demand became its de facto norm. Its TFR plummeted from 6.33 in 1955–1960 to a very low 1.6 by 1985–1990, and abortion played a significant role in the decline. Currently, an estimated 350,000 abortions are being performed each year while births are averaging about 450,000. South Korea has adopted a strong pronatalist policy over the last decade but it has not succeeded in increasing its very low fertility rate (1.22). On March 1, 2010 the Health Ministry, in an apparent response to worries about population decline, suddenly announced that it was establishing a "call center" to report illegal abortions (AFP 2010b). Informants will receive payments and obstetricians performing abortions will be referred to prosecutors for criminal charges. It is too early to know how many prosecutions have taken place or if an increase in births will result, but there are reports that the cost of an abortion has increased significantly (Yoon 2010).

Clearly policymakers in pronatalist states with liberal abortion policies already are being confronted with demographic arguments to reconsider their abortion policies. But the world has yet to truly experience what the current fertility transition has in store for it.

8.9 What the Future Holds: Low Fertility in the Twenty-First Century

States begin to worry about population decline and rapid population aging when their TFR falls noticeably below replacement levels. For this analysis "low fertility" will mean living in a country with a TFR of 1.9 or less. Currently there are 58 low fertility countries and 57 % of them have adopted pronatalist population policies. Many of the non-adopters are new arrivals to this low fertility group who until recently had much higher fertility and often active antinatalist campaigns. China is one such non-adopter. It has only recently changed its policy from one of "lowering" fertility to one of "maintaining" its current low fertility (1.7). Others, such as Iran, still have an official policy to "lower" its fertility even though its current TFR of 1.8 no longer appears to need lowering. These countries' fertility declines have been some of the most rapid ever experienced. But their cohorts of reproductive aged women have sizes that still reflect past high fertility, and therefore their populations will continue to increase for a time. China is projected to begin experiencing population decline by 2030, by which time its median age will be over 40. South Korea, which has completed a fertility transition during which its official government positions on the country's fertility level have shifted from "lower" to "maintain" to "increase," is expected to begin its period of population decline by 2025 with a median age of over 45. Predicting the eventual relationship between pronatalism and abortion policy is especially difficult for these new, largely Asian, arrivals to the low fertility group. Many have had a very rapid fertility transition which translates

Table 8.6 Percent of the world's population living in countries with total fertility rates (TFRs) of 4 or more and 1.9 or less, 1975–2035

TFR	1975[a] (%)	1985[a] (%)	1995[a] (%)	2009[a] (%)	2020–2025[b] (%)	2030–2035[b] (%)
4 or more	71.9	46.6	20.4	15.5	6.2	1.3
1.9 or less	2.4	16.0	37.6	40.0	48.1	69.1

Sources: [a]UN (2010) *World Population Policy 2009*; [b]UN (2009) *2008 Revision of World Population Prospects*

to rapid population aging and the relatively quick arrival of population decline. Their recent history of having significant government antinatalist population policies, often synchronized with liberal abortion policies, suggest policymakers with a pragmatic attitude toward abortion policy.

An unprecedented world-wide fertility transition is underway and over the next 25 years an additional 34 countries, with about 30 % of the world's population, will join the ranks of low fertility countries (Table 8.6). In 1975 72 % of the world's population was living in countries with a TFR of 4 or more, while only 2.4 % was living in countries with a TFR of 1.9 or less. Currently 15.5 % of the population is living in countries with a TFR of 4 or more, while 40 % is living in countries with a TFR of 1.9 or less. The UN projects that by 2035 just 1.3 % of the population will be living in countries with a TFR of 4 or more and 69.1 % will be living in countries with a TFR of 1.9 or less. Changes happening over the next 25 years will alter greatly the character of the low fertility country.

Currently 37 out of the 58 countries with a TFR of 1.9 or less are European (Table 8.7). In fact only two European countries have a TFR higher than 1.9: Iceland (2.1) and Ireland (2.0).[2] Even today, however, it would be incorrect to think of the world's low fertility population as being European or even as residing primarily in "more developed" countries. The 12 Asian low fertility countries actually contain well more than twice the population of all European low fertility countries (Table 8.7). Even when China's 1.35 billion are subtracted from Asia's current low fertility population, there are still 363 million Asians living in other low fertility countries. Contrary to the popular image of the low fertility country, only a third of the world's current low fertility population resides in "more developed" countries; two-thirds resides in "less developed" countries. Over the next 25 years an additional 34 countries are expected to have TFRs of 1.9 or less, and "low fertility" will assume an even greater "less developed" hue. Nineteen of these countries will be Asian, and this population will constitute 80 % of all the new additions. By 2025 Indonesia, Mongolia, Turkey and Viet Nam are projected to reach low fertility

---

[2]In addition to the 37 low fertility European countries these 21 countries currently have a TFR of 1.9 or less: Australia, Barbados, Brazil, Canada, Chile, China, Cuba, Cyprus, Georgia, Iran, Japan, Lebanon, Mauritius, North Korea, Singapore, South Korea, Thailand, Trinidad and Tobago, Tunisia, United Arab Emirates, and the United Kingdom.

Table 8.7 Countries with a total fertility rate (TFR) of 1.9 or less by region: 2009, projected new additions between 2009 and 2035, and in 2030–2035

Region	2009		New additions		2030–2035	
	Countries (N)	% world population (2009)	Countries (N)	% world population (2035)	Countries (N)	% world population (2035)
Europe	37	10.7	2	0.1	39	8.4
Asia	12	25.1	19	28.4	31	49.9
LA & Car.	5	3.3	10	2.2	15	5.2
Africa	2	0.2	1	0.1	3	0.3
North America	1	0.5	1	4.4	2	4.9
Oceania	1	0.3	1	0.1	2	0.4
Total	58	40.0	34	35.3	92	69.1

Sources: UN (2010) *World Population Policy 2009*; UN (2009) *2008 Revision of World Population Prospects*

levels. By 2035 fertility in Bangladesh, India, Malaysia, Myanmar, and Uzbekistan is expected to fall that low.[3]

By 2035 69 % of the world's population is projected to be living in low fertility countries, 73.7 % of which reside in countries currently classified as "less developed," 4.6 % in "least developed" countries, and only 21.7 % in "more developed" countries. What will this dramatically altered low fertility population mean for the makeup of countries adopting pronatalist policies? What will it mean for women's ability to have uncomplicated access to abortion?

8.10   A New Challenge for Reproductive Rights Movements

Table 8.8 examines current and projected low fertility countries in terms of their 2009 abortion policy. There is no way of "projecting" what will happen to a country's abortion policy in the future so this table is of limited predictive value. However, it does tell us the abortion policy "starting points" of countries that either have, or in the future are projected to have, low fertility. As countries experience population decline and significant population aging they will be doing so with this range of preexisting abortion policies.

At the present 45 of the 58 countries (78 %) with a TFR of 1.9 or less, containing 82 % of the low fertility population, grant women an uncomplicated access to

---

[3]Fifteen countries are projected to have a TFR of 1.9 or less by 2025: Bahamas, Bahrain, Brunei Darussalam, Costa Rica, Indonesia, Ireland, Maldives, Mexico, Mongolia, New Zealand, Saint Lucia, Turkey, United States, Uruguay, and Viet Nam. Nineteen additional countries are projected to reach that fertility level by 2035: Argentina, Azerbaijan, Bangladesh, Belize, Bhutan, Grenada, Guyana, Iceland, India, Kazakhstan, Kuwait, Kyrgyzstan, Libya, Malaysia, Myanmar, Saint Vincent and the Grenadines, Sri Lanka, Turkmenistan, and Uzbekistan.

Table 8.8 Countries with TFR ≤ 1.9 in 2009, countries projected to attain a TFR ≤ 1.9 between 2009 and 2030–2035, and countries with a TFR ≤ 1.9 in 2030–2035 by whether they permitted abortion on request or for economic or social reasons in 2009

| | | Abortion permitted on request or for economic or social reasons, 2009 | | |
		Yes	No	Total
58 countries with TFR ≤ 1.9 in 2009	Countries (n)	45	13	58
	% of countries	77.6	22.4	100
	% of population	81.8	18.2	100
34 new additions to TFR ≤ 1.9 by 2030–2035	Countries (n)	16	18	34
	% of countries	47.1	52.9	100
	% of population	77.0	23.0	100
92 countries with TFR ≤ 1.9 in 2030–2035	Countries (n)	61	31	92
	% of countries	66.3	33.7	100
	% of population	78.8	21.2	100

Sources: UN (2010) *World Population Policy 2009*; UN (2009) *2008 Revision of World Population Prospects*

abortion (Table 8.8). Since only 37 % of all countries, containing 62 % of the world's population, grant women such an access (Table 8.1), there seems to be a connection between low fertility and liberal abortion policies. However this connection, at least at the population level, is less definitive than it first appears. Much of it is due to presence of one country: China. It currently has a liberal abortion policy, a TFR of less than 1.9, and 1.35 billion people. Although only one of the 58 low fertility countries, China's population constitutes 49 % of the entire low fertility population. Only 64 % of the population of the remaining 57 low fertility countries lives with an uncomplicated access to abortion, a percentage similar to the world's average. Numerous relatively small European low fertility countries with liberal abortion policies are counterbalanced by a smaller number of populous developing countries with officially restrictive abortion policies, most notably Brazil, Iran, and Thailand.

When the current abortion policies of the 34 countries that the UN projects will enter the low fertility group by 2035 are examined (Table 8.8), a majority of them (18) restrict access to abortion. The data, however, still indicates that 77 % of the "new addition" population lives in countries with liberal abortion policies. Once again this connection of low fertility and liberal abortion policy is due to the presence of one country, in this case India. It currently has a liberal abortion policy and by 2035, it is projected to have 1.5 billion people and low fertility. India's population constitutes slightly more than half of the entire new addition population. Remove India from the new addition group and only 53.3 % of the population of the remaining 33 countries currently lives with an uncomplicated access to abortion, a percentage well below the world's average. In this remaining group there are a small number of more developed countries, most notably the United States, with liberal abortion policies, and a large number of less and least developed countries, such as Bangladesh, Indonesia, Malaysia, and Argentina, with restrictive abortion policies.

A similar observation can be made about the connection between low fertility and a liberal abortion policy data for all 92 low fertility countries projected to exist in 2035. Although 79 % of the projected low fertility population lives in countries with current liberal abortion policies, this high percentage is mainly due to two countries: China and India. The UN projects that they will have three billion people in 2035, more than half of the entire 5.9 billion projected low fertility population. Remove China and India from the group and only about 57 % of the population of the remaining 90 countries lives in a country that currently allows women an uncomplicated access to abortion in 2009.

What can we expect to happen to these countries' abortion policies as fertility decline and its consequences take hold? There is unlikely to be a single story. For example, consider China and India. China experienced a dramatic drop in its TFR from 5.9 in 1965–1970 to 2.6 in 1980–1985. After implementing its one-child campaign in 1979, fertility continued to drop to 2.0 by 1990–1995 and then to 1.7 by 2000–2005. This very rapid fall in fertility has already produced significant population aging: the median age increasing from 19.7 in 1970 to 34.2 in 2010. By 2035 the UN projects that China's population will be in decline and have a median age of 43. By 2050 the population over the age of 60 is expected to be 441 million, 31.1 % of the population. Chinese policymakers currently are considering removing restrictions from having second children, and it is unclear if ending such restrictions will have a significant effect on fertility (Morgan et al. 2009). Preliminary studies of women of childbearing age who themselves are only children, a class that is permitted to have second children under one-child regulations, indicate that their ideal family size is 1.46 and that 55 % of them think that a single child is best (Hvistendahl 2010). Even though China has long given women an uncomplicated access to abortion, its commitment to reproductive rights principles is suspect. Women have been pressured to abort wanted fetuses, for instance. State needs, not individual desires, always have determined Chinese policy. If over the course of the next 20 years Chinese policymakers determine that a fertility increase is needed, which is a likely possibility, what might happen to Chinese women's easy access to abortion? If China imposes restrictions on access to abortion, the impact on global reproductive rights would be monumental in demographic terms and could also spur efforts to delegalize abortion elsewhere. If it happened today, for instance, only 42 % of the world's population would be living in countries granting an uncomplicated access to abortion, not the current 62 %. India is a different story. Its policymakers are unlikely to feel any demographic pressure to reconsider its liberal abortion policy since it is projected to experience population decline and significant aging only in the second half of this century.

At the present, some of the lowest TFRs in the world are being experienced in more developed Asian areas, most notably in Taiwan (.94), Hong Kong (1.1), South Korea (1.2), Japan (1.3), and Singapore (1.3). They have experienced fertility levels well below replacement levels for several decades and extremely low fertility for the last decade. They have implemented substantial pronatalist programs that have yet to result in significant fertility increases (Suszuki 2009). Hong Kong and Singapore experience enough net in-migration to preclude population decline, but Japan is currently experiencing both population decline and rapid population aging; its median age is already 45. South Korea is expected to experience such changes shortly. The problems associated with their very low fertility have been extensively studied and are well known by both policymakers and the general public. Both Japan and South Korea have a past experience of harmonizing an abortion policy with an antinatalist population policy in order to facilitate fertility decline. Now there is pressure on policymakers to take effective action to increase fertility. Their tradition of viewing abortion policy in an instrumental way and the real problems associated with current very low fertility make some additional policy initiative likely, perhaps an incrementalist program of adding restrictions to women's uncomplicated access to abortion.

Most Western European countries have liberal abortion policies that originated from the presence of strong reproductive rights movements. Their current pronatalist policies are formulated to not conflict with reproductive rights principles. They seek to ensure that every woman has the means to have all the children that she desires. These countries have instituted programs that allow women to more easily participate in the labor force and have children, or that provide them with a portion of the costs associated with rearing a child. Such programs, sensitive to reproductive rights issues, are expensive and until recently have not been associated with much evidence of success. However, as "postponement" of childbearing has reached its outer limits in these countries, especially in those with "lowest low" fertility rates of 1.3 and below, there recently has been a several tenths of a child increase in fertility rates (Goldstein et al. 2009). The UN also projects a future increase, but never above 1.85. This increase works to lessen the pressure on policymakers to reassess current abortion policies. Unless the effects of the 2008–2009 global financial crisis results in a lasting period of stagnant economic growth and a return to lowest low fertility levels, then most Western European policymakers are not likely to succumb to pressures to revisit their liberal abortion policies in the near future.

In many post-socialist eastern European countries the story is different. After the breakup of the Soviet Union they have experienced fertility collapses and the early onset of actual population decline. Their current economic circumstances are not amenable to a sustained fertility revival and few governments have the resources needed to pursue meaningful non-coercive pronatalist programs. The UN projects continued significant population decline for these countries, a future that can be exploited by religious and nationalist critics of liberal abortion policies. The 2008–2009 global financial crisis has seriously impacted these countries' economies, making policymakers more susceptible to pressure from those who conflate economic and demographic decline.

About 80 % of Latin American and Caribbean countries, containing 79 % of the population, have restrictive abortion policies (Table 8.3). Only in Cuba might policymakers experience some demographic pressure to change current liberal abortion policies. Its population is projected to decline beginning in 2015; its median age is expected to be 40 in 2015 and to rise to 52 by 2050. Brazil and Uruguay also are projected to experience population decline and rapid aging during the first half of this century. However, these countries currently restrict access to abortion. Problems associated with population decline can only motivate their policymakers to keep restrictive policies in place. If Brazil and Uruguay adopt a pronatalist policy they will find their abortion policies already in harmony with it.

As low fertility becomes more widespread over the course of this century the first harmonizing of population and abortion policies will be by policymakers feeling a demographic pressure not to change restrictive abortion policies. Table 8.8 indicates that there are 31 countries whose total fertility rates are expected to be 1.9 or less in 2035 that currently have restrictive abortion policies. Fifteen are in Asia and nine are in Latin America and the Caribbean. In 2035 they are projected to include 20 % of the Asian low fertility population and 68 % of the Latin American and Caribbean low fertility population. If they keep their restrictive abortion policies these policymakers will encounter no policy "stress point" when considering a pronatalist policy. Whatever the prior reason for their restrictive abortion policies, there will now be an added demographic reason for them.

The rapid global transition from problems of population growth to problems of population decline means that the alliance between antinatalist policymakers and reproductive rights advocates is likely to quickly lose its potency. As fertility continues to decline the need for antinatalist programs diminishes, as does the ability of reproductive health advocates to use demographic arguments to extract added state resources for their programs. The window for exploiting the antinatalist stress point is short, even for Africa. Of Africa's 52 countries, 48 currently have restrictive abortion policies. The TFR of their population is 4.9. Over 70 % of these countries currently have an explicit policy to lower their fertility. Right now African policymakers are feeling the policy stress point associated with simultaneously having an antinatalist population policy and a restrictive abortion policy. By 2035 the TFR of these 48 countries is projected to fall to below 3.0. Policymakers then will be feeling noticeably less demographic pressure to liberalize their abortion policy, especially in a world where problems of low fertility hold center stage.

8.11 Responding to the Challenge

Historically, a number of states have adopted coercive pronatalist policies that stripped women of access to both contraception and abortion. Over the course of the twentieth century a consensus has developed about individuals having the right to practice contraception to control their fertility. Few states are likely to now adopt a coercive pronatalist policy that restricts access to contraception. However, no consensus has developed about women having an uncomplicated access to abortion. Abortion policies vary widely among states and have changed over time. This volatility and lack of consensus allows policymakers greater latitude in shaping abortion policies to further population goals. In an era of intensifying low fertility, population aging, and population decline, this presents a new challenge to reproductive rights movements. Increasing numbers of states that have no history of permitting women an easy access to legal abortion will be adopting pronatalist policies and their policymakers now will find it demographically advantageous to preserve restrictions. Others states that might have adopted liberal abortion policies as part of their former antinatalist stance, but that have a weak commitment to reproductive rights principles, are likely to reconsider their abortion policies under conditions of population decline. Even states with long traditions of support for reproductive rights principles might find that the growing social and economic consequences of population decline will make abiding by these principles more difficult.

There will be no simple solution to this threat to reproductive rights. Greater access to modern contraception is unlikely to eliminate unwanted births. A new low fertility regime is sweeping the world in which childbearing is taking place at later ages. More women are finding themselves in a situation comparable to that currently experienced by women in more developed countries: sexual activity is initiated well before children are wanted; childbearing is being postponed to later ages; and the desired number of children is falling to low levels. The number of years in which women are fecund and sexually active but want no children is increasing. Abortion has played a far from trivial role in how women in more developed countries have accomplished their new fertility goals. Currently, compared to those in less developed countries (Singh et al. 2010: 244), women in more developed countries have both a higher proportion of pregnancies that are said to be unintended (47 % vs. 40 %) and a higher proportion of their unintended pregnancies ending in abortion (53 % vs. 48 %). This is true even though their contraceptive prevalence rates are higher than those of women in less developed countries. There will be a continual need for an uncomplicated access to abortion as women in less developed countries enter more fully into this new low fertility regime.

Of course better access to more effective contraception is a good thing. But the threat to women's access to legal abortions to end unwanted pregnancies needs to be met by directly advocating clear reproductive rights principles, not simply by calling for more and better contraceptives. Ideologically, every pronatalist abortion policy is necessarily coercive and needs to be labeled as such. Requiring a woman to bring an unwanted pregnancy to term in order to increase a birth rate is a deliberately coercive population control policy. While it is true that past implementations of pronatalist abortion policies have had devastating effects on the health of pregnant women and the wellbeing of the many unwanted children who were abandoned or abused after birth, more than health arguments need to be made when criticizing these programs. These policies are wrong primarily because they take away a woman's right to determine whether and when to bear a child. This right requires a woman to have access to effective contraceptives *and* to safe abortions. What needs to be promoted now is a deep commitment by policymakers to the right of the individual woman to determine her own fertility. Only if policymakers have a clear history of a commitment to this right will they be able to resist the strong demographic pressures to adopt pronatalist abortion policies that they are likely to face in the future.

References

AFP. (2010a, January 18). Russia should cut abortions to boost population: Minister. *Agence France-Presse.* http://www.google.com/hostednews/afp/article/ALeqM5hhJEe6ViM4HNO Dw5vsHlgVc_i5lQ

AFP. (2010b, March 1). S. Korea clamps down on abortion to boost birthrate. *Agence France-Presse.* http://www.google.com/hostednews/afp/article/ALeqM5j_bk9WlSxA1ZubHhho4_ QiYiEQkQ

Arnold, C. (2008, June 28). *Abortion remains top birth-control option in Russia.* Radio Free Europe/Radio Liberty. http://www.rferl.org/content/Abortion_Remains_Top_Birth_Control_ Option_Russia/1145849.html

Baban, A. (1999). Romania. In H. P. David & J. Skilogianis (Eds.), *From abortion to contraception: A resource to public policies and reproductive behavior in central and Eastern Europe from 1917 to the present* (pp. 191–222). Westport: Greenwood Press.

BBC News. (2007, March 20). *Polish woman wins abortion case.* http://news.bbc.co.uk/2/hi/ europe/6470403.stm

Benedict XVI. (2006). *Address of his holiness Benedict XVI to the participants in the Plenary Assembly of the Pontifical Council for the Family.* http://www.vatican.va/holy_father/bene-dict_xvi/speeches/2006/may/documents/hf_ben-xvi_spe_20060513_pc-family_en.html

Benedict XVI. (2007a). *Address of his holiness Benedict XVI to the participants in the convention organized by the Commission of the Bishops' Conferences of the European Community (Comece).* http://www.vatican.va/holy_father/benedict_xvi/speeches/2007/march/documents/ hf_ben-xvi_spe_20070324_comece_en.html

Benedict XVI. (2007b). *Apostolic journey of his holiness Benedict XVI to Austria on the occasion of the 850th anniversary of the foundation of the Shrine of Mariazell: Meeting with the authorities and the diplomatic corps.* http://www.vatican.va/holy_father/benedict_xvi/speeches/2007/ september/documents/hf_ben-xvi_spe_20070907_hofburg-wien_en.html

Benedict XVI. (2007c). *Address of his holiness Benedict XVI to the participants in the General Assembly of the Pontifical Academy for Life.* http://www.vatican.va/holy_father/benedict_xvi/ speeches/2007/february/documents/hf_ben-xvi_spe_20070224_academy-life_en.html

Benedict XVI. (2008). *Address of his holiness Benedict XVI to the bishops of Hungary on their 'Ad Limina' visit.* http://www.vatican.va/holy_father/benedict_xvi/speeches/2008/may/documents/ hf_ben-xvi_spe_20080510_hungarian-bishops_en.html

Benedict XVI. (2009). Encyclical letter *Caritas in Veritate* of the Supreme Pontiff Benedict XVI. http://www.vatican.va/holy_father/benedict_xvi/encyclicals/documents/hf_ben-xvi_enc_ 20090629_caritas-in-veritate_en.html

David, H. P. (1992). Abortion in Europe, 1920–91: A public health perspective. *Studies in Family Planning, 23*(1), 1–22.

Davis, K., & Blake, J. (1956). Social structure and fertility: An analytic framework. *Economic Development and Cultural Change, 4*(3), 211–235.

Frejka, T. (1985). Induced abortion and fertility. *Family Planning Perspectives, 17*(5), 230–234.

Goldstein, J. R., Sobotka, T., & Jasilioniene, A. (2009). The end of lowest-low fertility? *Population and Development Review, 35*(4), 663–699.

Himes, N. E. (1932, March). Birth control in historical and clinical perspective. *The Annals of the American Academy of Political and Social Science, 160,* 49–65.

Hodgson, D. (2009). Abortion, family planning, and population policy: Prospects for the common-ground approach. *Population and Development Review, 35*(3), 479–518.

Hodgson, D., & Watkins, S. C. (1997). Feminists and neo-Malthusians: Past and present alliances. *Population and Development Review, 23*(3), 469–523.

Hvistendahl, M. (2010). Has China outgrown the one-child policy? *Science, 329*(5998), 1458–1461.

John Paul II. (2002). *Visit to the Italian Parliament (Palazzo Montecitorio in Rome).* http://www. vatican.va/holy_father/john_paul_ii/speeches/2002/november/documents/hf_jp-ii_spe_ 20021114_italian-parliament_en.html

Kulczycki, A. (1999). *The abortion debate in the World Arena*. New York: Routledge.

Morgan, S. P., Zhigang, G., & Hayford, S. R. (2009). China's below-replacement fertility: Recent trends and future prospects. *Population and Development Review, 35*(3), 605–629.

Myers, S. L. (2003, August 24). After decades, Russia narrows grounds for abortions. *New York Times*: http://www.nytimes.com/2003/08/24/world/after-decades-russia-narrows-grounds-for-abortions.html?pagewanted=2&src=pm

New York Times. (2007, April 14). Poland: Parliament rejects move to ban abortion. http://www.nytimes.com/2007/04/14/world/europe/14briefs-abortion.html?_r=0

Sedgh, G., Singh, S., Shah, I. H., Åhman, E., Henshaw, S. K., & Bankole, A. (2012). Induced abortion: Incidence and trends worldwide from 1995 to 2008. *Lancet, 379*, 625–632.

Singh, S., Wulf, D., Hussain, R., Bankole, A., & Sedgh, G. (2009). *Abortion worldwide: A decade of uneven progress*. New York: Guttmacher Institute.

Singh, S., Sedgh, G., & Hussain, R. (2010). Unintended pregnancy: Worldwide levels, trends, and outcomes. *Studies in Family Planning, 41*(4), 241–250.

Suszuki, T. (2009). Fertility decline and governmental interventions in Eastern Asian advanced countries. *Japanese Journal of Population, 7*(1), 47–56.

Titkow, A. (1999). Poland. In H. P. David & J. Skilogianis (Eds.), *From abortion to contraception: A resource to public policies and reproductive behavior in Central and Eastern Europe from 1917 to the present* (pp. 165–190). Westport: Greenwood Press.

Trujillo, C. A. L. (2003). *The family and life in Europe*. http://www.vatican.va/roman_curia/pontifical_councils/family/documents/rc_pc_family_doc_20030614_family-europe-trujillo_en.html

UN. (2002). *Abortion policies: A global review* (Vols. 1–3). New York: United Nations. http://www.un.org/esa/population/publications/abortion/

UN. (2009). *World population prospects: The 2008 revision*. New York: United Nations. http://www.un.org/esa/population/publications/wpp2008/wpp2008_text_tables.pdf

UN. (2010). *World population policies 2009*. New York: United Nations. http://www.un.org/esa/population/publications/wpp2009/wpp2009.htm

WHO. (2003). *Safe abortion: Technical and policy guidance for health systems*. Geneva: World Health Organization.

WHO. (2004). *Abortion and contraception in Romania: A strategic assessment of policy, programme and research issues*. Geneva: World Health Organization.

WHO. (2011). *Unsafe abortion: Global and regional estimates of the incidence of unsafe abortion and associated mortality in 2008* (6th ed.). Geneva: World Health Organization.

World Bank. (2009). *World development indicators database*. http://databank.worldbank.org/data/views/variableSelection/selectvariables.aspx?source=world-development-indicators

Yoon, S. (2010, March 17). South Korean women caught in abortion limbo. *Seattle Times* (Associated Press). http://seattletimes.com/html/nationworld/2011366974_apasskoreaabortiondebate.html

Chapter 9
Climate Change Science, Policy and Programming: Where Are Population and Reproductive Health?

Karen Hardee

9.1 Introduction

Climate change is among the most pressing issues facing the world today. Its severity, causes, consequences and solutions are the subject of continued scientific scrutiny and policy discourse. Evidence overwhelmingly implicates human activity in the rise of greenhouse gas emissions that is leading to climate change (IPCC 2007). With their high past and present consumption rates, affluent populations have undoubtedly contributed most to climate change to date; however, ongoing rapid population growth in other world regions exacerbates scarcity of food and water, vulnerability to natural disasters and infectious diseases, and population displacement, which are all linked to climate change (UNFPA 2009; Jiang and Hardee 2010). Fertility rates have fallen in much of the world; yet the global population is still growing and more than half (27) of the world's 49 least developed countries are projected to at least double their current population by 2050, according to UN population projections. If, as Cohen (2010) suggests, people are part of the problem and part of the solution, where does population, and particularly reproductive health, fit into climate science and into the climate change policy discourse? Is reproductive health being factored into programs to address climate change and if so, how, and how could it be better considered in the equation?

The potential effects of climate change are enormous and stem from an accumulation of greenhouse gas emissions that trap heat in the atmosphere. Over the last 100 years, the temperature of the earth's surface has risen 0.74 °C (IPCC 2007) and the pace of temperature rise is increasing. Rising temperatures are leading to sea level rise, and greater variability in weather, including droughts in some places and severe storms and flooding in other places. While the industrialized world has

K. Hardee, Ph.D. (✉)
Center for Policy and Advocacy, Futures Group, Washington, DC, USA
e-mail: KHardee@futuresgroup.com

A. Kulczycki (ed.), *Critical Issues in Reproductive Health*, The Springer Series on Demographic Methods and Population Analysis 33, DOI 10.1007/978-94-007-6722-5_9,
© Springer Science+Business Media Dordrecht 2014

contributed most to the buildup of greenhouse gases in the atmosphere, it is the developing world, where most of the world's people live, that will suffer the worst effects, even though those countries have contributed least to climate change. The impacts of climate change are already being felt and are most likely to get worse in the future (IPCC 2001). Responding to climate change will require multifaceted responses to keep global temperatures from rising beyond which catastrophic outcomes could result (IPCC 2007).

This chapter examines the evidence linking climate change with population and reproductive health, and addresses three challenges to incorporating population and reproductive health into climate change programming. The chapter also reviews current programming on mitigation and adaptation to climate change to assess how population, and specifically how reproductive health could be included. In the process, we also briefly address how this important, complex and poorly understood topic has been presented in often confusing terms to publics through both the media and policy discourse.[1]

9.2 Evidence Linking Population, Reproductive Health and Climate Change

Population, defined in its broadest sense to include a range of demographic factors such as size and growth, age composition, geographic distribution, household size and migration patterns, is potentially linked to climate change in three ways. First, population serves as a potential driver of carbon emissions. Second, population growth translates into increasing numbers of people exposed to the impact of climate change. Third, population dynamics influence adaptation to changes in climate. Reproductive health, a good in its own right, helps women control their own fertility and is hypothesized to strengthen their ability to cope with changes in climate – for themselves and their families. Reproductive health, to the extent that access to family planning is expanded and women choose to have fewer children, is linked to climate change mitigation through affecting fertility rates. Micro fertility decisions add up to macro populations.

9.2.1 Population, Reproductive Health and Mitigation

Current attention to addressing climate change is based on climate models projecting greenhouse gas emissions into the future. The 2007 Intergovernmental Panel on Climate Change (IPCC) Special Report on Emission Scenarios identified population growth, economic growth, technological change, and changes in patterns of energy

---

[1] For example, even by the occasional sensationalist standards of the media, prominent U.S. and English newspapers have also often reduced the topic to emotive levels by turning out headlines such as: "Can condoms combat climate change? *Los Angeles Times*, September 17, 2009; and "Stop Blaming the Poor: it's the wally yachters who are burning the planet," *Guardian*, September 28, 2009.

and land use as the major driving forces of the growth in greenhouse gas emissions (Nakicenovic et al. 2000). This report paid significant attention to population size, the only demographic factor currently included in emissions scenario modeling related to climate change. Including only population size and growth has introduced an erroneous assumption of homogeneity in consumption patterns within a population. Instead, studies conducted over the past two decades have found that urban–rural residence, age structure, and household size are demographic characteristics associated with different patterns of energy consumption (Jones 1989; Yamasaki and Tominaga 1997; Pachauri and Jiang 2008). Projections of future population also suggest that total population size, aging, urbanization and declining average household size will be important demographic trends in the coming decades (Lutz and Samir 2010).

Given the UN population projections that show the world's population in 2050 could range between roughly 8 and 11 billion people, some researchers have asked what difference those trajectories make to carbon emissions. Using climate modeling techniques,[2] O'Neill and colleagues (2010: 17521) show that "slowing population growth could provide 16–29 % of the emissions reductions suggested to be necessary by 2050 to avoid dangerous climate change." Their model included urbanization, age structure and household size in addition to population size and growth. They found that while urbanization is the predominant demographic feature related to climate change in developing countries, aging is the dominant demographic feature in the industrialized world.

Building on the analysis by O'Neill and colleagues, Wheeler and Hammer analyzed the contribution that family planning could make to addressing mitigation. Their analysis showed that "both female education and family planning are highly cost-competitive with almost all the existing options for carbon emissions abatement via low-carbon energy and forestry/agriculture" (Wheeler and Hammer 2010: 4) Such other options include wind, and nuclear power, second-generation biofuels, and carbon capture and storage. In their analysis, family planning cost $17 per ton of carbon abated, far less than other options. An earlier, less rigorous analysis, which received wide media coverage, likewise concluded that family planning can make a highly cost-effective contribution to addressing climate change (Wire 2009).

Another line of research related to fertility, reproductive health and climate change has attempted to measure the "carbon legacy" of childbearing. Large differences in fertility levels and emission rates exist between the 11 most populous countries in the world, namely China, India, the United States, Indonesia, Brazil, Pakistan, Bangladesh, Russia, Nigeria, Japan and Mexico (Murtaugh and Schlax 2009).[3] In the United States, where half of all pregnancies (49 %) are

---

[2]Their analysis uses the Population-Environment-Technology (PET) model, "a nine-region dynamic computable general equilibrium model of the global economy with a basic economic structure that is representative of the state of the art in emissions scenario modeling" (O'Neill et al. 2010: 17521).

[3]In this analysis, "each legacy is the sum of the lifetime emissions of the ancestral female subject to the 2005 fertility rate, plus the weighted emissions of her descendants, assuming all future reproduction follows the medium-variant projection of fertility for her home country" (Murtaugh and Schlax 2009: 18).

Table 9.1 Lifetime emissions of CO_2 saved by various actions, for the United States, 2007

Action	CO_2 saved (metric tons[a])
Increase car's fuel economy from 20 to 30 mpg	148
Reduce miles driven from 231 to 155 per week	147
Replace single-glazed windows with energy efficient windows	121
Replace ten 75-W incandescent bulbs with 25-W energy-efficient lights	36
Replace old refrigerator with energy-efficient model	19
Recycle newspaper, magazines, glass, plastic, aluminum, and steel cans	17
Reduce number of children by one	
Constant-emissions scenario[b]	9,441
Optimistic scenario[c]	562
Pessimistic scenario[d]	12,730

Source: Murtaugh and Schlax (2009: Table 3, p. 18)
See Murtaugh and Schlax (2009) for more detail on the methodology
[a] One metric ton equals 2205 lb; mpg = miles per gallon; 2 = watts
[b] Optimistic scenario: Per capita emission rate changes linearly from its 2005 value to a global target of 0.5 t CO_2 per person per year by 2100, and emissions continue at that rate indefinitely
[c] Constant scenario: Per capita emission rates remain indefinitely at their 2005 values
[d] Pessimistic scenario: Per capita emissions rate increases linearly from its 2005 value to 1.5 times its 2005 value by 2100, and emissions continue at that rate indefinitely

unintended (Finer and Henshaw 2006), the average emissions added by having a single child is 9,441 metric tons compared to 56 metric tons in Bangladesh. Table 9.1 shows, for the United States, the relative contribution of changing fertility behavior compared to other behavior change related to climate change. This line of research has spawned a new label – GINK – green inclination, no kids, which Hymas (2010: 1) describes as "a luxurious indulgence that just so happens to cost a lot less for me and weigh a lot less on the carbon-bloated atmosphere." This research reinforces that fertility choices of individuals and couples have implications for carbon emissions and climate change. Of course, fertility choices in the United States have much more impact on carbon emissions than the fertility decisions in the developing world.

9.2.2 Population, Reproductive Health and Adaptation

While most effort has focused on reducing carbon emissions through mitigation, over the past decade it has become increasingly clear that adaptation to the inevitable effects of rising global temperatures is also critical. The prevailing focus in the research and discourse on population and climate change mitigation obscures discussion of the role that addressing population and demographic factors, and incorporating reproductive health, might play in adaptation. Definitions of adaptation, vulnerability and resilience focus on systems. Adaptation includes initiatives and measures to reduce the vulnerability of natural and human systems against actual or expected climate change effects. Vulnerability is characterized as how a system is exposed to climate change and variation, its sensitivity to the effects, and its adaptive capacity (IPCC 2007). Resilience is the inverse of vulnerability. Vulnerability and adaptive capacity of individuals are not included in definitions related to climate change adaptation. Research on impacts, vulnerability and adaptation continues to be dominated by the natural rather than the social sciences (Malone 2009). Schensul and Dodman (2010: 1) contend that "current approaches to vulnerability and adaptation are based on a model with hidden gaps in understanding, which results in the links between population dynamics and vulnerability being ignored, assumed, or glossed over." McLeman (2010) offers a typology of the interactions between population change and vulnerability to climate change that addresses conditions of population increase, decrease and stability, and high volatility (for example rapid changes in population triggered by climatic or non-climatic events).

Studying adaptation in small communities in eastern Ontario, Canada, (McLeman 2010: 312) found that "adaptive capacity at the community level can change over time, and can be very sensitive to changes in the demographic composition of the community" Writing about the impacts of climate change for the United States, Karl et al. (2009) noted that demographic factors as well as aging infrastructure, buildings, and air pollution, will exacerbate climate change impacts. Assessment of migration in relation to climate change is beginning.

There is an emerging literature on the links among population, fertility and reproductive health and adaptation to climate change (UNFPA 2009; Hoepf Young et al. 2009; Jiang and Hardee 2010; Mogelgaard 2010; Stephenson et al. 2010). Poor reproductive health contributes to one-third of the burden of disease among women (WHO 2005) and can be exacerbated by climate change. Providing women and couples with the ability to have their desired number and spacing of children can contribute to promoting adaptive capacity within families and communities. Analysis of National Adaptation Programmes of Action (NAPAs), developed under the auspices of the United Nations Framework Convention on Climate Change (UNFCCC) by 49 of the world's least developed countries and small island states, found that among 41 NAPAs completed by May 2009, fully 37 mentioned rapid population growth as a factor exacerbating the effects of climate change (Mutunga and Hardee 2009; Bryant et al. 2009).

A study from several areas of Ethiopia sought to determine if people living under changing climate conditions considered population and fertility pressures to be related to climate change. The study also explored the potential roles of family planning and reproductive health in increasing resilience to climate change impacts. Women and men both described the increasing challenges they face in adapting to climate change. Specifically, they recounted how rising temperatures, more frequent draughts, increased flooding, receding agricultural grazing land and diminishing forests, were making it more difficult for their families and communities to cope. They linked population pressure to the effects of climate change and reported that families should consider having fewer children to avoid as much hardship in making a living and in utilizing natural resources for survival. As one young rural woman from Ethiopia explained:

... if a family has limited children, he will have enough land for his kids and hence we can protect the forests.... In earlier years we had a lot of fallow lands, but now as a result of population growth we don't have adequate fallow land. Therefore, limiting number of children will help us to cope with the change in climate (Kidanu et al. 2009: 3).

An assessment of vulnerability to glacier ice melts in Asia also noted that "existing vulnerabilities in human health status, population pressure, degraded ecosystems and – especially – water stress make societies and ecosystems vulnerable to any changes in water availability as glacier melt accelerates in the coming decades" (Malone 2010: 5). The need to address population pressure, including through meeting family planning needs, was one of nine cross-sectoral approaches recommended to addressing glacier melt.

9.3 Population and Reproductive Health in Climate Change Programming

Analysis of the links between NAPAs and national development plans, using population as an example, shows that critical issues such as population pressure and dynamics are falling through the cracks in both climate change adaptation programming and in development assistance (Hardee and Mutunga 2009). In all, 85 % of the countries that wrote NAPAs cited population pressure as an issue exacerbating the effects of climate change, only six suggested that addressing population should be part of the country's adaptation strategy, two proposed projects that included family planning/reproductive health and no projects were funded. While NAPAs are not the only climate adaptation programming, they may give an instructive representation of such programming, which focuses on addressing climate change adaptation through technological solutions to climate change systems (e.g. building seawalls). Among the 448 projects proposed in 41 NAPAs, half address three issues: food security (21 %), water resources (16 %) and terrestrial ecosystems (15 %). The social sectors are hardly addressed. The health sector accounts for about 7 % of the total projects and the education sector is not represented. Reasons for these omissions are discussed below.

Community-based adaptation (CBA), a newly emerging type of climate adaptation programming, offers a potential for integrated programming that focuses on natural and human systems. CBA fosters community-engagement and projects are developed based on climate science and local knowledge about weather trends and ways to adapt to the trends (Reid et al. 2009). CBA is supposed to be designed to meet community needs, therefore if a community identifies population growth or lack of access to reproductive health services or education as issues related to their ability to adapt to climate change, CBA projects should be able to accommodate these issues. A number of international organizations, including the United Nations Development Program (UNDP) and non-governmental organizations (NGOs) have embraced CBA; however, analysis of projects to date suggest that the bias against social sector programming continues. For example, although UNDP's CBA project activities are designed to increase the resilience of land and biodiversity resources to the impacts of climate

Table 9.2 Unmet need[a] for contraception in ten countries with CBA projects

Country	Unmet need among married women (%)	Year
Bangladesh	17.1	2007
Bolivia	20.2	2008
Guatemala	27.6	2002
Jamaica	11.7	2002/3
Kazakhstan	8.7	1999
Morocco	10	2003/4
Namibia	6.7	2006/7
Niger	15.8	2006
Samoa	45.6	2009
Vietnam	4.8	2002

Source: National surveys, various years. Compiled by author and colleagues at the Population Reference Bureau
[a] Unmet need is the percent of married women who are fecund and who desire to postpone or stop childbearing, but who are not currently using a contraceptive method

change (UNDP 2010a), none of the projects include components related to reproductive health, despite high levels of unmet need for family planning in a number of the countries in which UNDP is supporting CBA projects (Table 9.2).

9.4   Challenges to Incorporating Population and Reproductive Health into Climate Change Programming

While population size, growth and dynamics, are among the factors contributing to greenhouse gas emissions, I argue that there are three challenges to incorporating population and reproductive health into climate change programming. The first challenge is the continued sensitivity of the term "population," which makes it difficult to consider population variables in climate change programming. The second challenge relates to the architecture that has been built to respond to climate change, which is not conducive to addressing population and reproductive health. The third challenge is that the evidence base on the links between reproductive health and climate change is only slowly emerging.

9.4.1   Population Continues to Be a Highly Sensitive Topic

Since 1995, the world's nations have been convening through annual Conference of the Parties (COP) under the UNFCCC to address global policy responses. Controversy surrounding population and climate change was again evident at the

16th COP held in Cancun, Mexico, 2010, indicating the contested place of population thinking in the policy discourse. When the results of a recent analysis about the effects of population on global greenhouse gas emissions were presented (O'Neill et al. 2010), Ted Turner, an American media mogul and philanthropist who established the UN Foundation and is known for his gifts to environmental and population causes, "urged world leaders to institute a global one-child policy to save the Earth's environment" (McCarthy 2010). In response, Mary Robinson, former president of Ireland, UN High Commissioner for Human Rights and Chair of the International Institute for Environment and Development, warned that such radical prescriptions would ensure that population would be left off the agenda of international climate talks.

At the time of COP 15 in Copenhagen, 2009, an Australian Member of Parliament wrote, "People who believe that we can meet serious carbon targets without curbing population growth are...delusional" (Thompson 2009). Prior to the meeting, the head of the UNFCC had reportedly said: "A lot of people say population pressure is a major driving force behind the increase in emissions, and that's absolutely true but then to say, 'OK, that means we need to have a population policy that reduces emissions,' takes you onto shaky ground morally" (Casey 2008). India's Minister for the Environment warned that population should be kept off the table in Copenhagen (Crossette 2009).

After all, per capita emissions in the developing world are far lower than in the industrialized world. In 2007 per capita emissions in North America were 15.8 metric tons of CO_2 per capita, compared to 1.0 in Africa (US Energy Information Administration 2010). And yet, virtually all population growth is taking place in the developing world. In 2010, 82 % of the world's population lived in today's developing nations, a percentage that will likely rise to 85 % in 2035 (UN Population Division 2010). As people in those countries progress economically, as they should, emissions will grow. Already, total emissions from China outstrip those of the United States. At the 2009 COP, the Chinese government added fuel to the discussion by claiming that its one-child policy had resulted in 400 million fewer births since 1979, with a concomitant reduction in carbon dioxide emissions of 1.8 billion tons per year (McCarthy 2010), raising the ire of critics of China's strict population policy. A prominent *New York Times* foreign affairs correspondent, who covered population issues for many years, concluded that population will not be included in climate talks because "family planning is a toxic subject in too many places, best buried as a malingering relative of Malthusian population 'control'" (Crossette 2009: 1).

In addition to the policy discourse, a robust debate has emerged among the population and sexual reproductive health and rights communities about linking "population" with climate change. Some researchers and advocates have also joined the critique, identifying "advocates for population control" seeking to "regain ground–and capture new resources—by taking advantage of international concern about climate change" (Silliman 2009). Some have even called proponents of population and climate change programming as racist, saying that to

Table 9.3 Illustration of core development, climate resilient development and adaptation activities and eligible financing

Action	Financing	Example
Core development	Domestic budgets plus Overseas Development Assistance (ODA)	Investments in education and health, income-generation programs; etc.
Climate resilient development	Increased ODA plus additional climate finance	Accelerated agricultural diversification; climate resilient road construction and irrigation systems, climate forecasting; capacity building, etc.
Adaptation	New and additional climate finance	Seawalls; dikes; additional shelters and water storage

Source: World Bank (2010a)

mention population in this context implies "the 'new' population control craze" (Hartmann 2009: 1). Still others caution that the topic should be approached cautiously and in an ethical manner (Petroni 2010) with an environmental justice frame (Mazur 2009).

9.4.2   The Architecture to Address Climate Change Is not Conducive for Incorporating Population and Reproductive Health

The second challenge for incorporating population and reproductive health into climate change programming is that the global architecture that has been built under the auspices of the UNFCCC to respond to climate change is designed to augment but not be integrated into development assistance. Climate change programs are supposed to take development strategies into consideration but not to replace development programming. NAPAs, for example, are to be developed in alignment with national development plans. The issue is "additionality," or the principle that climate funding is not supposed to replace development assistance, but be provided to countries in addition to development funding (Agrawala and Fankhauser 2008; Huq and Ayers 2008). Calls to link climate change and development programming tend to focus on "climate-proofing development" with continued development funding for traditional development activities, with the addition of climate funding to pay for ensuring that climate change is considered. Analysis from the World Bank (2010a) illustrates additionality through showing what types of programming are eligible for climate financing verses development financing (Table 9.3). Programming to address population issues, including reproductive health and related activities such as girls' education, which could build resilience in women, are currently solely in the "core development funding" category. To date, few voices from the climate change adaptation community are calling for

Table 9.4 Additional resource needs for female education and family planning: 2000–2050

Year	School-age females not in school (millions)	% of school-age females not in school (millions)	Additional resources for 100 % enrollment ($ millions)	Women not served by family planning (millions)	Women not served as % of fertile age women	Additional resources for service extension ($ millions)
2000	216	30	21,735	145	13	2,669
2010	180	24	23,143	148	11	1,853
2020	152	20	25,150	144	10	1,453
2030	122	15	26,014	138	9	1,132
2040	94	12	26,801	130	9	913
2050	74	10	28,642	127	8	809

Source: Wheeler and Hammer (2010: 28)
See Wheeler and Hammer (2010) for explanation of methodology

inclusion of population and reproductive health into climate change programming. Those calls are coming from some in the population and reproductive health community.

9.4.3 Evidence on Reproductive Health and Climate Change Is Slowing Emerging

As noted above, the evidence base linking reproductive health and climate change adaptation is scant and only recently remerging. More analyses and especially country studies are urgently needed to show the effects of reproductive health programming – in addition to other social sector programming such as promoting girls' education – on building resilience and helping people and communities adapt to climate change.

Emerging research is stimulating calls for renewed commitment to fully funding reproductive health and family planning programs, in addition to other notable social programs. Responses related to demographic issues that affect climate changes include universal secondary education, voluntary contraception, maternal health services, and smarter urban design and construction. These have also been noted as "effective responses to the twin challenges of reducing poverty and reducing greenhouse gas emissions" (Cohen 2010: 179). It has also been observed that "family planning policies would have a substantial environmental co-benefit" (O'Neill et al. 2010: 17525) and that, if unmet need for family planning were satisfied in all countries, world population growth would fall between the UN's low and medium projections (Moreland et al. 2010).

Wheeler and Hammer (2010) found a strong synergy between the potential contribution of family planning and female education to emissions reductions. Further, they concluded that given the benefits of both interventions to sustainable development and climate change, their low cost and the likely funding shortfall for both (see Table 9.4), "the evidence is strongly consistent with an allocation of some carbon mitigation resources to the population policy options" (p. 16).

9.5   Population, Health and Environment Programming as a Model for Community-Based Adaptation (CBA)

Population, Health and Environment (PHE) programming, which acknowledges and addresses the complex connections between humans, their health, and their environment, offers a promising approach to climate change adaptation, most notably CBA. PHE programs in the Philippines (D'Agnes et al. 2010), Ethiopia (Worku 2007; Hardee et al. 2010), Cambodia (Conservation International 2008); Tanzania (Torell et al. 2010), Nepal (D'Agnes et al. 2009), and Madagascar (Mohan 2009), among other countries, illustrate the effect of addressing natural resources, livelihoods, population and health simultaneously. In Palawan province in the Philippines, for example, programming that integrated coastal resources management (CRM) and reproductive health services in one municipality, compared to separate programming (reproductive health in one municipality and CRM in another municipality), "generated higher impacts on human and ecosystem health outcomes compared to the independent coastal resources management and reproductive health interventions" (Table 9.5). Project beneficiaries also perceived the integrated programming approach as more realistically addressing their needs. Youth, for example, were encouraged to become stewards of the environment and of their sexuality (D'Agnes et al. 2010).

In Nepal, a PHE project in the Terai Region tested whether forest user groups could include family planning and education with programming addressing conservation, health and sustainable livelihood activity (D'Agnes et al. 2009). Over a 2 year period, the project taught women and girls about reproductive health, family planning and environmental issues, provided education and services to promote safer sex and condom use, conducted media campaigns and promoted energy efficiency in homes.

Table 9.5 Statistically significant trends on selected indicators (2001–2007) from integrated reproductive health and coastal resources management project in the Philippines

Indicators	CRM + RH	RH only	CRM only
RH and food security indicators			
Youth contraceptive use during first sexual intercourse	+	−	−
Proportion of young (15–24) males sexually active	+	−	−
Proportion of households dependent on fishing	+	−	−
Community knowledge of dynamite use in fishing	+	−	−
Community knowledge of cyanide use in fishing	+	−	−
CRM indicators			
Coral reef: conditions index	+	−	−
Reef fish: target species richness	−	−	+
Reef fish: total species density	−	+	−
Mangrove: volume	+	O	O
Mangrove: density	+	O	O
Mangrove: mean diameter at breast height	−	−	−
Mangrove: regeneration	O	−	O

Source: D'Agnes et al. (2010: 10)

CRM costal resources management project components, *RH* reproductive health components

Key: +, trend in the desired direction; O, trend in undesired direction; −, no trend

Contraceptive use in the project area rose from 43 % to nearly 73 %. The project helped shift attitudes towards the benefits of family planning from simply improved health to also contributing to resource management. Similarly in the coastal reserve Velondriake on the southwest coast of Madagascar, integrated programming that protects coral reefs, mangroves, seagrass beds, baobab forests and other threatened habitats, in addition to providing family planning at the request of women in the 25 villages in the reserve, has improved both natural resource management and increased use of family planning (Mohan 2009). Tanzania is experiencing climate change, including altered precipitation and increased sea surface temperatures that are affecting coastal communities. In preparing community-based climate change vulnerability and adaptation action plans for a project in the Bagamoyo district, attention is being given to environmental impacts and to population, health, equity and food security – all issues that arose during preparatory discussions with the communities (Torrell et al. 2010).

Including an expanded focus in climate change adaptation assessments is not automatic; indeed, population is virtually absent in most adaptation assessment tools. UNDP (2010b) guidelines for implementing gender-sensitive adaptation programming do not mention reproductive health. Given its attention to both the human and natural aspects of systems that are supposed to be the focus on climate change adaptation programs, PHE programs should be eligible for climate change adaptation funding, including funding for CBA programming (Bremner et al. 2011).

9.6 Discussion

Emerging evidence highlights both the link between macro population trends and climate change as well as the benefits of promoting rights-based, voluntary reproductive health programs to contribute to building resilience in women to the effects of climate change. Increasing calls are being made to address population factors, often with a focus on reproductive health, as part of climate change programming, and with climate funding.

Despite this mounting evidence, evidence-based policymaking on this topic is fraught with sensitivity. Population dynamics are related in complex ways to climate change. How many people there are on earth, where they live, their age structure and household composition, their fertility, their education and health status, their patterns of movement, their use of energy and consumption levels all matter, and should be well understood to address climate change.

While evidence is emerging, there is a need for continued research on the links between demographic factors, reproductive health and climate change. Climate change adaptation is a new area and the literature on impacts, vulnerability and adaptation contains little on population issues (Malone 2009). Emerging evidence shows that a range of demographic factors need to be considered in climate change programming. There is a need to develop and evaluate the effects of programs that do address demographic factors and integrate reproductive health with other interventions to address climate change.

Both in climate science and in the policy discourse, the term population has been narrowly framed by many to mean size and growth – with a policy prescription to "control" numbers, through controlling women's fertility in developing countries. This framing has also resulted in a focus on mitigation and the role addressing population can play, to the neglect of understanding factors related to building resilience for adapting to climate change. Country studies can contribute to the policy discourse, because if "the affected countries themselves identify [population] as a local priority [it] avoids the conflict that comes from framing population regulation as a way of reducing global greenhouse emissions" (Campbell-Lendrum and Lusti-Narasimhan 2009: 807). For example, countries themselves identified population as an exacerbating factor for climate change adaptation in their NAPAs. If the sensitivity around population were reduced, perhaps reproductive health programming related to climate change could follow.

It will be necessary to reframe the discourse on population and climate change in at least two key ways. First, such discourse should incorporate a broader view of how demographic processes both affect and are affected by climate change. Secondly, there is need for explicit recognition that reproductive health care in the context of climate change programming needs to be rights-based and voluntary – refuting calls for a global one-child policy. Campbell-Lendrum and Lusti-Narasimhan (2009) call this "Tak[ing] the heat out of the population and climate debate." It is both possible and essential to discuss and address population and climate change topics and interactions in a just and ethical manner. Prior to the Copenhagen COP in 2009, an editorial in *The Lancet* noted the tensions between some representatives of both the population and the sexual and reproductive health communities, and asked whether "it is time for the sexual and reproductive health community to use the climate change agenda to gain the traction women's health deserves" (Lancet 2009).

To reframe the issue, détente is needed between SRHR advocates and those working on reproductive health who also advocate addressing population factors more broadly associated with climate change. The roots of this toxicity date back to the 1960s and 1970s when programs were based on demographic targets rather than individual rights, and the desire among the sexual reproductive health and rights community to maintain gains made at the International Conference on Population and Development (ICPD) in Cairo (Stephenson et al. 2010). Yet, the ICPD's Programme of Action (PoA) has 15 other chapters. In addition to promoting reproductive rights and reproductive health, the PoA draws attention to both macro population and development issues. Climate change was linked to unsustainable production and consumption patterns, and the preamble noted that:

> The 1994 Conference was explicitly given a broader mandate on development issues than previous population conferences, reflecting the growing awareness that population, poverty, patterns of production and consumption and the environment are so closely interconnected that none of them can be considered in isolation (Para 1.5) (UN 1995)

Upholding all aspects of the ICPD's PoA would be beneficial for addressing climate change. The vilification of individuals and groups discussing population and reproductive health is unhelpful.[4] A unified effort is needed among those working to implement all aspects of the ICPD's PoA.

Furthermore, the architecture that has been built to address climate change, based on interventions that are exclusive of or "additional" to development initiatives, has resulted in programs that have focused on natural systems over human systems. The result has meant that addressing population and reproductive health issues has largely been left out of climate change programming. It is important to fully understand the global architecture being built to respond to climate change, including grasping financing issues and the potential for using climate funding or a mix of climate and development funding for programs that address population factors and reproductive health. Given the complexity of climate change impacts on both people and the natural environment, programming that integrates social and natural systems, or people and their environment, is likely to show the most promise in meeting needs to increase resilience and promote adaptation; and population, health and environment (or PHE) approaches offer lessons for community-based adaptation programming. Documenting the effects on climate change outcomes of programming that addresses population issues and reproductive health in addition to natural systems, the environment and livelihoods, will be critical, as will be advocacy for inclusion of integrated programming in climate change policies and programs.

References

Agrawala, S., & Fankhauser, S. (Eds.). (2008). *Economic aspects of adaptation to climate change: Costs, benefits and policy instruments*. Paris: OECD.
Bremner, J., Hardee, K., Mogelgaard, K., & D'Agnes, H. (2011, October). Is there a link between population, health and environment (PHE) and climate change adaptation? Forthcoming in UNFPA monograph from the *Population dynamics and climate change II: Building for adaptation workshop*, Mexico City, 2010.
Bryant, L., Carver, L., Butler, C. D., & Anage, A. (2009). Climate change and family planning: Least developed countries define the agenda. *Bulletin of the World Health Organization, 87*, 852–857.
Campbell-Lendrum, D., & Lusti-Narasimhan, M. (2009). Taking the heat out of the population and climate debate. *Bulletin of the World Health Organization, 87*, 807. doi:10.2471/BLT.09.072652.
Casey, M. (2008, December 12). Population growth contributes to emissions growth. *FoxNews.com*. http://www.foxnews.com/printer_friendly_wires/2008Dec12/0,4675,ASClimateConferenceBoomingPopulation,00.html
Cohen, J. E. (2010). Population and climate change. *Proceedings of the American Philosophical Society, 154*(2), 158–182.
Conservation International. (2008). *Health and conservation in the Cardamoms in Cambodia*. Phnom Phen: Conservation International and CARE.

[4]Such incidents still occur at prominent international fora. For example, at the NGO Forum on Sexual and Reproductive Health and Development in 2009, Dr. Musimbi Kanyoro, the director of the Population Program at the Packard Foundation, and an African woman, was greeted with boos by a few participants when she gave a presentation, "Where is the P in ICPD."

Crossette, B. (2009, September 28). Factoring people into climate change. *The Nation*. http://www. thenation.com/article/factoring-people-climate-change. Accessed 3 June 2013.

D'Agnes, L., Oglethrope, J., Thapa, S., Rai, D., & Gnyawali, T. P. (2009). Forests for the future: Family planning in Nepal's Terai Region. *Focus, 18*, 1–10.

D'Agnes, L., D'Agnes, H., Schwartz, J. B., Amarillo, M. L., & Castro, J. (2010). Integrated management of coastal resources and human health yields added value: A comparative study in Palawan (Philippines). *Environmental Conservation, 37*(4), 398–409. doi:10.1017/S0376892910000779.

Finer, L. B., & Henshaw, S. K. (2006). Disparities in rates of unintended pregnancy in the United States, 1994 and 2001. *Perspectives on Sexual and Reproductive Health, 38*(2), 90–96.

Hardee, K., & Mutunga, C. (2009). Strengthening the link between climate change adaptation and national development plans: Lessons from the case of population in National Adaptation programmes of Action (NAPAs). *Mitigation and Adaptation Strategies for Global Change*. doi:10.1007/s11027-009-9208-3.

Hardee, K., Deribe, S., Teklu, N., & Edmonds, J. (2010). The contribution of a PHE approach to climate change adaption in Ethiopia. *BALANCED Newsletter, 1*(2), 19–21.

Hartmann, B. (2009, Fall). The 'new' population control craze: Retro, racist, wrong way to go. *On the Issues*. http://www.ontheissuesmagazine.com/2009fall/2009fall-hartmann.php. Accessed 3 June 2013.

Hoepf Young, M., Malone, E., Madsen, E., & Coen, A. (2009). Adapting to climate change: The role of reproductive health. In L. Mazur (Ed.), *A pivotal moment: Population, justice and the environmental challenge*. Washington, DC: Island Press.

Hymas, L. (2010, March 31). The GINK Manifesto: Say it loud — I'm childfree and I'm proud. Blog post on *Grist*. http://grist.org/article/2010-03-30-gink-manifesto-say-it-loud-im-childfree-and-im-proud/

Huq, S., & Ayers J. (2008, November). Taking steps: Mainstreaming national adaptation. *IIED Briefing*. International Institute for Environment and Development (IIED), London.

Intergovernmental Panel for Climate Change (IPCC). (2001). *Climate change 2001: Impacts, adaptation, and vulnerability, contribution of Working Group II to the third assessment report of the IPCC*. Cambridge: Cambridge University Press.

IPCC. (2007). *Climate change 2007: Impacts, adaptation and vulnerability. Contribution of Working Group II to the fourth assessment report of the intergovernmental panel on climate change*. Cambridge: Cambridge University Press.

Jiang, L., & Hardee, K. (2010). How do recent population trends matter to climate change? *Population Research and Policy Review, 30*(2), 287–312. doi:10.1007/s11113-010-9189-7.

Jones, D. W. (1989). Urbanization and energy use in economic development. *The Energy Journal, 10*, 29–44.

Karl, T. R., Melillo, J. M., & Peterson, T. C. (Eds.). (2009). *Global climate change impacts in the United States*. Cambridge: Cambridge University Press.

Kidanu, A., Rovin, K., & Hardee, K. (2009). *Linking population, fertility and family planning with adaptation to climate change: Views from Ethiopia*. Washington, DC: Population Action International.

Lancet. (2009, September 19). Sexual and reproductive health and climate change. Editorial. *Lancet, 347*, 949.

Lutz, W., & Samir, K. C. (2010). Dimensions of global population projections: What do we know about the future population trends and structures? *Philosophical Transactions of the Royal Society, 365*, 2779–2791.

Malone E. L. (2009). *Vulnerability and resilience in the face of climate change: current research and needs for population information* (PNWD-4087). Washington, DC: Pacific Northwest Division, Battelle.

Malone, E. (2010). *Changing glaciers and hydrology in Asia. Addressing vulnerability to glacier ice melt impacts*. Washington, DC: USAID.

Mazur, L. (Ed.). (2009). *A pivotal moment. Population, justice and the environmental change challenge*. Washington, DC: Island Press.

192   K. Hardee

McCarthy, S. (2010, December 5). Ted Turner urges global one-child policy to save planet. *Globe and Mail*. http://www.theglobalmail.com/news/national/ted-turner-urges-global-one-child-policy-to-save-planet/article1318451. Accessed 3 June 2013.

McLeman, R. (2010). Impacts of population change on vulnerability and the capacity to adapt to climate change and variability: A typology based on lessons from "a hard country". *Population and Environment, 31*, 286–316.

Mogelgaard, K. (2010, Summer). Reproductive health and solutions to climate change: Connecting the dots. *Global Health Magazine*, 18–20.

Mohan, V. (2009). *Providing sexual and reproductive health services for communities in Velondriake, southwest Madagascar: Project Development Plan 2009–2011*. Also see https://blueventures.org

Moreland, S., Smith, E., & Sharma, S. (2010). *World population prospects and unmet need for family planning*. Washington, DC: Futures Group.

Murtaugh, P. A., & Schlax, M. G. (2009). Reproduction and the carbon legacies of individuals. *Global Environmental Change, 19*, 14–20.

Mutunga, C., & Hardee, K. (2009). Population and reproductive health in National Adaptation Programmes of Action (NAPAs) for climate change. In J. M. Guzman, G. Martine, G. McGranahan, D. Schensul, & C. Tacoli (Eds.), *Population dynamics and climate change*. New York/London: International Institute for Environment and Development/UNFPA.

Nakicenovic, N., Alcamo, J., Davis, G., de Vries, B., Fenhann, J., Gaffin, S., et al. (2000). *Special report on emissions scenarios: A special report of Working Group III of the intergovernmental panel on climate change*. Cambridge: Cambridge University Press.

O'Neill, B. C., Dalton, M., Fuchs, R., Jiang, L., Pachauri, S., & Zigov, K. (2010). Global demographic trends and future carbon emissions. *Proceedings of the National Academy of Sciences, 107*(41), 17521–17526. doi:10.1073/pnas.1004581107.

Pachauri, S., & Jiang, L. (2008). The household energy transition in India and China. *Energy Policy, 36*, 4022–4035.

Petroni, S. (2010). Policy review: Thoughts on addressing population and climate change in a just and ethical manner. *Population and Environment*. doi:10.1007/s11111-009-0085-1.

Reid, H., Alam, M., Berger, R., Cannon, T., Huq, S., & Milligan, A. (2009). Community-based adaptation to climate change: An overview. In *Participatory learning and action 60* (pp. 11–33). London: IIED.

Schensul, D., & Dodman, D. (2010). Populating adaptation: Incorporating demographic dynamics in climate change adaptation policy and practice. *Population dynamics and climate change II: building for adaptation workshop*, Mexico City: UNFPA. Forthcoming in a UNFPA and IIED book.

Silliman, J. (2009). In search of climate justice: Refuting dubious linkages, Affirming right. *Arrows for Change, 15*(1), 1–3.

Stephenson, J. K., Newman, K., & Mayhew, S. (2010). Population dynamics and climate change: What are the links? *Journal of Public Health, 32*(2), 150–156.

Thompson, K. (2009, October 1). Leaders need to admit population is the problem. *Science Alert*. Australia & Newzealand. http://www.sciencealertcom.an/opinions/page-12.html. Accessed 3 June 2013.

Torell, E., Tobey, J., Mahenge, J., Mkama, W., & Robadue, D., Jr. (2010). Climate change along the North Coast of Tanzania – Community-based adaptation planning with a population, health, and environment (PHE) lens. *BALANCED Newsletter, 1*(2), 12–15.

UNDP. (2010). *Gender, climate change and community-based adaptation: A guidebook for designing and implementing gender-sensitive community-based adaptation programmes and projects*. New York: UNDP.

UNFPA. (2009). *Facing a changing world: Women, population and climate. State of the world population report 2009*. New York: UNFPA.

United Nations (UN). (1995). *Report of the international conference on population and development*. A/CONF.171/13/Rev.1. New York: United Nations.

United Nations Development Programme (UNDP). (2010a). *Community-based adaptation*. Available at: http://www.undp-adaptation.org/projects/websites/index.php?option=com_content&task=view&id=204. Accessed 12 Oct 2010.

United Nations Population Division. (2010). *World population prospects. The 2008 revision. Online database*. http://esa.un.org/UNPP/p2k0data.asp. Accessed 23 Dec 2010.

US Energy Information Administration. (2010). *International energy outlook 2010*. http://www.eia.doe.gov/oiaf/ieo/emissions.html#3. Accessed 23 Dec 2010.

Wheeler, D., & Hammer, D. (2010). *The economics of population policy for carbon emissions reduction in developing countries* (CGD working paper, 229). Washington, DC: Center for Global Development.

Wire, T. (2009). *Fewer emitters, lower emissions, less cost*. M.Sc. dissertation submitted to the London School of Economics and Political Science. Sponsored by The Optimum Population Trust.

Worku, M. (2007). The missing links: Poverty, population and the environment in Ethiopia. *Focus, 14*, 8.

World Bank. (2010a). *Monitoring climate finance and ODA*. Washington: The World Bank.

World Bank. (2010b). *Development and climate change: World development report 2010*. Washington, DC: The World Bank.

World Health Organization. (2005). *The world health report 2005: Make every mother and child count*. Geneva: WHO.

Yamasaki, E., & Tominaga, N. (1997). Evolution of an aging society and effects on residential energy demand. *Energy Policy, 25*, 903–912.

Chapter 10
Reproductive Health Aid: A Delicate Balancing Act

Hendrik P. van Dalen and Maja Micevska Scharf

10.1 Introduction

"All countries should take steps to meet the family planning needs of their populations as soon as possible and should, in all cases by the year 2015, seek to provide universal access to a full range of safe and reliable family planning methods and to related reproductive health services which are not against the law." (UN 1995, par. 7.16) With this emphatic statement, 179 governments expressed their commitment to the Programme of Action (PoA) at the International Conference on Population and Development (ICPD) held in Cairo, 1994. Targets were also set for funding the costs of implementing the PoA, with donor governments promising to finance one-third of the total amount of resource flows needed for population activities in developing countries. The ICPD PoA was lauded with praise and depicted as "a turning point in humanity" and "a quantum leap to a higher state of energy" (McIntosh and Finkle 1995).

Today, the program is near its end date and commentators, policy makers and advocates are worried by the unbalanced attention given to specific population issues within the ICPD agenda, and by the gap between the actual disbursements of funds and those that were promised. Specifically, many within the family planning

H.P. van Dalen (✉)
Department of Economics, Tilburg School of Economics and Management (TISEM), Tilburg University, P.O. Box 90153, 5000 LE Tilburg, The Netherlands

Netherlands Interdisciplinary Demographic Institute (NIDI), P.O. Box 11650, 2502 AR The Hague, The Netherlands
e-mail: dalen@nidi.nl

M. Micevska Scharf
Department of Social Sciences, Roosevelt Academy, P.O. Box 94, 4330 AB Middelburg, The Netherlands

A. Kulczycki (ed.), *Critical Issues in Reproductive Health*, The Springer Series on Demographic Methods and Population Analysis 33, DOI 10.1007/978-94-007-6722-5_10, © Springer Science+Business Media Dordrecht 2014

movement are concerned by the dominance of STDs/HIV/AIDS programs[1] and the comparative neglect of family planning and other aspects of reproductive health care in the Millennium Development Goals (MDGs) (cf. Cleland and Sinding 2005). As Steven Sinding has stated: "If you're not an MDG, you're not on the agenda. If you're not a line item, you're out of the game" (cited in Crossette 2005: 77).

Ever since its approval, the PoA has been plagued by many of the same kinds of problems that bedevil international development aid, aptly depicted by William Easterly in his book *The White Man's Burden* (Easterly 2006). In designing and executing the grand plans of bringing welfare and development to poorer countries, the only thing which seems to count is the movement of money. In the social engineering mindset of planners, the money should flow to places where the reproductive health status of women is threatened and family planning needs cannot be met due to a lack of resources. In this chapter, we will take up the question of how the funding efforts to achieve the ICPD's goals have fared since 1994, and what lessons can be learned from this experience so far.

10.2 Tracking the Good Intentions of Donors

Compromises have to be drawn at population conferences, whose overall good intentions are often stated in such high spirits that some disappointment is inevitable in the years that follow, when attempts are made to put the grand ambitions of conference negotiations into practice. To understand the PoA, one first needs to consider the diverging views on population policies and the different schools of thought that surfaced at the Cairo conference (Potts 2004). These ranged from groups traditionally opposed to organized family planning programs such as the Vatican, which continued its hard-line stand against any form of 'artificial contraception' and condemned the use of condoms; to those who had launched national family planning programs in many developing countries during the 1960s and thereafter, and who continued to maintain their concern about rapid population growth and emphasized that fertility would fall rapidly if only the unmet need for family planning was met in a respectful way. Other groups were also present at Cairo. They included the women's health advocates who focused on the needs of the individual woman and downplayed demographic forces, often portraying family planning programs as coercive; as well as groups emphasizing the inequalities between the global North and South and the need to redistribute the world's wealth more equally. Given such diverse views on population policies, the ICPD achieved a remarkable degree of consensus. Its PoA underscored the heavy burden of social and cultural injustice that falls on many women in the world. The conference considered

---

[1] The ICPD PoA frames all funding in for this category under the heading of Sexually Transmitted Diseases (STDs) including HIV/AIDS. Throughout the text we will use the shorter term HIV/AIDS and wherever UN figures are presented on HIV/AIDS, these also include STDs.

Table 10.1 Proportions of demand for family planning satisfied (in percentage terms) by modern contraceptive use by wealth quintile (Q1 poorest, Q5 wealthiest), selected major world regions, 1990–2000

	Period	Q1	Q2	Q3	Q4	Q5	All quintiles
Sub Saharan Africa	1990–1995	12.9	16.0	17.7	24.7	36.9	22.9
	1996–2000	23.7	25.2	29.1	37.2	48.0	33.9
Latin America	1990–1995	29.4	40.7	49.0	57.4	65.3	50.0
	1996–2000	38.1	48.8	57.3	61.7	68.0	56.4
Asia	1990–1995	48.2	51.0	57.5	57.5	67.6	57.1
	1996–2000	50.0	57.1	59.8	63.7	70.7	60.9
North Africa/Middle East	1990–1995	36.8	45.7	53.7	58.2	65.4	53.8
	1996–2000	49.7	59.0	62.0	67.5	70.5	62.7
Global average	1990–1995	29.2	35.8	40.4	46.2	55.6	42.7
	1996–2000	37.9	44.4	49.3	54.7	62.1	50.8

Source: Ross et al. (2005: 52). Regional averages are unweighted averages for countries within these regions. The original data are from the Demographic Health Survey program

sexually transmitted diseases (STDs) and HIV/AIDS, condemned female genital mutilation, and set family planning in a broad context of reproductive health care.

But how has the PoA fared in the terms that matter most for the citizens receiving the aid? It is almost impossible to review the entire field of reproductive health and the progress that has been made. Instead, we focus on the three most important elements of reproductive health and, specifically, discuss developments in: (1) family planning, which is key to increasing household wealth and to improving overall reproductive health; (2) maternal health, which is central to the health of women during pregnancy, childbirth and the postpartum period; and (3) HIV/AIDS, which destroys not only the human capital of those infected but also, as a potent infectious disease, involves a host of global public governance and program design problems in the provision of a global public good that entails more sophistication than top-down development planners seem ready to admit (Sandler 2004).

In general, contraceptive use has increased over time, even in sub-Saharan Africa (SSA), and yet despite the considerable progress made during the 1990s in particular, services are still finding it hard to reach the poorest families. Table 10.1 presents some data from the Demographic Health Survey (DHS) program on how the demand for modern contraception across families of different wealth statuses is satisfied in the various regions of the world. In most countries the wealthiest 20 % (Q5 in Table 10.1) of families are using family planning when they want no more children or want to space children at least 2 years apart. More recent evidence (Bernstein 2006) shows that despite continued overall progress, the poorest families (Q1) still lag behind in SSA in particular, and less than a third of the poorest families can satisfy their demand for family planning.

The importance of this failure to access family planning in this part of the world becomes evident by taking account of the robust evidence on the relationship between contraceptive use and fertility. Experience shows that as contraceptive prevalence rises, so the total fertility rate falls. A host of studies has documented the spread of fertility decline throughout the developing world, including SSA. Recently, however, concerns have emerged that the ongoing fertility decline has stalled in a number of African countries. For example, Ezeh et al. (2009) examined the stalling fertility transitions in four Eastern African countries (Kenya, Tanzania, Uganda and Zimbabwe) over two decades. They found that fertility decline has been highly selective among specific subgroups of women, especially the most educated and urban, whereas the fertility rate actually rose for women with little or no formal education. Acceptance of family planning as a legitimate way of controlling births may have even fallen; the proportion of Kenyan youth (15–19 years) who disapproved of family planning increased between 1998 and 2003 from 13 to 22 % (Ezeh et al. 2009: 3005).

Maternal health is the second major element of reproductive health that we shall consider. Although motherhood is widely seen as a positive and fulfilling experience, for too many women in developing countries, it is also associated with suffering, ill-health and even death. In May 2008, WHO's Executive Director acknowledged that progress had stalled towards reaching the MDGs, particularly MDG 5 (improving maternal health), and that continued progress would be "slow and uneven". Beyond the major direct causes of maternal morbidity and mortality (hemorrhage, infection, high blood pressure, unsafe abortion, and obstructed labor) maternal health may also be compromised by harmful behaviors. In Africa these include female genital mutilation. The most recent prevalence data indicate that 91.5 million African girls and women above 9 years old are currently living with the consequences of female genital mutilation (Yoder and Khan 2008); and according to a consortium of UN agencies, 100–140 million girls and women worldwide have undergone female genital mutilation/cutting, with more than three million girls at risk for cutting each year in Africa alone (WHO 2008b). The measurement and monitoring of maternal health are difficult, but we know that the divergence in maternal mortality rates throughout the world is very large. Although the most recent estimates indicated an overall decline in maternal deaths, the lifetime risk of dying from pregnancy and childbirth ranges from 1 in 4,300 in developed countries, to as high as 1 in 31 in SSA (Hogan et al. 2010). Many more women are estimated to suffer pregnancy-related illnesses (9.5 million), near-miss events (1.4 million), and other potentially devastating consequences after birth (20 million long-term disabilities) (Fillippi et al. 2006). Access to antenatal and delivery care received varies widely. Also, about 19 million unsafe abortions are practiced annually worldwide and were estimated to account for 68,000 (or 13 % of all) maternal deaths in 2000. The prevalence of unsafe abortion differs across regions and is higher in South America, many areas of SSA, and South Asia. Progress, however, is slow to achieve. Although some progress occurred in Latin American and the Caribbean over the period 1990–2000, most developing countries saw no appreciable change in their rates of unsafe abortion (Grimes et al. 2006).

Finally, HIV/AIDS is the element of reproductive health which has received most attention over the period discussed. For 2009 it was estimated that 31–35 million people globally were living with HIV, 2.6 million people were newly infected (down from a peak of 3.2 million in 1997) and approximately 1.8 million people died from AIDS-related causes (down from a peak of 2.1 million in 2004) (UNAIDS 2010). The prevalence rate varies greatly, from 0.1 % among adults aged 15–49 years in East Asia to 5 % in SSA, which continues to be the region most affected by the pandemic. It is still hard to speak of major progress in this field, but it is encouraging that the global AIDS pandemic appears to have stabilized. However, levels of new infections remain high and the number of people living with HIV worldwide has increased given the progress made in reducing mortality rates among those infected.

10.3   Whatever Happened to Cairo's Good Intentions?

The ICPD's participants set themselves an ultimatum (the year 2015) for achieving the goals they had agreed upon in Cairo. Much has happened between 1994 and 2010, but it does not take an expert's eye to see that the ambitions of 1994 have not been realized and will probably also not be realized by the year 2015. The developed nations are trying to cope with the huge financial problems that have resulted in the aftermath of the 2008–2009 economic crisis; and given that population assistance is highly elastic with respect to income developments within donor countries (cf. Van Dalen 2008), the financing of reproductive health aid is bound to be affected negatively. It is timely, therefore, to take stock of what may underlie the gap between intentions and actions. To unravel the reasons for the divergence between Cairo's ambitions and the day-to-day practice in matters of reproductive health, it may help to look at a number of different causes, ranging from the probable and simple to the more complex causes of development failure.

10.3.1   No Sense of Urgency

The first and most plausible reason goes to the heart of the issue of population assistance. Although women's reproductive rights figure prominently in the ICPD agenda, in the minds of decision makers, the concerns of economic growth, sound fiscal policy, and the miracle of making markets work, all outrank the more abstract issues of reproductive rights or reproductive health when thinking about development. As Peter Piot, the former head of UNAIDS, has once said: "I asked myself what political leaders really care about. The truth is, it's not health. It's economics and security. Health is what they talk about if there's money left at the end of the day." It is tempting to view the lack of attention to issues of reproductive health as a reflection of this so-called 'Washington Consensus' among policy makers and advisors (Williamson 1990).[2] We venture that there are two other and more important factors which explain the lack of urgency.

First of all, the very success of the industry of family planning may have diminished the sense of urgency among policy makers in supporting family planning. Fertility rates have been falling in developing countries and this decline has been pivotal in mitigating the feared consequences of a population explosion (Lam 2011). It remains, of course, an empirical question whether the fall in fertility rates can be ascribed to family programs. Bongaarts and Sinding (2009, 2011) provide ample evidence in response to critics that family planning has been instrumental in bringing fertility rates down and that the need for family planning remains of utmost importance in curbing population growth. Despite these efforts, the image seems to stick in the minds of the public and policy makers that the population problem is a thing of the past (Wattenberg 1997).

The second factor can be traced to the lack of consensus about the importance of the population issue, and specifically about whether (global) population growth really is a problem. For policymakers, the decision to support reproductive health programs is far easier when consensus is high among experts that high fertility rates and rapid population growth are indeed a problem. As Sinding (2000) makes clear in his review of grand population debates of the past, the debate about *whether* population growth is a problem remains unsolved. This conclusion also resounds in a survey carried out by Van Dalen and Henkens (2012) among demographers around the world, who were quite divided on the importance of the population problem. For instance, approximately half of the demographers did not agree with the statement: "The current size of the world population exceeds the carrying capacity of the earth." This agnostic attitude is also reflected in the policy orientation of demographers: those who firmly disagree that the world population exceeds the carrying capacity of the earth are also far more set on a laissez-faire population policy. In short, if the low level of consensus on this particular issue among experts is also present among policy makers, one can better understand why the sense of urgency is not all that strong and why achieving a consensus at global population conferences is such a difficult matter.

10.3.2   Insufficient Funding

A second reason for not achieving the goals of the ICPD is often aired by UNFPA and NGOs involved in matters of family planning and reproductive health: the funds to finance the PoA are insufficient. The latest evaluation of financial resource flows assisting the PoA was conducted in 2009; it noted that the ICPD target for donor countries was met in 2005 (UN 2009). This achievement was unforeseen, not least because development aid generally does not meet promises. Indeed, it may even have

[2]The term "Washington Consensus" was first coined by John Williamson to describe the policy prescriptions promoted for crisis-ridden developing countries by Washington, D.C.-based institutions like the IMF, World Bank, and the US Treasury Department. It refers more generally to an orientation towards free market policies followed by both advanced and emerging economies. This mindset dominated economic thinking and the views of many politicians and journalists during the 1990s, but then ended with the outbreak of the 2008–2009 financial crisis.

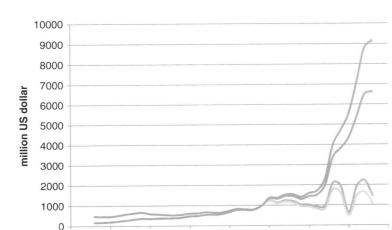

Fig. 10.1 Development of primary funds for population assistance programs, 1973–2008 (million US dollars, nominal and at constant 1994 prices) (Source: Van Dalen and Reuser (2005) and UNFPA/NIDI database (UNFPA/NIDI 2010))

caused some concern at the head offices of the UN, NGOs and government bureaus dealing with foreign aid for reproductive health, because continued flows for any development assistance project may partly depend on an ability to show that there is a gap between what is needed and what is available. For a long time, such gaps were visible and real in the case of reproductive health care (Potts et al. 1999). However, while the ICPD PoA may have seemed a logical contract from the layman's point of view, for the accountant who has to keep track of the good intentions, the financial paragraphs made for a nightmare. They included different commitments; targets for donors were set in real terms with nothing said about which deflator should be used (consumer price, the price of health care); targets for developing countries were stated in nominal terms; out-of-pocket expenditures for reproductive health care were delegated to an appendix; and the distribution across reproductive health categories remains arbitrary, perhaps because the dividing lines between those categories are in practice not as clear as they were in the heads of the conference delegates.

If one takes a longer term perspective on population assistance (see Fig. 10.1), the Cairo conference appears as a turning point in the short history of collective action on population issues. In nominal terms, funds have increased by a factor of ten since 1994 and in real terms, the increase, by a factor of 7.4, is less pronounced but still considerable.

This increase may be explained by a number of plausible factors. Both the number of donors – not only governments but also private donors like the Bill and Melinda Gates Foundation – and the 'wealth' of donors have increased. However, two additional reasons may help explain why the achievement of the original PoA is to some extent illusory. We will discuss these under the headings of *shifting* priorities and *diverging* priorities over time.

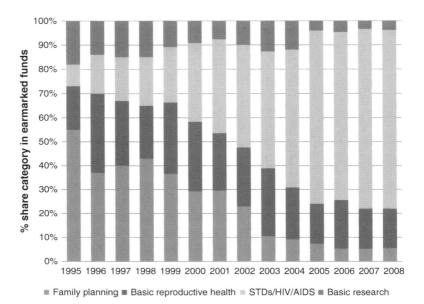

Fig. 10.2 Development assistance for reproductive health (DARH) from 1995 to 2008 by share of reproductive health category in total (excluding general contributions) (Source: UNFPA/NIDI 2010)

Shifting Priorities

Certain developments were unforeseen in the design of the PoA. The clearest example is, of course, the steep increase in HIV/AIDS prevalence. The enormous increases in funds allocated to HIV/AIDS programs obscures the fact that funds for other components of reproductive health are far below target and, in the case of family planning, have declined over time. The category of HIV/AIDS was allotted 7 % of the funds allocated to all ICPD categories at the start of the PoA in 1994, a proportion that grew to as much as 74 % in 2008 (see Fig. 10.2). This shift in emphasis has been so strong that the funds allotted to non-HIV/AIDS categories has remained more or less the same since 1994 (see Fig. 10.1).[3]

Two factors have been pivotal in causing this shift in priorities. The first and more down-to-earth observation is that at the time they made their pledges, the

---

[3]The share of general contributions in total development assistance for reproductive health (DARH) also decreased. This is somewhat surprising in view of the current debates among donors emphasizing the importance of funds that are not linked to specific projects or diseases. Advocacy of the new agenda for aid effectiveness embodied in the 2005 Paris Declaration and its follow-up, the Accra Agenda for Action, reflects a view that provision of unrestricted funds is the best funding method for alignment with the priorities of recipient countries and improved harmonization among donors. As a result, donors have pledged to move away from project-related aid in favor of general and sector budget support. Clearly, this has not happened in the domain of DARH.

ICPD participants obviously did not realize how strong the spread of the HIV/AIDS epidemic would become, especially in SSA. The story of HIV/AIDS is, however, not only one about an infectious disease; it is also about technological progress, which has lengthened the remaining life expectancy of those infected. These two elements resulted in a strong increase in the number of people living with HIV/AIDS. Global awareness of the HIV/AIDS pandemic mounted steadily and was expressed in the UN Millennium Declaration adopted in September 2000. Nevertheless, the huge increase in funds that became available to fight the rapidly spreading pandemic should be primarily ascribed to the initiative of U.S. President George W. Bush, who started in 2003 what became known as the PEPFAR program (US President's Emergency Plan for AIDS Relief).[4]

This global collective action was underpinned by the second factor that explains the strong increase in funds: the emergence of the MDGs. Besides halving the proportion of the world's people whose income is less than one dollar a day by the year 2015, the MDGs also sought to reduce by the same date under-five child mortality by two-thirds (MDG 4) and maternal mortality by three-quarters (MDG 5); and to halt, and begin to reverse, the spread of HIV/AIDS and the scourge of malaria and other major diseases (especially tuberculosis) (MDG 6). Although highly complementary to the ICPD's PoA, this new UN initiative was also, to some extent, competing with it.[5]

The ICPD PoA urged the international community to take steps towards ensuring universal access to reproductive health services. The ICPD agenda for reproductive health has been considered its most comprehensive element, broadening the spectrum of reproductive health services and influencing many countries to embark upon initiatives to improve the reproductive health status of their populations. However, with the ratification of the MDGs, the focus of most countries shifted from concepts highlighted by the ICPD towards achieving the MDGs. Presently, the term 'ICPD' is hardly mentioned anymore and all categories are interpreted within the 'MDGs.' To be sure, although there is not a direct convergence between the ICPD's PoA and the MDGs, there is a significant overlap, especially with regard to MDGs 5 and 6. Nevertheless, the health-related MDGs are less comprehensive than the ICPD categories: they do not include family planning or related program elements such as information, education and communication campaigns, and other health programs. Moreover, as the MDGs have become increasingly important for setting donor priorities, the fact that family planning does not feature as one such distinct MDG goal would put at risk efforts aimed at securing enough funding for improving this category.

---

[4]The remarkable increase of funds allocated to STDs/HIV/AIDS between the years 2004 and 2005 is due to the implementation of PEPFAR, which holds a place in history as the largest effort by any nation to combat a single disease.

[5]In his address to the fifth Asian and Pacific Population Conference in 2002, the former Secretary-General of the UN, Mr. Kofi Annan, made the following remark: "The MDGs, particularly the eradication of extreme poverty and hunger, cannot be achieved if questions of population and reproductive health are not squarely addressed" (UNFPA 2004).

Diverging Priorities

Shifting priorities may not trouble the 'madmen in authority' as long as the course set is right and that there exists a consensus on the direction and intensity of the shift. However, another distinguishing mark of global collective action and reproductive health in particular is that priorities may shift in unpredictable ways. In general, three reasons can be put forward why priorities may shift in making donations. These include diverging preferences and ideologies, a growing inability to pay, and the problem of 'free riders,' as discussed below.

Diverging Preferences and Ideologies

The provision of funds is a matter of 'taste': a taste for caring about others, or a preference for certain programs which are in line with one's religious beliefs or *Weltanschauung*. In this respect, one can expect some donor countries to be more sensitive than others towards the fate of people living in the less developed world when (population) programs are more in line with their preferences or political ideology; or because of geographic proximity or historical ties such as to former colonies (Alesina and Dollar 2000). Furthermore, governments of, for example, Scandinavian countries and the Netherlands are known to be more egalitarian than Anglo-Saxon countries in their national economic policies, and such preferences tend to carry over towards attempts to reduce income differences in the world at large. But differences in taste may also be reflected in religious and other belief systems and such differences may surface at distinct points in time. For instance, diverging views on the importance of reproductive health were a hurdle of some significance in the adoption of the MDGs. Due to the increased concern with mass poverty in the 1990s, the international community adopted the international development goals (IDGs), one of which focused exclusively on providing access to reproductive health for all women of appropriate age.[6] With the transformation of IDGs to MDGs at the UN Millennium Development Summit in 2001, the reproductive health goal was dropped from the agenda, mostly because of opposition from conservative developing nations and North American right-wing groups (Crossette 2005; Campbell-White et al. 2006). However, after lobbying by many governments, NGOs and others, world leaders endorsed incorporating universal access to reproductive health as a target within MDG 5 (improving maternal health).

Perhaps the most significant policy which illustrates the diverging views on family planning refers to the U.S. government's so-called 'Mexico City Policy,' first introduced by President Reagan in 1984 and re-imposed by successive Republican Party presidents. This ruling, dubbed by its opponents 'the Global Gag Rule,' restricted foreign NGOs that received USAID family planning funds from

---

[6] For further information see, for example, the description given in the Asian Development Bank's donor report on "Fighting Poverty in Asia," available at: http://www.adb.org/Documents/Reports/ADF/VIII/adf0200.asp

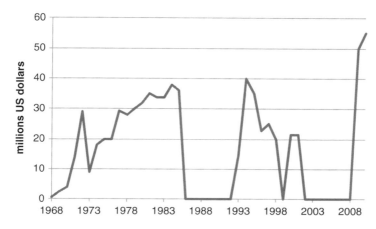

Fig. 10.3 Funding of UNFPA from USAID, 1968–2010 (in millions of U.S. dollars) (Source: Population Action International (2010))

using their own, non-USAID funds to provide any abortion-related activities. The policy was rescinded by President Clinton in 1993, reintroduced by President George W. Bush, and rescinded again by President Obama in 2009. It is not surprising that ideology matters in making choices, but what made this U.S. foreign aid policy different from other textbook public choices is that it may have had substantial spillovers in the decisions and actions of other donor countries and aid recipients, and at some points it may even have affected researchers' freedom of speech.[7] Even though it is extremely difficult to gauge the actual effects of the policy, it likely increased the number of abortions where the US government's imposed restrictions disrupted the provision of family planning activities (Crane and Dusenberry 2004).

Dominance is seldom healthy, be it in private or public affairs. The recent Global Gag Rule is a powerful reminder of the overpowering dominance of the United States and the ideological values held by many Republicans in setting the rules of the game in global health programs (Kulczycki 2007; Crimms 2007; Van Dalen 2008). Perhaps this is most clearly illustrated by the erratic funding pattern received from USAID over the past four decades by UNFPA, the key player charged with keeping track of the ICPD agenda (Fig. 10.3). This leads to potentially far-reaching consequences. In short, U.S. dominance disrupts the global public governance of the reproductive aid process.

---

[7]*International Perspectives on Sexual and Reproductive Health* (formerly known as *International Family Planning Perspectives*), one of the most influential peer-reviewed journals on reproductive health, inserted from 2002 to March 2008 the following restriction in its guidelines to authors: "Because the journal receives funding from the US Agency for International Development, it is prohibited under the Helms amendment (P.L. 93–189) from publishing material that promotes abortion." As with all scientific research, however, it remains an open question whether the publishing policy guideline affected actual decisions implemented.

Lack of Ability to Pay

Donor governments themselves often make this argument when funds are not forthcoming and the press or a consortium complains about members not living up to their promises. Foreign aid is part of the budget deliberations of national governments, and when a business cycle downturn occurs or when other unexpected demands on government spending emerge, ambitions have to be toned down and priorities changed. The emergence of the credit crunch in 2008 made it inevitable that donor governments would reappraise their priorities and slash official development assistance. The income elasticity of government donations with respect to reproductive health is unity (Van Dalen and Reuser 2006), implying that a fall in national income by 10 % implies more or less an equal fall in reproductive health aid.

'Free Rider' Behavior in Financing Global Public Goods

The ideal world of social planners is destroyed by free riders. This includes individual governments who benefit from collective action but who do not contribute, or who do not contribute sufficiently, such that goods are either not provided or in inadequate amounts. Reproductive health aid poses a collective action problem for the international community not unlike many other foreign aid programs. Many developing nations must rely on other nations to provide them with resources and cash to finance population activities like family planning, investments in reproductive health, HIV/ AIDS programs and basic research. By increasing the welfare of a recipient country, foreign aid serves as a collective global good for all donor countries. The U.S. government has been the largest donor of public development assistance for reproductive health (DARH) throughout this time, accounting on average for 40 % of the total amount of DARH. Following its entry into the DARH arena in 1998, the Bill & Melinda Gates Foundation became the largest private donor, but the continued dominance of the U.S. government's contribution to the DARH has allowed the US government to push its own priorities in global health programs (Van Dalen 2008). Dominant parties have the unattractive feature of not only dominating the agenda, but also encouraging free riding by smaller countries. The reproductive health agenda is a case in point. This mechanism is akin to a host of collective action failures in foreign aid and may well explain why promises are rarely met. Detecting free rider behavior is, however, far more difficult than stating the problem of free riders. Van Dalen (2008) has shown that free riding is not present for each and every category.

10.3.3 Misalignment of Donor Funds

A final reason why the good intentions have not fully realized pertains to a misalignment between needs and funds. In an analysis using multiple waves of data from 41 Demographic Health Surveys (DHS) conducted between 1988 and 2006, Case and

Paxson (2009) document how strong the impact of the HIV/AIDS pandemic has been on non-AIDS related health services. They found a clear deterioration in the quality of care received by women and children as measured by indicators of antenatal care, birth deliveries and children's immunization in this specific period. The real root of this problem cannot be detected using DHS data, but Case and Paxson show that this divergence in quality of non-HIV related services between low and high prevalence HIV regions started in the mid-1990s. Ideally one would expect governments to donate and allocate resources efficiently so as to achieve the 'biggest bang for the buck', or to rephrase this in the language of the 2004 Global Forum for Health Research: health research and development priorities should be set according to, among other factors, reduction in the burden of disease per dollar spent. As funding for HIV/AIDS has come to dominate the ICPD agenda, it is natural to ask whether this dominance could be justified by the concern of donor countries about the needs of developing countries. One way to answer this question is to link donor funding to the burden of disease in developing countries, as measured by disability adjusted life-years (DALYs).[8]

If it is assumed that donors respond in proportion to the scale of health problems in the developing world, one would expect a certain level of correspondence between donor funding for a health category (e.g. HIV/AIDS) and the corresponding burden of disease. At a rudimentary level, this link can be established using data on DALYs from the Global Burden of Disease (GBD) project,[9] so that funding levels for the project's disease categories should be directly comparable to two of the four ICPD-costed population package categories: (1) STDs, including HIV/AIDS; and (2) reproductive health diseases, mainly maternal and perinatal conditions.[10]

As can be distilled from Table 10.2, donor dollars spent per healthy life-year lost differ significantly between these two ICPD categories. This indicates that by this criterion, the principles of efficiency are not obeyed. In the late-1990s, the category 'reproductive health' received more funding per DALY relative to HIV/AIDS. This situation was reversed in the following decade: the category HIV/AIDS was heavily favored relative to the burden it caused, receiving US$76 per DALY relative to only US$18 per DALY received by reproductive health. While funding per DALY due to HIV/AIDS increased more than tenfold between the late-1990s (1995–1999) and c. 2004 (2000–2007), funding per DALY due to maternal

---

[8]Researchers developed the DALY measure explicitly in recognition of resource scarcity to aid policy-makers in making difficult allocation decisions (World Bank 1993; Murray and Lopez 1996).

[9]The data are available for the following years: 1990, 1998, 1999, 2000, 2001, 2002, and 2004 (World Bank 1993; WHO, various years).

[10]We have also included reproductive cancers in this category. These account for a negligible share both in the total burden of disease due to reproductive conditions and in the donor funding (a detailed project description search revealed only a handful of projects targeted at reproductive cancers). However, it should be realized that reproductive cancers in developing countries are significantly underreported. Excluding this category from our calculations does not change the results.

Table 10.2 Donor funding levels for STDs/HIV/AIDS and reproductive health diseases, c. 1998–2004

	DALYs (millions)		Donor funding (millions of US$)		Donor dollars per DALY	
	Late 1990s	2000s	Late 1990s	2000s	Late 1990s	2000s
STDs including HIV/AIDS	188	315	1,371	23,887	7.29	75.86
Reproductive health diseases	209	435	2,042	8,023	9.78	18.46

Sources: WHO (various years); UNFPA/NIDI (2010)
Notes: Donor funding for the late 1990s is a sum of funding levels in current US$ over the years 1995–1999; donor funding for the 2000s is a sum of funding levels in current US$ over the years 2000–2007. DALYs for the late 1990s are averaged over the years 1998 and 1999; DALYs for the 2000s are averaged over the years 2000, 2001, 2002, and 2004. Reproductive health diseases include maternal and perinatal conditions, and reproductive cancers

and perinatal conditions – disease categories that are of particular concern to vulnerable groups, namely women and infants – increased by only 89 %. Altogether, this suggests that HIV/AIDS as a category received more donor funding than can be explained by its share in the burden of disease.

Table 10.2 highlights the prominence of HIV/AIDS on the donor agenda in the first years of the new century. Although other research has come to similar conclusions (UNFPA 2004; Van Dalen and Reuser 2006), the new results presented here additionally show that the increased funding for HIV/AIDS activities cannot be explained by its share in the burden of disease. Reproductive health problems have received relatively less funding, although they pose a significant burden in terms of DALYs in developing countries.

Ethiopia is a typical example of how the foreign aid priorities of donor nations are not always aligned with local health needs. A large portion of foreign aid to Ethiopia goes towards HIV/AIDS even though its national prevalence rate is relatively low (2.3 %) and its maternal mortality rate is among the highest in the world. The biggest needs of the Ethiopian population, which is largely rural, include safe water, transportation, and more doctors, nurses, and midwives (Loewenberg 2010). Yet all of these basics receive little attention from foreign donors. Given the lack of health insurance, Ethiopians pay a large share of their health expenditures – including expenditures for reproductive health – out of their own pocket. Although maternal health services delivered at public facilities are free in principle, about half of the mothers delivering at public hospitals reported making out-of-pocket expenditures to get needed healthcare services (Micevska Scharf 2010). The highest amounts were spent on drugs and medical supplies, with transport, accommodation, food, and other indirect expenses also accounting for a large fraction of out-of-pocket expenditures by mothers giving birth. Overall, the combined direct and indirect cost of the supposedly 'free' maternity care services is significant in Ethiopia and may deter utilization of health services, especially by poor mothers.

The global burden of disease is increasingly shifting from infectious diseases to non-communicable diseases. As a result, WHO predicts that mortality due to maternal and perinatal conditions in developing countries may feature even more prominently in the global picture of health over the next 20 years (WHO 2008a). These predictions are debatable for various reasons, for example, some maternal and perinatal conditions are due to HIV/AIDS, and there may be more progress made than anticipated to combat maternal and perinatal conditions. Nevertheless, if funding for family planning and reproductive health is not increased, it will undermine efforts to prevent unintended pregnancies, and reduce maternal and infant mortality in the years to come.

10.4   Lessons from Inside and Outside the Money Machine

If the participants of the ICPD would meet again in 2015, would they do things differently? What lessons would they draw from 20 years of development experience? These type of questions will certainly have to be faced when the final date of 2015 approaches. In this closing section we will draw together a number of lessons that emerge from the history of development so far.

The first lesson is that a strong focus on monetary targets – as set in 1994 at Cairo – is impractical: resource tracking has proven to be extremely difficult. To be sure, the transparency of donor organizations and recipient governments should be a guiding principle for their day-to-day operations; and given the frequently disappointing results of foreign direct assistance, it would be enlightening to examine the day-to-day practice of development aid, and simply 'follow the money' and see how funds are spent in countries of destination. Furthermore, observers of development aid should guard against over-simplifying the complexity of reproductive health aid, household behavior and welfare; viewing them as simply regressions may give policy makers the illusion that such policies have large social external benefits, whereas closer examination of the richness of the relationships between fertility and human capital formation within households shows far smaller effects of policies on family outcomes (Schultz 2008). The provision of reproductive health aid should be guided by more than the maxim 'it is the thought that counts'. Nevertheless, the quality of data on the type of health expenditures that recipient governments spend is both weak and incomplete, and the lack of reliable data gives significant leeway for various agencies and pressure groups to claim more and more resources for their goals. In this line of development work, it is often hard to distinguish between the words of an independent scholar and that of a compassionate policy advocate. For health policies to work best, it may be best to formulate goals in the terms that matter most, that is, the health outcomes and demographic indicators which capture the essence of the intentions of participants. The MDGs go a long way in capturing the essence of reproductive health aid, but they have the drawback that essential services that complement efforts to reduce the spread of HIV/AIDS have been left out.

A second lesson concerns the need for more attention to be paid to incentives and the benefits of social insurance. Overall, citizens in developing countries pay a large share of their health expenditures out of their own pocket. Access to health care is intimately tied to the resources and incentives in health insurance and production.[11]

A third lesson, which is related to the previous two, concerns the need for a comprehensive approach to the evaluation of reproductive health policy (Van Dalen and Reuser 2008). The apparent success of fertility decline seems to have made many policy advisers and advocates over-confident that fertility levels and maternal health are no longer a problem. They have shifted their focus almost exclusively to HIV/AIDS, which received only 7 % of funding at the time of the 1994 Cairo pact. With the benefit of hindsight, the various categories of allocation (basic research, family planning, reproductive health and HIV/AIDS) used by the PoA quickly became outdated. A major factor that led donors to reconsider their priorities was the course of the HIV/AIDS pandemic. This seemed to rapidly escalate and required more attention than was envisioned in Cairo. Also, the ICPD's budgetary targets were set too low to significantly advance goals such as to "provide universal access to a full range of safe and reliable family planning methods." According to ICPD projections at the time, reproductive health costs in developing countries and countries in transition would likely total 17 billion US dollars in the year 2000 and 21.7 billion US dollars in 2015 (at 1993 US dollars).[12] The latest revision of the total package that is needed to fulfill the dreams of Cairo amounted to 64.7 billion in 2010, a sum expected to reach 69.8 billion US dollars in 2015 (UNFPA 2009).

There are two main reasons why the crowding out of family planning and maternal health investments in favour of HIV/AIDS assistance is worrisome. First, HIV/AIDS programs would profit considerably from a more balanced approach, as maternal health and family planning investments go to the heart of the problems of SSA – in particular, that high population growth rates keep numerous countries trapped in poverty (Cleland and Sinding 2005). In most SSA countries, the TFR hovers around five, far above the replacement rate of 2.1 children. Judging from the DHS surveys carried out in developing countries, desired fertility rates fell faster over time than actual rates, as reflected in high levels of unmet need and high proportions of births that are ill-timed or unwanted. High fertility leads to rapid population growth rates, exacerbating scarcities in health care, education, land for farmers, and all other public domains of life. Family planning might alleviate some of these problems, but evidently it is no longer the "hot" subject it was for such a long time at many a population conference. Insiders to these negotiations claim that family planning seems even to have become "morally suspect" again (Blanc and Tsui 2005). This is particularly unfortunate because the evidence of progress in maternal health has been relatively weak and investment is very much needed.[13]

---

[11] The faltering experiment in the provision and insurance of health care in China (WHO 2005; Meng et al. 2000; Liu et al. 2000) may provide ample evidence of outright market failure and highlights that government should play a pivotal role in setting up a basic form of health insurance.

[12] This clause was made explicit for donor countries in the ICPD PoA (par. 14.11), and it was once explicated for developing countries in one of the preparatory committees (UNFPA 1994).

[13] It should be noted with respect to the latter shortcoming that a recent initiative launched by the Bill and Melinda Gates Foundation and others (at the Women Deliver conference 2010) intends to invest much more money into efforts to reduce maternal mortality.

Second, the unprecedented rise of HIV/AIDS funds is disrupting fiscal policy and local health care systems, whereas a more balanced investment in reproductive health and HIV/AIDS would make use of the existing infrastructure. Vertical programs such as HIV/AIDS erode primary health care systems in developing nations. The substantial new levels of HIV/AIDS funding are swamping public health budgets, in some cases exceeding 150 % of the government's total allocation to health care (Lewis 2005). Too much money must be spent in too short a time. Such a situation, particularly in the conditions of extreme poverty and poor governance prevalent in SSA, easily results in the "poaching" of health care workers and bureaucrats from other worthy public projects. Large "white elephant" investment projects signal to donors that money is being spent (Robinson and and Torvik 2005), but chances are that resources are not spent wisely. When public governance systems are weak, these large but volatile sums of "easy money" promote corruption, moonlighting, and absenteeism in delivering health care (World Bank 2004).

The short history of reproductive health aid is not a story of grand successes: collective action is an intricate and delicate balancing act. Spending large aid budgets on HIV/AIDS is a delicate cocktail, and an unbalanced mixture may do more harm than donors imagine. Foreign aid ought to be guided not by ideas or ideologies that have lost touch with reality or that are used opportunistically, but by evidence and true engagement, aiming at long-term sustainable solutions.

References

Alesina, A., & Dollar, D. (2000). Who gives foreign aid to whom and why? *Journal of Economic Growth, 5*, 33–63.

Bernstein, S. (2006). *The impact of population growth on the attainment of the millennium development goals and other consensus international development goals.* New York: UNFPA.

Blanc, A., & Tsui, A. (2005). The dilemma of past success: Insiders' view on the future of the international family planning movement. *Studies in Family Planning, 36*, 263–276.

Bongaarts, J., & Sinding, S. (2009). A response to critics of family planning programs. *International Perspectives on Sexual and Reproductive Health, 35*(1), 39–44.

Bongaarts, J., & Sinding, S. (2011). Population policy in transition in the developing world. *Science, 333*, 574–576.

Campbell-White, A., Merrick, T. W., & Yazbeck, S. A. (2006). *Reproductive health: The missing millennium development goal.* Washington, DC: The World Bank.

Case, A., & Paxson, C. (2009). *The impact of the AIDS pandemic on health services in Africa: Evidence from Demographic and Health Surveys* (Working Paper No. 15000). Cambridge: NBER.

Cleland, J., & Sinding, S. (2005). What would Malthus say about AIDS in Africa? *The Lancet, 366*, 1899–1901.

Crane, B. B., & Dusenberry, J. (2004). Power and politics in international funding for reproductive health: The US Global Gag Rule. *Reproductive Health Matters, 12*(24), 128–137.

Crimms, N. J. (2007). The Global Gag Rule: Undermining national interests by doing unto foreign women and NGOs what cannot be done at home. *Cornell International Law Journal, 40*, 587–633.

Crossette, B. (2005). Reproductive health and the millennium development goals: The missing links. *Studies in Family Planning, 36*, 71–79.

Easterly, W. (2006). *The white man's burden: Why the West's efforts to aid the rest have done so much ill and so little good.* New York: The Penguin Press.

Ezeh, A. C., Mberu, B. U., & Emina, J. O. (2009). Stall in fertility decline in Eastern African countries: Regional analysis of patterns, determinants and implications. *Philosophical Transactions of the Royal Society, Biological Sciences, 364*, 2991–3007.

Fillipi, V., et al. (2006). Maternal health in poor countries: The broader context and a call for action. *The Lancet, 368*(9546), 1535–1541.

Grimes, D. A., et al. (2006). Unsafe abortion: The preventable pandemic. *The Lancet, 368*(9550), 1908–1919.

Hogan, M. C., Foreman, K. J., Naghavi, M., Ahn, S. Y., Wang, M., Makela, S. M., Lopez, A. D., Lozano, R., & Murray, C. J. (2010). Maternal mortality for 181 countries, 1980–2008: A systematic analysis of progress towards millennium development goal 5. *The Lancet, 375*(9726), 1609–1623.

Kulczycki, A. (2007). Ethics, ideology, and reproductive health policy in the United States. *Studies in Family Planning, 38*(4), 333–351.

Lam, D. (2011). How the world survived the population bomb: Lessons from 50 years of extraordinary demographic history. *Demography, 48*, 1231–1262.

Lewis, M. (2005). *Addressing the challenges of HIV/AIDS: Macroeconomic, fiscal and institutional issues* (Working Paper No. 58). Helsinki: Center for Global Development.

Liu, X., Liu, Y., & Chen, N. (2000). The Chinese experience of hospital price regulation. *Health Policy and Planning, 15*, 157–163.

Loewenberg, S. (2010). Ethiopia struggles to make its voice heard. *The Lancet, 376*, 861–862.

McIntosh, C. A., & Finkle, J. L. (1995). The Cairo conference on population and development: A new paradigm? *Population and Development Review, 21*(2), 223–260.

Meng, Q., Liu, X., & Shi, J. (2000). Comparing the services and quality of private and public clinics in rural China. *Health Policy and Planning, 15*, 349–356.

Micevska Scharf, M. (2010). *Examining out-of-pocket expenditures on sexual and reproductive health in rural Ethiopia*. Mimeo. The Hague: NIDI.

Murray, C. J. L., & Lopez, A. D. (1996). *The global burden of disease*. Cambridge, MA: Harvard School of Public Health, World Health Organization and World Bank.

Population Action International. (2010). *Trends in U.S. population assistance*. Washington, DC: Population Action International.

Potts, M. (2004). *Family planning programs: Development and outcomes. International encyclopedia of the social and behavioral sciences* (pp. 5332–5336). Amsterdam: Elsevier.

Potts, M., Walsh, J., McAninch, J., Mizoguchi, N., & Wade, T. J. (1999). Paying for reproductive health care: What is needed, and what is available? *International Family Planning Perspectives, 25*, S10–S16.

Robinson, J. A., & Torvik, R. (2005). White elephants. *Journal of Public Economics, 89*, 197–210.

Ross, J., Stover, J., & Adelaja, D. (2005). *Profiles for family planning and reproductive health programs* (2nd ed.). Glastonbury: Futures Group.

Sandler, T. (2004). *Global collective action*. Cambridge: Cambridge University Press.

Schultz, T. P. (2008). Chapter 52: Population policies, fertility, women's human capital, and child quality. In T. P. Schultz & J. Strauss (Eds.), *Handbook of development economics* (Vol. 4). Amsterdam: North-Holland.

Sinding, S. W. (2000). The great population debates: How relevant are they for the 21st century? *American Journal of Public Health, 90*(12), 1841–1845.

UN. (1995). *Report of the international conference on population and development* (A/CONF.171/13/Rev.1). New York: United Nations.

UN. (2009). *Flow of financial resources for assisting in the implementation of the programme of action of the international conference on population and development* (Economic and Social Council, E/CN.9/2009/5). New York: United Nations.

UNAIDS/WHO. (2010). *Report on the global HIV/AIDS epidemic 2010*. Geneva: UNAIDS and WHO.

UNFPA. (1994). *Background note on the resource requirements for population programmes in the years 2000–2015* (Working paper prepared for the ICPD). New York: UN.

UNFPA. (2004). *Investing in people: National progress in implementing the ICPD programme of action 1994–2004*. New York: United Nations.

UNFPA. (2009). *Revised cost estimates for the implementation of the programme of action of the international conference on population and development: A methodological report*. New York: United Nations.

UNFPA/NIDI. (2010). *Resource flows database*. New York/The Hague: UNFPA/NIDI.

Van Dalen, H. P. (2008). Designing global collective action in population and HIV/AIDS programs, 1983–2002: Has anything changed? *World Development, 36*(3), 362–382.

Van Dalen, H. P., & Henkens, K. (2012). What is on a demographer's mind? A worldwide survey. *Demographic Research, 26*, 363–408.

Van Dalen, H. P., & Reuser, M. (2005). *Assessing size and structure of worldwide funds for population and AIDS activities* (NIDI report). The Hague: NIDI.

Van Dalen, H. P., & Reuser, M. (2006). What drives donor funding in population assistance programs? Evidence from OECD countries. *Studies in Family Planning, 37*, 141–154.

Van Dalen, H. P., & Reuser, M. (2008). Aid and AIDS: A delicate cocktail. *Vox – research-based policy analysis and commentary from leading economists*, 07-07-2008. http://www.voxeu.org/article/aid-and-aids-delicate-cocktail

Wattenberg, B. (1997, November 23). The population explosion is over. *New York Times Magazine*, pp. 60–63.

WHO. (2005). *China: Health, poverty and economic development*. Beijing: WHO Representative in China. http://www.who.int/macrohealth/action/CMH_China.pdf

WHO. (2008a). *Eliminating female genital mutilation: An interagency statement*. Geneva: World Health Organization and other UN agencies.

WHO. (2008b). *World health statistics 2008*. Geneva: World Health Organization.

Williamson, J. (1990). What Washington means by policy reform. In J. Williamson (Ed.), *Latin American adjustment: How much has happened?* Washington: Institute for International Economics.

World Bank. (1993). *World development report – investing in health*. Oxford: Oxford University Press.

World Bank. (2004). *World development report – Making services work for poor people*. Oxford: Oxford University Press.

Yoder, P. S., & Khan, S. (2008). *Numbers of women circumcised in Africa: The production of a total*. Calverton: Macro International Inc.

Chapter 11
Looking Back and Looking Ahead to Where Are We Going: A Round-Table Symposium on the Past, Present, and Future of Reproductive Health

Panelists: Daniel E. Pellegrom, Marleen Temmerman, Neil Datta, Jill Sheffield, Stan Bernstein, and Elizabeth Lule

11.1   Look Over Your Shoulder and Prepare for More: It's About Sex After All

Daniel E. Pellegrom

The central challenges that face the reproductive health movement are neither medical nor technical. While a more perfect contraceptive would be a welcomed addition, such a development does not rise to the level of a central challenge. More valuable than a new contraceptive method would be a new metrics that all could agree upon as a more accurate and durable device to measure the success of interventions like those employed by Pathfinder International and its partners. Even as helpful as a new measuring stick would be, neither does it rise to a prominent level.

Indeed the challenges faced by this great social movement are more fundamental and far trickier; they are conceptual, political and they are controversial.

D.E. Pellegrom
Pathfinder International, Newtown, MA, USA

M. Temmerman
Department of OB/GYN, ICRH, Ghent University, Ghent, Belgium

N. Datta
European Parliamentary Forum (EPF) on Population and Development, Brussels, Belgium

J. Sheffield
Women Deliver, New York, NY, USA

S. Bernstein
ReGeneration Consulting LLC, New York, NY, USA

E. Lule
Regional Integration Department, Africa Region World Bank, Washington, DC, USA

A. Kulczycki (ed.), *Critical Issues in Reproductive Health*, The Springer Series on Demographic Methods and Population Analysis 33, DOI 10.1007/978-94-007-6722-5_11, © Springer Science+Business Media Dordrecht 2014

I have a troubling recollection to share from a conversation that occurred more than a decade ago. The setting was a conference room in Washington, D.C., where about three dozen CEOs of U.S. based humanitarian organizations were deliberating on recent U.S foreign assistance policies. These NGO organizational leaders turned to each other and pondered what their diverse organizations had in common. (Represented in the room were faith-based organizations and secular ones, child sponsorship organizations, some focused on refugees, and others that do development or provide health care.) I was the only one in the room representing family planning and reproductive health and most knew my views on the big issues, like abortion, to be unequivocal. Nevertheless, I offered an opinion on what we all had in common, which seemed to surprise my humanitarian colleagues.

I said that while there was much that separated us—Catholic Relief Services and Pathfinder International hardly could keep secret their differences—there was one single, underlying passionate and fundamental claim that unified us. Each of us had utter disdain for poverty and its grip on about one in every three people on earth. We were to a person—to an organization—united in our conviction that poverty was abhorrent and equally united in our compassion for those who were in poverty's grip. I think I went on about the feminization of poverty and maternal mortality among the poor before I became aware that I had surprised many in the room. A coffee break soon followed where upon I was nearly swarmed with people—colleagues—expressing that I had startled them; they conveyed that they would never have expected a family planner to express these sentiments. I was stunned by this and pressed them to tell me why they seemed so surprised that a family planner was passionately disturbed by poverty. I did not need to probe for long. What I discovered has bothered me ever since: our cause—our social movement—was viewed as defenders of women, but not as defenders of the impoverished.

It is tempting for me to criticize them. Why didn't they see that defending women in a less developed country typically means standing face to face with the poorest of the poor? But I think it is more productive to be introspective than to be defensive. I reflected upon my conversation and it took me all the way back to Margaret Sanger. Providing the poorest women the ability to space, time and plan their pregnancies was her driving concern. Poverty, and its hold on women in particular, is what drove Sanger to challenge the Comstock Laws.[1] Sure, she believed that women in general could never be truly free to take their rightful place in society if they remained captives of their fertility, and as a public health nurse, she devoted this conviction toward providing service to the poorest women in her society.

We are a movement born of our compassion for those who live in the slums. We are not the defenders of the elite; we are the defenders of the impoverished.

---

[1]The 1873 Comstock Act, named after a zealous crusader against what he viewed as obscenity, was part of a campaign for legislating public morality in the United States. Specifically, it was used to prosecute those who sold or distributed birth control literature, including information on contraceptives or abortion. Collectively, state and federal restrictions on distributing such materials became known as the Comstock laws. Those targeted included Margaret Sanger, founder of the U.S. birth control movement, and her husband, who was convicted of selling a single copy of her *Family Limitation* pamphlet. Her case was dismissed in 1938, effectively ending use of the Comstock Law to target birth control information and devices.

The voice of the family planner needs to be loud, but it is our message, not our voice, that must be heard. And, our message is that poverty is not something to be made more palatable. The family planner doesn't just want to alleviate poverty; the family planner wants to obliterate poverty. Poverty is unacceptable and what it does to people is abhorrent. That is what we believe.

If that is the conceptual concern, my political concern follows and attaches itself to it. Whenever someone assails family planning, they are assailing the poorest, most vulnerable people on earth.

Have you ever heard someone, even a family planner or reproductive health volunteer or professional, say something like this: "Why is what we do so controversial after all these years?" Maybe the person saying it is just suffering from momentary fatigue. Maybe you have thought this in a weak moment. But I am afraid that when this occurs, it is not only a weak moment, but a dangerous one. If we do not understand why our work is not controversial, then the opposition understands our work better than we do, and that is dangerous. What we do has always been controversial. We do not mostly provide preventative medical care. Not really. We do not mostly cure diseases or prevent them. What we do is social change. We are determined to call for a fundamental change in the social order. We believe that women deserve to be completely enfranchised in society, each to be as free to determine her place as any male, and that girls deserve protection from predators. Period. We believe that people should have control over their own most basic and personal decisions and we suggest that none is more personal than the decision if and when to bear a child.

We don't equivocate about who should have access to family planning information and services. The answer is anyone. No, everyone. We believe that people who are free to make these decisions—and have available to them the wherewithal to make truly informed choices—will far more often than not make good choices. And, we believe that people who are free to make their own choices are probably also apt to create freer communities and freer societies.

What have I said? I think I have said that the family planner is willing to challenge traditional assumptions about the roles of women in society, willing to challenge traditional assumptions about sex and gender, and willing to challenge barriers to personal freedom of choice whether religious, political or cultural.

If that's not controversial, I'm not sure what controversial is. Isn't that what the family planner signed on for? I fear that too many in our ranks have allowed themselves to succumb to the notion that the controversy in our midst is caused whenever the word "abortion" is uttered. In fact, in her remarkable book, *Abortion and the Politics of Motherhood*, published in 1984, Kristin Luker handily dispelled the idea that abortion was the source of the controversy. It isn't about abortion; the divide, in fact the chasm, according to Luker, is that there are those who believe that women deserve to be equal in society and others who believe that the one thing that separates women—puts them on a pedestal—is their ability to become mothers. One group believes that women ought not to be put on pedestals—they should just be treated right. The other, I suppose, accepts that women will never be treated equally and so wishes them to be treated separately.

Just after the January 22, 1973 Roe v. Wade decision by the U.S Supreme Court, in the early days of what we now know as the Right to life movement, their early publications essentially acknowledged that their opposition was always there. We just didn't quite know it. Their literature referred to the U.S Supreme Court as having "nationalized" their movement. They wrote then about how they were just not galvanized, coordinated and connected into a movement. But the Roe v. Wade decision offered them their "May pole" around which to rally. It wasn't even abortion that rallied them; it was a decision by the Court about abortion. The point is Luker's point; here are two spectacularly divergent views regarding the role of women in society. To one of these divergent views abortion stands to symbolize the divergence in a most egregious way. To this group, it is blasphemous; indeed the most contemptuous symbolism imaginable. Hence, it has been used to mobilize that constituency and to manipulate politicians. But make no mistake; their goal is not to obliterate abortion. Their goal is to restore women to separate, but equal status; to put them on a pedestal. Hence, they oppose everything that we stand for and, if we are not wise to this, we fail ourselves and the cause we claim to serve.

I have observed reproductive health providers over 40 years. In my case, that means mostly domestic providers from the late 1960s through the mid-1980s and since then, mostly overseas providers. Those organizations which have gotten into serious trouble have rarely done so because of poor patient care. Rarely has difficulty occurred due to poor medical practices. When serious problems develop, it is far more likely to be caused by poor political judgement or mishandling of money. I point this out because it is tempting to focus and fund technical assistance in those areas when transgressions are the least numerous or onerous rather than on the areas where the problems are most frequent and egregious—politics and finance.

I point this out because it serves to illustrate how frequently experts who are drawn to the field are technical experts and how this frequently results in providing technical assistance where exposure is least likely rather than providing it where the vulnerability is greatest—fiscal and political. Again, we slip up when we fail to realize that our work is less medicine than political. Some of us protest too loudly because we want the controversy to disappear. An illustration of this can be lifted from the Congressional Record, February 24, 1969:

> We need to make population and family planning household words. We need to take the sensationalistm out of this topic so that it can no longer be used by militants who have no real knowledge of the voluntary nature of the program, but, rather, are using it as a political stepping stone. If family planning is anything, it is a public health matter.

Congressman George Bush of Texas was a supporter of family planning until he ran for Vice President in 1980 on his party's ticket with Ronald Reagan, who, using it as a "political stepping stone", turned an issue which had been largely bi-partisan toward a partisan divide that has lasted for three decades. Congressman Bush was a supporter of family planning funding both through the domestic Title X program and internationally through USAID. The same man, when Vice President and President, enforced the Global Gag Rule as though it was his position to begin with.

Recently in the U.S. Congress, Republican Latta (R-OH) filed an amendment to eliminate $440 million for international family planning and reproductive health assistance in the FY11 continuing budget resolution. Meanwhile, others in Congress, using budget austerity as their cover, are trying to eliminate Title X funding (which is the principle family planning funding source for providing family planning services in the U.S.) as well as eliminating financial support for family planning within the U.N. (UNFPA). None of this has anything to do with abortion except that it will cause it to increase. It has everything to do with women and children; everything to do with fanning the flames of old political struggles.

It is dangerous to underestimate one's opposition. Those opposed to us are opposed to our view of the world, to our view of the role of women in that world. They are adversaries of social justice, as we view it. Abortion is an implement to be used by them. Make no mistake, the prize to them goes way beyond abortion; it always has been about more. They have revealed this over and over again, just as current proposed legislation in Congress demonstrates.

We must recognize that ours is a reform movement and social change always incites opposition. This is not about public health; it is about public policy. It is about politics. And, when your politics involves defending women, among them the poorest and most vulnerable, we should not just expect controversy, we should embrace it.

11.2 The Exceptionality of Family Planning and Sexual and Reproductive Health and Rights

Marleen Temmerman and Neil Datta

"Sure, I know what a diaphragm is. I make them at home with some tissue and plastic." This comment was made by a female sex worker from Mombasa, Kenya in an acceptability study on the use of female barrier methods in the prevention of HIV in 2002. This 44-year-old woman used a home-made diaphragm that consisted of a piece of cloth and some folded polythene for 16 years to protect herself from pregnancy and sexually transmitted infections (STIs). This survey marked the start of a pilot study directed by the Kenyan branch of the International Centre for Reproductive Health (ICRH), and she was the first female participant who expressed any knowledge of the diaphragm.

"I know my husband is moving around, but what can I do to protect myself when he comes home?" was a frequently heard cry from the nurses and female staff in Nairobi in 1990. These women were healthcare professionals, working on a research project on HIV transmission, who were very aware of the dangers of unsafe sex. But despite being married women, who were educated and employed, they had very little 'sexual power' as a consequence of societal, cultural and relational factors. As women they had to stand by their men and their family and undergo whatever their husbands subjected them to, even if this would lead to unplanned pregnancies, unsafe abortions and STIs or HIV infection. Meanwhile the men *"moved around"* as much as they wanted.

These stories vividly illustrate the challenges faced by women from all walks of life in the developing world, the limitations of current female-controlled methods of protection against unwanted pregnancies and STIs, and the huge need for additional research to improve these methods and to expand their use. Solutions are needed that can be used without male knowledge and co-operation, such as vaginal microbicides and cervical barriers against infection, including the diaphragm. Political support from the international community is essential for this to come about.

Despite having the support of the scientific community, and clearly benefitting the rights of the world's most vulnerable and disadvantaged citizens, family planning and sexual and reproductive health and rights (SRHR) face unprecedented political opposition from small – and yet highly vocal – interest groups in Europe, the USA and beyond. And this opposition is hampering efforts to protect the rights and the health of women like those referred to above. They desperately need the help of the international community: help which would be greatly facilitated if the international community would recognise the exceptionality of family planning and SRHR.

11.2.1 The Context

The HIV pandemic has had an enormous impact on health and societies in the last 30 years, and the reaction of the international community to it has been strong. Since the late 1990s we have become accustomed to hearing about the exceptionality of HIV/AIDS in public discourse, and the attention that the pandemic must receive from the international political, development and medical communities. The response from the international community to this call to action has been spectacular. Over the last decade funding for development assistance projects dealing with HIV/AIDS has increased by 1,400 %: a rise in public spending rarely seen in the funding of any international cause, which demonstrates the undeniable success that health activists and HIV/AIDS advocates have had.

During this period the ICPD was held and its Programme of Action (PoA) laid out an impressive and ambitious set of goals for improving SRHR all over the world by the target date of 2015. However, since this event, initiatives in the field of family planning have experienced a funding increase of just 34 %. Despite being an area of public health, social policy, and education that is as central to human wellbeing and development as fighting HIV/AIDS, family planning and SRHR have been neglected.

The apparent "exceptionality" of HIV/AIDS has helped to facilitate this increase. It is clear that much more still needs to be done to curb and control the pandemic, but we can draw satisfaction from the fruits of the attention it has received, and from being within range of achieving the results that the international community desires. However, regarding the problems caused by inadequate family planning and SRHR, we are far from achieving the aims set out in the Millennium Declaration (and more specifically in Development Goals 3, 4 and 5). These rights are fundamental to the human rights of half of the world's population and of the world's largest generation of young people ever as they enter their reproductive age. They concern some of the most devastating and pervasive human rights abuses which still are practiced today systematically and with near impunity. These include child marriage, female genital mutilation, sex trafficking, gender-based violence, and maternal mortality.

It is therefore time to build on the example set by the HIV/AIDS community, and to achieve similar results for family planning and SRHR. These areas are not only central to the health and well-being of the people they affect, but they are also central to allowing these people their human rights; for it is every woman's right to have control over her fertility. Moreover, family planning and SRHR are also central to slowing population growth that is too rapid to enable a population to be fed and adequately supplied by the resources that are available to it. Just meeting the unmet family planning needs will have major impact on the health of this planet.

11.2.2 The Challenge

All deaths resulting from poverty-related health inequities are tragic. In the twenty-first century, nobody should die prematurely as a result of diseases such as diarrhoea, tuberculosis and malaria (among many others) and their complications, which can be simply avoided and treated when the resources are available. The international community is aware of this, and it is generally unified in its political and ideological approach to the eradication of these diseases. For this reason it has devised cost-effective and carefully targeted approaches that are based on scientific principles and are designed to be as efficient as possible.

For family planning and SRHR, however, this unified political will from the international community does not exist. Even though the solutions that are required to stop the deaths caused by complications of pregnancy – from the schoolroom to community centres, clinics and hospitals – are clearly known, and have been proven by countless researchers, these issues cannot be dealt with in the same way as those that were outlined above as the more simple by-products of poverty. For the deaths that occur owing to inadequate SRHR are not only caused by economic poverty, but also by culturally ingrained inhumanity.

This causal link with social practices and ideology makes SRHR more politicised than any other area on the development agenda. At the European Union (EU) level, for example, a Commission employee recently remarked that EU Member States find it easier to agree on the conflict between Israel and Palestine than on family planning and SRHR. This extreme politicisation is caused by a range of factors, including societal and cultural factors, religious ideology, and inherently patriarchal and chauvinistic mindsets that dominate national decision-making in some donor countries. And it is readily demonstrated in the EU and the USA, which contribute 85 % of all international funding for the field.

In Brussels, no other global health issue mobilises entire delegations and political parties in the European Parliament in the same way as SRHR. Staunchly Christian Members of the European Parliament (MEPs) are fighting against what they label as "discrimination against Christians." They claim to be suffering from laws that protect the rights of homosexuals, for example, which they say are hindering Christians from living according to their faith. Sexuality education is seen as an intrusive indoctrination of the secular agenda in schools, and as a result is also being strongly opposed. Looking overseas, opposition forces choose to see China's one-child policy as being closely aligned with the pro-choice ideology of the European SRHR camp, and will often refuse to distinguish between the coercive abortion carried out in China and the legal, voluntary abortion carried out in most European countries. In addition, SRHR has become the single most difficult issue for EU coordination at the UN, where the EU regularly fails to agree and support a common position on SRHR.

Despite these challenges, the voice of Europe consists of an overwhelming majority of 25 countries who are pro-choice and respect the human rights of individuals to determine their reproductive choices. These countries should not be stopped in their efforts to achieve this by a small number of staunchly Catholic anti-choice countries.

Similarly, in the USA when the Republican Party gains positions of influence in the US Congress or takes control of the White House, their first action is to work to re-instate the Global Gag Rule, de-fund UNFPA and cut funding to voluntary family planning and comprehensive SRHR. In terms of human suffering, this is equal to de-funding vaccination programmes in developing countries, or de-funding the Global Fund for AIDS, Malaria and Tuberculosis, or UNICEF. Yet, for reasons of culture, religion and ideology, this negligence and abuse of human rights is viewed as legitimate.

Culture and religion play a huge role in determining the health-based development spending in donor countries. This role has meant that among all global health interventions, SRHR and FP are treated according to cultural and religious principles and ideals, rather than scientific and evidence-based facts. As a result, these poorly conceived policies are effectively deemed an acceptable development approach, and women are dying as a consequence.

Furthermore, the cause of SRHR opponents is strengthened by the simplified, emotive and manipulative way in which its supporters are able to influence casual and uninformed members of public. Exaggerated campaigns relating to issues such as abortion frequently harness the emotional reactions of the general public to persuade them about an issue that is far more complex than the appearance that they give it. Pro-choice decision-makers are therefore also confronted with a more complex story to tell than the opposition, and need to combat the emotional blackmail that the opposition has potentially at its disposal.

11.2.3   The Solutions

SRHR advocates have an incredibly strong and persuasive message that has the backing of the scientific, the public health and the human rights communities. This message should also have the support of the largely moderate religious mindsets that prevail across the developed world, which is apparent in the morality and charity that are demonstrated in most areas of public life. The solution for depoliticizing SRHR, therefore, lies in communication: the world must hear our message clearly and simply.

Since public opinion is so vulnerable to the messages of populist cultural and religious influences, it is important for people to continue to see family planning as a free-standing issue that is as linked to individuals' overall human rights as it is to their SRHR. For if we only considered family planning when it is referred to as being part of SRHR, then we would run the risk of over-complicating a simple issue, and in doing so playing into the hands of the opposition and their emotive and propagandist advocacy. Therefore we must firstly always consider family planning as an issue in its own right to make it more understandable and recognisable.

An important way in which we can spread the SRHR message is to inform the world clearly and publicly about misunderstandings that they appear to have of the SRHR agenda. Anti-choice MEPs were recently seen to have a poor understanding of the role played by the United Nations Population Fund (UNFPA) in China, for example, and also do not seem to distinguish between coercive and selective abortion. Both facts are crucial to the public legitimacy of the SRHR community towards the audience for opposition communicative activities, and should be publicly addressed in the most suitable arena. Other key messages that must be clearly communicated are:

1. At least 200 million women want to use safe and effective family planning methods, but are unable to do so because they lack access to information and services or the support of their husbands and communities.
2. More than 50 million of the 190 million women who become pregnant each year have abortions, many of which are clandestine and performed under unsafe conditions.
3. The need for voluntary family planning is growing fast and it is estimated that the 'unmet need' will grow by 40 % during the next 15 years.
4. Even though it is an economically sound investment, family planning has been losing ground as an international development priority. Funding is not increasing on a par with demand, yet the gap between the need and the available resources is growing.
5. Slowing population growth can reduce the range of pressures placed on the world by humans. Family planning can have a positive effect on the world's resources and its ecology. For example, it can help reduce demand for scarce and critical natural resources that – if unchecked – would undermine the ability of agricultural economies to absorb the available labour pool, promote landless poverty, upset the ecological balance, and accelerate the growth of urban slums.

11.2.4 Conclusion

Advancing SRHR, and specifically family planning, is one of the most important steps we can make in supporting human rights and democratic values, and for providing multiple long-term contributions to environmental concerns and sustainable development. Few other global health interventions have such powerful knock-on effects as family planning. Neutralizing the politicization around SRHR should be the priority in our work to advance the ICPD PoA and the MDGs. We can start by recognising how exceptional SRHR and family planning really are and by following the model that has been made by work to defeat HIV/AIDS.

To bear fruit, our messages should reach policy-makers from both ends of the political spectrum, and they should do so by both political and public means. Organisations such as the European Parliamentary Forum on Population and Development are vital in this process; for they bring together politicians from all major political parties who are united by their belief in the need to protect and strengthen the rights of the victims of ingrained and culturally propagated human rights abuses. This work helps to create and inform SRHR champions in parliaments across Europe, who are vital actors in ensuring that substantive efforts are made in the field of SRHR by the international community.

Women are suffering and dying as a result of inhuman practices that are being spread by long-held dogmas and ideologies that disadvantage women. We must find a solution so that the cultural and religious hypocrisy which touches both sides of the Atlantic can no longer hold the lives of women in developing countries as hostage. Tradition and culture have their value, but in the twentyfirst century, no national or cultural setting with traditional practices that are harmful to girls and women should be accommodated or promoted.

As we look to the future, it would be easy to be alarmed about the voluble opposition that the pro-choice, pro-human rights SRHR community is facing. But if we look at the progress that humanity has made in recent decades, then we can reassure ourselves that the opposition is so voluble because it is losing. Across the world, from Malta to Mozambique, humanity is slowly progressing and allowing humans to improve their SRHR. Whether this is the right of Maltese citizens to get divorced, of Portuguese same-sex couples to get married, or of girls in any one of the countries in the developing world to make an informed decision about the number of children they will have, we are making progress. We have an example to follow; we have the solutions; so let's take action.

11.3   Championing MDG5: Invest in Women, It Pays

Jill Sheffield

In the early 1980s while I was volunteering at a family planning clinic in Kenya, a young woman, my age, came to the clinic. She was carrying a newborn baby on her front and an older baby on her back. In her 27 years, she had had 11 pregnancies and six living children. She had been on a bus since 4 a.m. and was told that she needed her husband's permission to get birth control. "Not on my watch," I said to myself, and she left the clinic with protection in hand.

That is how and where my life-long battle to improve maternal health and reproductive rights began. Today, I am the President of Women Deliver, a global advocacy organization that seeks to promote and improve the health of girls, women, and mothers and works toward achieving Millennium Development

Goal 5 ("MDG5")—reducing maternal mortality, improving women's health and guaranteeing access to universal reproductive health. And, to this day, it is still the same motto: "Not on my watch." Not on my watch will girls and women continue to die from pregnancy-related conditions when these conditions are preventable. Not on my watch will girls and women be denied choices on when to be pregnant. Not on my watch will girls and women be silenced, neglected, or ignored.

Five years ago, one woman died every minute from complications of pregnancy and childbirth, and millions more suffered from serious injuries. MDG5 was making little progress and receiving the least financial support of all the UN global health goals. To ignite change and focus attention on MDG5, Women Deliver held a global conference in London in 2007. This conference brought to light a new case for supporting MDG5: *US $15 billion is lost every year due to maternal and newborn mortality.* This estimate was from 2001 data, and many believe too low, even then. But even so, the number was astounding – imagine $15 billion annually in lost productivity – this made some ears hear the issue for the first time.

And today, *Invest in women, it pays* has become a collective rallying call. That is not to say we neglect the social justice issue– *no girl or woman should die giving life.* But we have become realistic at framing a message which resonates with political leaders. The facts are simple: women deliver, not only babies, but stable societies and healthy economies.

By bringing these economic facts to light, Women Deliver moved the issue of maternal health beyond the global health context, linking it to broader economic and development issues, human rights, gender issues, and sexual and reproductive health. Funds started to flow, and the political will to invest in girls and women began to grow. The maternal and reproductive health communities came to consensus on the solutions, and the estimates of maternal deaths began to decline from 500,000 to 350,000.

Are we happy about the numbers? You bet, but we must do more. One woman dying every 90 seconds is not good enough. We have solutions. We know what to do. It's a fact where governments have had the political will to invest in meeting girls' and women's needs, the number of deaths decrease and many lives improve. Where governments have not made those investments, as in much of sub-Saharan Africa and South Asia, pregnancy continues to be a life-threatening event, families are threatened, and progress for girls is difficult.

One of the many things that I have learned in these 30 years plus in this field is that we cannot be complacent about our successes. Building global and sustaining momentum requires vigilance and continuous effort. Advocates exulted in the aftermath of the 1994 Cairo International Conference on Population and Development and the 1995 Beijing World Conference on Women. We believed that the world had agreed that a woman's journey from poverty to self-sufficiency and from oppression to equality started with her sexual and reproductive health and rights. But such feelings were short-lived. Soon after 1995, family planning and reproductive health were put out to pasture in the difficult years of the gag rule. And, it would be many more years before these issues would again regain momentum and take the international stage.

There is much we can do and must do to keep MDG5 on track, and global advocacy is an essential part of the effort. This is where Women Deliver will devote its energies in the next 4 years.

We will make sure that girls and women are not ever left out of the equation. Their second-class status in many areas of the world make them especially vulnerable in times of economic distress. The media has become our ally in our effort to keep the global focus on girls and women. We take advantage of every opportunity to remind the world on the value of investing in girls and women. The 100th Anniversary of International Women's Day in March 2011 was an opportunity to recognize 100 outstanding individuals who have delivered for girls and women across sectors and across the globe. We chose not to highlight only the global stars, but a combination of people, global stars and local heroes who are truly delivering for women. Their stories were not only heralded in the international press, but in their local newspapers. The continual demand for 24-hour news helps us get coverage. Messaging is also an important part of our media work – messages that are positive, simple, and memorable. *Blog 4* named Women Deliver 2010, our global conference, a top 2010 health communications strategy: *"The successful Women Deliver Conference in Washington got coverage global health advocates usually only dream of — it was covered by 235 reporters and generated 295 news stories."*

Special events and conferences are a trademark of Women Deliver and serve as an important launch pad for new funding, new thinking, and policy initiatives. Global conferences have proven to be galvanizing events, propelling action on the world stage and broadening the base of support. We have actively planned for the 2013 Women Deliver conference in Kuala Lampur. We cannot wait until 2014 or 2105 to check on our progress or to plan post ICPD and post MDGs. As a lead-up to the conference, we held regional consultations to identify regional barriers and to inform our 2013 agenda.

We will continue to promote solutions that can be implemented now. Our 2010 conference was all about solutions, and there are so many good projects that are making a difference. Short-term solutions can help us reach our long-term goals of strengthened health systems and adequate health personnel. While we need to keep our eye on the long-term, we must remember that girls and women don't wait for the perfect system to get pregnant!

We will continue to reach out to unlikely allies. Healthy girls and women are central to every aspect of development – education, labor, finance, gender equality, HIV/AIDS, economy, environment, etc. We used to believe different development sectors shared different goals and that we were in competition for scarce development dollars. As a result there were winners and losers. But the truth is MDG5 today has allies in nearly all sectors because we have shown that it is important, if not critical to their cause, that girls and women neither die nor suffer injuries from complications of pregnancy and childbirth. It is an absolute truth that MDG5 is the heart of all MDGs, or as the Dutch say, the mother of all MDGs.

We will focus on family planning. I am ashamed to say that at our 2007 global conference, family planning was hardly mentioned. Three years later, we devoted a full-day technology symposium to contraception. Family planning is like girls' education, a silver bullet to achieve a significant drop in maternal mortality. The unmet need for family planning alone is huge. More than 215 million women want to avoid pregnancy, but are not using modern contraception, and demand is expected to grow 40 % by 2050 as history's largest generation of young people ages. While there are many obstacles, stock-outs, transportation barriers, tariffs, attitudes, etc., we have great organizations and coalitions working on these issues.

We will focus on youth. Young people make up a major portion of the global population, particularly in the developing world, and the truth is that too many mothers are just girls. We need to focus explicitly on their unique needs. And we need to engage, and count on young people to help us deliver for girls and women. Their perspectives, their experiences, and their willingness to question offer the greatest hope for challenging the social norms and decades-old policies that harm girls and women. One only has to look at how young people harnessed social media to bring dramatic change to the Egyptian and Tunisian governments to understand this amazing untapped power.

We have learned in our work with young people that the language of maternal health is a significant barrier to their engagement. We cloak our messages in medicalized terms devoid of any emotional appeal: "family planning", "birth control", "family-life education", "safe motherhood", "maternal health", and "fertility regulation". We tuck abortion under the term "reproductive health". We rally for solutions that are complicated and difficult to explain: "health systems strengthening" and "achieving sexual and reproductive health and rights".

When young people are aware of the facts, the dangers they face, and their lack of rights, they are motivated and passionate. Women Deliver saw this first hand when we recruited a global group of 100 Young Leaders to attend a special advocacy skills-building session just before the Women Deliver conference in June 2010. Once engaged, these young advocates have written blogs, addressed the media, developed You-Tube videos, and continually tried to connect to us and the issue. As they have become better informed and more skilled advocates, they have spread the message that maternal deaths are a tragedy that can and must be prevented. In the next 3 years, Women Deliver will work on identifying the issues and words that engage young people and seek with partners across the globe to build a cadre of young people speaking out for MDG5.

We will engage the private sector. The potential contribution of the private sector to achieving MDG5 is largely untapped. Whereas the HIV sector has reached out to embrace business and to capitalize on what business can offer, by and large the maternal and reproductive health sectors have kept at arms length the international business community. Yet private sector products such as vaccines, medicines, medical supplies, supply chain services, and communications are all part of the essential package to improve the health of girls and women. Doing business and doing good for girls and women are not incompatible. We need to help corporations get their life-saving products to market and to develop better and more effective products.

Women Deliver has created the C-Exchange, a forum to promote enhanced collaboration between the private and public sectors, including, but not limited to, corporations, governmental organizations, civil society, foundations, and institutions of higher learning. Over the next 3 years, the C-Exchange will concentrate on four technological solutions, all of which are available today and can significantly reduce maternal mortality and morbidity. They are (1) contraception; (2) postpartum hemorrhage prevention and treatment; (3) HPV vaccination, testing, and cervical cancer treatment; and (4) communications technology such as mobile telephones.

We will bring the topic of unsafe abortion out of hiding. Although globally there have been significant changes including less restrictive laws, increased use of contraception, including emergency contraception and growing use of medical abortion, deaths from unsafe abortion extract an enormous toll on girls and women and their families. Their deaths are preventable, yet unsafe abortion tends to receive less attention that any other sexual and reproductive health component.

We need to peel away the rhetoric and emotion that surrounds legalizing abortion services by focusing tightly on the issue of safety. Legal abortion can be and often is unsafe, and on the other hand, illegal abortion can be safe. By reframing the discussion to safety, we will guide the conversation to how and what governments can do today– right now– to reduce maternal mortality and morbidity from unsafe abortion. Strategies can entail ensuring access to contraceptives (including emergency contraception), scaling up post-abortion care, and promoting safe abortion services where legal. With our end goal as safety, we allow those who oppose abortion to be part of the conversation. We all share a common goal of saving lives of girls and women.

We will promote accountability. Above all, we need to hold ourselves and each other accountable at each step of the way. Donor governments must make good on their pledges; countries must not only pass laws that advance the health and well-being of girls and women, but implement them. NGOs must show results and value in their work. Accountability is a test of our tools and our willingness to hold everyone's feet to the fire. We have never been better equipped as we have new technologies to help us collect information and almost universal agreement that this is something that must be done. The Commission on Information and Accountability for Women's and Children's Health is a positive step with its two working groups, one on results and one on resources. Its accountability framework is expected to bring greater transparency and improvements in monitoring our progress. When we know where we have been, we can better plan where we should be.

The next 4 years offer great promise. There is no doubt in my mind that we are on the right path. So many great organizations are working on maternal and reproductive health. Sometimes I believe I am the luckiest person in the world to have made this my life-career, where one, dozens, hundreds and thousands of advocates can each personally make a difference.

11.4   A Driver Without Wheels: The Continued Relative Neglect of the Reproductive Health Agenda

Stan Bernstein

Reproductive health services and population dynamics, the former being a substantial determinant of the latter, remain an undervalued and underinvested portion of the development agenda. There has been some progress in recent years, but previous neglect and continuing debate still put women, children and families at risk.

A comprehensive understanding of the contribution of population dynamics to development prospects at local, national, regional and global levels is established but fades in and out of priority discussions over time. The cause of this ambivalence is more based on values conflicts than on evidence.

The recurrent gloss on population issues, whatever the topic of a relevant report, is tied to added numbers expected at various times. Whatever the publication, different interest groups – those supportive of reproductive health and rights, and those with a different set of priorities regarding sex and reproduction as individual concerns – stake out their own agendas. There are also some serious and deeply ingrained habits of thought, mental ruts, actually, that recur to no positive effect.

11.4.1 Bad Habits

The storyline on population, particularly in the mainstream media, is one of growing numbers of the aggregate total of people on Earth. Sometimes (when the UN's Population Division biennially revises its projections) the projections are revised upwards; sometimes downwards. The usual outcries result. When revised upwards, visions are offered of looming catastrophe; when downwards, accusations of earlier doom-mongering by biased interest groups (the population community or "industry") are leveled. Whichever the direction of adjustment, whatever the aggregate numbers offered, the right Reverend Robert Thomas Malthus is resurrected to suffer again. The broader development context is missed in a focus on numbers and an over-rehearsed set of scripts.

An example of this problem can be found in the annual response to the UNFPA *State of World Population Report*. Each year a different thematic topic is selected for examination. Recent years have addressed urbanization, displaced populations, population and environment links. In the years since ICPD, other themes have included reproductive rights, population and the environment, changing age structures (the "new generations" of the elderly and the adolescents), population and development relations, population and poverty. In 2011 the report addressed the population milestone of the 7 billionth person. The reporting was more heavy than usual, but differed little from non-milestone reports. Invariably a large share of the headlines and lead stories highlighted the total population number. The reports are always more nuanced.

11.4.2 Population and Development, Writ Larger

The broader development context in such discussions is, unfortunately, lost. Population and development linkages are multiple, multi-sectoral (i.e., related to institutional environments more usually organized for intra-sectoral linkages), influenced by various actors –both public and private- and addressing differing time schemes for their targets and evolution. Such confusion about evidentiary bases in the area of population and reproductive health isn't surprising. Even among professionals in population studies, evidence about immediate rewards and demonstrations of (often short-term) impact and influence trump longer-term perspectives.

Population and development dialogues remain impenetrable to non-specialized audiences because of the diversity of levels of discourse and linkages among these proliferating concerns that must be addressed. With specialists unable to unify their statements, people outside the fold, including policy makers, have little reason to accept their conclusions. The improving quality of technical reviews in the field might advance internal cohesiveness and address other audiences' needs. Recent publications have strengthened our knowledge of population and poverty relations[2] and of the efficacy of particular relevant interventions.[3]

11.4.3 A Path Late Taken

Hope for unification of development priorities was vested in the MDGs. But fears of political imbroglios kept both reproductive health and gender equality issues marginalized. Women's empowerment was given a goal but the monitoring was restricted to indicators related to education, parliamentary participation and non-agricultural employment. (Control of resources – credit, land tenure – and freedom from violence and physical and social mobility, among other concerns – could not be discussed). Reproductive health was denied either a goal or a target; among the accepted indicators, contraceptive prevalence was included, along with the proportion of contraceptive use represented by condoms, under the HIV/AIDS (and TB and malaria) Goal.

This official MDG road map definition occurred despite a June 2000 publication – signed by the UN Secretary General (on his own behalf and that of the heads of the major UN agencies), OECD, the IMF and the World Bank, entitled *A Better World for All: Progress Towards the International Development Goals*-- that contained a goal of "universal access to reproductive health", with component targets of HIV and maternal mortality reduction. It took 7 years of the 15 year MDG time horizon for universal access to reproductive health to be accepted as a target under the goal "Improve Maternal Health", with indicators related to family planning (contraceptive prevalence and unmet need for family planning), antenatal care (promoting attention to the full continuum of care for reproductive, maternal, newborn and child

---

[2]UNFPA. 2011. *Population Dynamics in the Least Developed Countries: Challenges and Opportunities for Development and Poverty Reduction* (New York: United Nations Population Fund).

[3]See, for example, Lisa Mwaikambo, Ilene S. Speizer, Anna Schurmann, Gwen Morgan, and Fariyal Fikree. "What works in Family Planning: A systematic review". *Studies in Family Planning* 2011; 42[2]: 67–82.

health) and adolescent fertility levels (pointing to a key under-served population group, whose entry into adult roles and responsibilities is greatly affected by when they choose – or are compelled – to start families). But the long delay before its adoption has granted the target less visibility than others.

11.4.4 New Concerns and Unseen Continuities

Just as HIV/AIDS "hijacked" all development attention on matters related to sex and reproduction (without politically or culturally sensitive indicators and with a concentration on treatment, not prevention), so has climate change now moved higher up development priorities. Both population and climate change share the characteristic of having gradual cumulative impacts, only occasionally punctuated by a tectonic shift, and are, therefore, hard to fit into the shorter-term reality of political election cycles. Climate change has gained attention because of the magnitude of the potential impacts, and because it fits within a long-standing narrative about the victimization of less developed countries by the rich consumers of the more developed countries (but with the added twist of faster progress towards adaptation and amelioration starting to take place within the BRICS).[4]

Development discourse continues to be shaped in a highly political environment, though some of the discussion is about technical matters (e.g., the relative costs and benefits of climate-promoting behavioral adjustments on various scales, the role of different health and social development attainments in changing family size and composition preferences, etc.) or, at least, couched in technical terms. Collective impacts predominate, however dramatic the impacts on individuals, in instrumental discussions of development priority setting. The focus on individuals and their prospects and welfare is more consistently maintained within discussions about reproductive health as a matter of human rights. As important as this bulwark of support for sexual and reproductive health is, a more instrumental mentality and approach is required to free the purse strings for the necessary investments to ensure that these rights are addressed and enforced.

Many publications about population and climate change now routinely include two elements: a recognition that population growth (without sufficient off-setting efficiency gains from new technologies) is a driving force behind increases in damaging greenhouse gas emissions and a concern for more equitable access to new technologies. Similarly, many publications about national and international security point to the role of population growth (particularly in poor settings with large under-employed young populations) as a driver of instability at national,

---

[4]The acronym BRICs refers to the four emerging economies of Brazil, Russia, India, China (with some commentators adding South Africa), which are at a similar stage of newly advanced economic development and are expected to become a much larger force in the world economy and polity over the next few decades. In particular, the BRICs may become as or more wealthy than most current major economic powers.

regional and global scales. However, in both these key areas, while population is recognized as a driver, calls are rarely made for investments in reproductive health programs that would enable people to implement their desires for smaller and better spaced families, as recognized in the high levels of unmet need for family planning. The driver lacks wheels: both those that steer the discussion and those that make contact with the day-to-day grounded reality of service availability, quality and barriers.

11.4.5   Mortality and the Rest of Health: Cure and Prevention as Contending Priorities

Though it is an area where it should not be considered exceptional or unusual, development dialogue concerning health is also flawed. Much of the discussion of health and monitoring of progress has been centered only on mortality. The WHO Charter's definition of health (adapted at the ICPD for the definition of reproductive health), "a state of complete physical, mental and social well-being and not merely the absence of disease or infirmity" has, in the context of international goals, largely been ignored, with greatest attention given only to mortality reduction. (The "Improve Maternal Health" goal of the MDGs originally only had a mortality target. The expansion of the HIV/AIDS related goal in 2008 only cited universal access to treatment. Technically, the UNGASS[5] recommendation for universal access to treatment, prevention, care and support occurred after the 2005 World Summit that legitimated MDG adjustments).

There have been exceptions to this myopia, but they have not been fully realized. The WHO's Commission on Social Determinants of Health was tasked to elucidate the range of social processes that impact the ability of people, and particularly the poor, to access health services. The value added from this effort, however, did not extend to a rich recognition of the complex social dynamics in the area of reproductive health. Again, an illness-focused health discussion dominated.

The dichotomy between prevention and curative approaches intruded once more. Barriers to treatments and cure got more recognition than the social barriers to prevention, with particular failure to address these in women's health. Earlier efforts to elicit the "voices of the poor" on the causes of their poverty were dominated by issues related to out-of-pocket expenditures forced by acute health crises. The short-term, admittedly catastrophic, impacts of dealing with

---

[5] UNGASS refers to the United Nations General Assembly 26th Special Session held in New York, 2001, which adopted a Declaration of Commitment on HIV/AIDS. Accordingly, all UN member states committed to reverse the HIV/AIDS epidemic by 2010 as well as specific and measurable measures by different years to achieve progress towards implementing this Declaration.

health crises got more attention than the cumulative impact of unintended pregnancies as a continuous drain on household resources and as a contributor to greater impacts on family wellbeing of lesser health emergencies. Families already living near the edge can be pushed into poverty by comparatively smaller emergency outlays than the catastrophic conditions that they and those better off may have to face.

11.4.6 What Comes Next?

The UN Secretary-General's Global Strategy on Women's and Children's Health[6] marks a new opportunity for reproductive health and population concerns to gain greater attention. At the outset, attending to "women's" and not just "maternal" health emphasizes that women have special health needs, and requirements for family, community and health system support even before they become, or intend to become, mothers. Similarly, the emphasis on health system strengthening provides the opportunity to address the integration of reproductive health, including family planning, with other health delivery. It is likely that any successor arrangement to the MDGs will not throw out the existing framework but will seek to fine tune and prioritize action to accelerate progress and link the past efforts to new concerns (e.g., non-communicable diseases, including mental health outcomes from unintended pregnancy; human resources for health; gender-based violence; a more inclusive strategy for women's empowerment; etc.). A broader focus on empowerment and agency, rather than the delivery of the "stuff" related to selected outcomes could emerge as a priority concern. Further, a deeper recognition of larger development issues that unfold beyond the timetable of decadal deadlines is likely to emerge.

In the area of reproductive health, a more comprehensive, ICPD-related, perspective on unintended pregnancy and the social conditions that lead to it and that follow from it would be a positive direction. The MDG indicators for Target 5B advanced the reproductive health agenda and pointed to an integrated view of relevant service delivery, but a more comprehensive understanding of the nexus of women's health, women's power and self-determination, and gender and generational relations would further speed progress on health and social outcomes that shape women's capabilities.

---

[6]See United Nations Secretary-General Ban Ki-Moon. 2010. *Global Strategy for Women's and Children's Health*. New York (accessible at http://www.who.int/pmnch/activities/jointactionplan/en/index.html). This effort describes a multi-actor, multi-level strategy to speed attainment of the MDGs related to reducing child mortality and improving maternal health by 2015 that was launched at the 2010 High Level review of progress on the MDGs. It includes a strategy to use $40 billion in pledges to address the full continuum of reproductive, maternal, newborn and child health.

   Significant progress has been made as well on appreciating the need to address
inequities and inequalities, as basic matters of social justice, as well as aggregate
outcomes. This developed through various rubrics related to different MDG goals
including "localizing the MDGs" (in the area of urban slums and labor issues),
power analyses (in the Millennium Project's Task Force on maternal and child
health) and civil society advocacy efforts.
   Finally, issues of intergenerational relationships provide an opportunity to incorporate issues related to population age structure changes and their implications for
social unity and progress.
   Recent developments are encouraging concerning development of a concerted
approach to reproductive health through the life cycle, a heightened concern about
improving family planning services, greater attention to unintended pregnancy and
a more nuanced attention to population dynamics and its role in social development.
These can be succinctly summarized as follows:

1. Further concern with service integration: a key component of the UN Secretary
   General's Global Strategy[7];
2. Greater priority to preparing and serving youth: statements of priority from the
   new UNFPA Executive Director, Babatunde Osotimehin;
3. Strengthening of commodity supply systems (and ensuring inclusion of family
   planning commodities), including the recommitments made and progress noted
   at a June 2011 meeting in Addis Ababa[8];
4. National, regional and global policy commitments to family planning services,
   including recommitments to the Maputo Plan of Action,[9] the Ouagadougou
   Declaration,[10] the recent Istanbul Call to Action at the Least Developed Countries
   meeting[11];

---

[7]The Secretary General's forward to his report (op.cit.) emphasized: "support for country-led health
plans, supported by increased, predictable and sustainable investment; integrated delivery of health
services and life-saving interventions – so women and their children can access prevention, treatment
and care when and where they need it; stronger health systems, with sufficient skilled workers at their
core; innovative approaches to financing, product development and the efficient delivery of health
services; improved monitoring and evaluation to ensure the accountability of all actors for results."

[8]For details, see http://www.unfpa.org/public/home/news/pid/7931.

[9]In 2010, the African Union extended the implementation of the 2006 Maputo Plan Of Action for
the Operationalisation of the Continental Policy Framework for Sexual and Reproductive Health
and Rights 2007–2010, for the period up to 2015. The Plan identified nine areas of action: integration of sexual and reproductive health (SRH) services into primary health care (PHC), including
integration of HIV/AIDS and SRH, repositioning family planning, youth-friendly services,
addressing unsafe abortion, quality safe motherhood, resource mobilization, commodity security,
and monitoring and evaluation. The review and extension document can be found at http://www.
docstoc.com/docs/38789919/MAPUTO-PLAN-OF-ACTION-REPORT-2010.

[10]Francophone West Africa identified family planning as an urgent development need. Information
about the meeting, and a summary report, can be found at http://www.respond-project.org/pages/
in-action/2011-05-18-west-africa-fp-conference.php.

[11]The call to action included a call to "Provide universal access to reproductive health by 2015,
including integrating family planning, sexual health and health-care services in national strategies
and programmes". Information on the conference and links to the documents can be found at
http://www.un-ngls.org/spip.php?page=aldc4&id_article=3507.

5. Dedicated research and dissemination efforts to strengthen the evidence base for programming: the international Family Planning meetings (first Kampala and then Dakar in 2011),[12] and the STEP UP Consortium[13] being supported by the UK's Department for International Development (DfID), and the Advance Family Planning project,[14] including parliamentary discussions, supported by these efforts;
6. Forging of a new coalition with the climate change community: appreciation that population dynamics (and particularly faster growth rates than peoples' self-reports suggest they desire) still matters, as at a recent Population Footprints meeting in the UK with participation from academia, foundations, international agencies, bilateral donors and civil society.[15]

How this return of concern will translate into policies and programs remains to be seen. As the ICPD Programme of Action approaches its 20th anniversary, and the MDGs their 15th (both approaching their final target dates), it might finally be time for the driver to be given access to all the wheels needed for further progress.

11.5   Adapting to Change to Achieve Universal Access to Reproductive Health

Elizabeth Lule

When I was born in Uganda several decades ago, its population numbered about 6 million people. It has since reached over 33 million and is projected to grow to 91.3 million by 2050. Although the family planning movement was launched in the 1950s, and the Ugandan government included family planning in its primary health care package in 1986, only 26 % of women of childbearing age used modern contraceptives in 2011. As a result, Ugandan women still have over six children each against a global average of 2.5 children per woman. Not surprisingly, Uganda has one of the world's highest unmet needs for family planning (41 %), with 40 % of the population under the age of 14 and 15 % of babies born to teenage mothers. Uganda's youthful population presents a challenge, as well as an opportunity.

Currently, maternal and child health conditions still carry a heavy disease burden, representing approximately 20.4 % of disability adjusted life years (DALYs) lost. For

---

[12]These meetings were technical conferences reviewing on-going research into policies and programmes. The Kampala meeting (International Conference on Family Planning: Research and Best Practices) was attended by over 1,500 participants: details can be found at http://www.fpconference2009.org/.

[13]The STEP UP research programme consortium is led by the Population Council, partnering with the London School for Hygiene and Tropical Medicine, ICDDRB, the African Population and Health Research Center, Marie Stopes International and Partners in Population and Development. The acronym stands for Strengthening Evidence for Programming on Unintended Pregnancy. A summary and fact sheet can be found at http://www.popcouncil.org/projects/325_STEPUP.asp.

[14]See details about this advocacy effort at http://www.advancefamilyplanning.org/toolkits/advancefp.

[15]See details at http://www.populationfootprints.org/.

women of childbearing age, the disease burden has been exacerbated by the HIV/AIDS epidemic, although prevalence has declined from 22 to 6.7 % today. However, we know that the lifetime risk of maternal death is a function of the number of pregnancies and the quality and utilization of health care services. As long as child mortality remains high, women will continue to desire more children, and as long as fertility remains high, progress towards reducing maternal and child mortality, as well as addressing the other Millennium Development Goals (MDGs), is likely to be slow.

Uganda has made some progress in poverty reduction, boosting education, and advancing gender equality, but much more needs to be done to get the multiplier effect for reproductive health. Improving access to reproductive and child health services has been too slow and family planning has proved controversial. Many more investments in girls and women are needed to achieve the MDGs. Despite an array of policies on population, reproductive health, adolescent health and a road map to improving maternal health, Uganda has yet to fully and successfully implement an appropriate policy framework that enables it to capitalize on the demographic dividend offered by its youthful population. Yet research shows that investing in youth – whether in access to reproductive health care, in education, employment or in other key areas of their lives – has synergistic effects that promote overall economic development, as occurred in parts of South East Asia (Birdsall, Kelley, Sinding 2001).[16] The shift to smaller families, that is taking place in developing countries and as their demographic transitions advance, presents a window of opportunity as workers have fewer old and young dependants to support. However, a demographic dividend is not a given, and making the most of it requires the right economic and social policy environment that facilitates flexible labor markets, market-based opportunities for investment, and macroeconomic stability with a thriving private sector to generate the jobs needed for the expanding working age group. Social policies must promote gender equality, female economic empowerment and skills development, as well as improved access to basic social services in education, health and social protection. However, not all countries have taken advantage of this window of opportunity. Whether Uganda captures this moment will depend on its level of political commitment and recognition that the effects of the age structure, not population numbers, will fuel its economic and social development.

Uganda's situation illustrates much of the unfinished agenda for achieving universal access to reproductive health. It also reflects the challenges and disparities that exist across regions and countries, between developed and less developed countries, and between the rich and the poor. Even in countries that have made progress, there are pockets of socially excluded groups and areas. Averages for regions and countries can be deceptive and mask dramatic disparities within each region and country, as well as between different population groups and geographic areas. While reproductive health rights advocates have passionately embraced individual rights, they have not always focused on the broader equity agenda so critical to their whole agenda.

---

[16]Birdsall, Nancy,. Allen .C. Kelley and Steven .W. Sinding, eds. 2001. *Population Matters: Demographic Change, Economic Growth, and Poverty in the Developing World*. New York: Oxford University Press.

There is growing consensus that we would make faster progress to achieving the MDGs if we provided more targeted services to the underserved, to the marginalized and most vulnerable populations, and to those otherwise lagging behind.

Poverty and inadequate health and community systems compound vulnerability to sickness and even to death. At the same time, poor health also exacerbates poverty by placing financial and social burdens on families, e.g., a catastrophic event such as a pregnancy complication that requires expensive health care, or a disease like HIV/AIDS that may kill people in their prime. For the poorest, an unwanted pregnancy is more threatening to their family resources. Yet, public services and subsidies benefit the wealthy more, partly because they have better health seeking behaviors and are more likely to have higher demand for reproductive health services. Research shows that the poorest of poor young women are between 1.7 and 4.0 times as likely to have an early birth as the richest 20 % of young women, and the poorest 20 % of women aged 15–19 have a total fertility rate almost double that of the richest 20 % (Macro International 1990–1998, unpublished raw data). Disparities in reproductive health between the rich and poor are worse than in any other area of health. To date, public subsidies are not sufficiently targeted to reach the most vulnerable or socially excluded, who make huge out-of-pocket payments for low quality services. Incorporating social justice and equity aspects in service delivery would make individual rights a reality for millions of women in both developing and developed countries.

I know from my experience of working in Africa and South Asia that no magic bullet will fix everything, in the same way, and everywhere. Myriad social, political and economic factors determine service access, quality, choices, and utilization. There are huge market failures in access to information and government failures abound in distributing equitable services. Financing is important but progress also depends on how effectively and efficiently investments are used to achieve long term results, which may be eroded by poor governance and corruption. Much also depends on how well social, legal and health systems work, how adequate are human resources, supplies and management capacity; and how equity and social protection mechanisms work.

In a recent consultation with ministers and civil society in Africa, I asked why their countries were making little progress in reproductive health. High on their list were cultural and social norms that result in gender inequalities; services not reaching rural areas and conflict zones; and insufficient financing and implementation capacity. Civil society groups highlighted non-accountability, corruption, limited scaling-up of effective interventions, and inappropriate youth policies and services. Youth unemployment came up as a risk factor. NGOs added their concerns about declining resources as donors increasingly shift to budget support. While ministers of health mentioned workforce and drug shortages, poor infrastructure, and challenges of decentralization, ministers of finance mentioned competing priorities and managing resources that are not channeled through government. They asked for better evidence and more rigorous analyses of the economic returns of government investment in reproductive health, more rigorous benefit-cost analyses that include multiplier effects from other sectors (e.g. the impacts of nutrition or ill-health), and experimental studies that show causal effects between interventions and outcomes.

238 — E. Lule

In the future we need to invest more in connecting research and policy, particularly in the area of economic returns to investment.

Family planning started off as a well-funded vertical program, but stalled in some regions as investments shifted to other vertical programs and global initiatives. Investments in vertical reproductive health and family planning programs focused more on short-term results, and not long-term outcomes. The importance of institutionalizing reproductive health services (especially family planning) in the primary health care system and investing in sustainable delivery systems with adequate human resources were underestimated. Since the Alma Ata Declaration of 1978, the development community has swung between vertical programs and strengthening health systems and primary health care. Investments in strengthening health systems, local capacity and institutions take longer to show results and may cost more in the long run, but donors and countries need to stay the course on both results and long term development sustainability. With the recent financial, food and fuel crises, the development community struggles with how to respond to emergencies without derailing existing programs and long term development.

The global AID architecture has changed dramatically and become more complex since Cairo. Although overall official development assistance (ODA) has increased to a record USD$129 billion in 2010, pledges made have not been fully materialized and program commitments, including those for achieving the MDGs, remain underfunded. Current ODA represents 0.32 % of the combined gross national income (GNI) of Organisation for Economic Co-operation and Development (OECD)/ Development Assistance Committee (DAC)[17] countries, but many donor countries have yet to reach the promised United Nations target of providing 0.7 % of GNI needed to meet development needs. The ongoing financial crisis in donor countries makes it less likely that they will realize these pledges.

While development assistance for health (DAH) also increased to almost USD$27 billion in 2010, the rate of annual growth fell from 13 % during 2004–2008 to 6 % annually during 2008–2010.[18] This financing has favored reproductive health as financing for HIV/AIDS and maternal, newborn and child health have also increased. However, maternal and child health received about half as much as financing for HIV/AIDS in 2008 and spending for family planning has declined despite increased demand. DAH does not always target countries of highest need or burden of disease. In addition, DAH will in the future be increasingly competing with emerging priorities like climate change, food security and infrastructure.

The global aid architecture is fragmented and unpredictable, with many uncoordinated players and global health initiatives. The development community has made commitments to coordinate better, align with country priorities, use country

---

[17] The OECD is an organization of 34 countries who work together to address economic, social and governance challenges of the globalizing World Economy. The DAC is a group of 24 World's main donors who seek international development cooperation and aid effectiveness.

[18] Institute for Health Metrics and Evaluation (IHME). 2010. *Financing Global Health 2010: Development Assistance and Country Spending in Economic Uncertainty.* Seattle, WA: IHME.

systems, and focus on results (see the 2005 Paris Declaration and 2008 Accra Agenda for Action on aid effectiveness), but progress in achieving these goals has been slow. Donors have also shifted from earmarking funds and to direct financing of country budgets and sector-wide approaches.[19] With these changes, the opportunity lies in understanding these new aid instruments and working more cohesively across all the areas of reproductive health to ensure they are prioritized and get a fair share of the national budgets.

Equally important are government's own domestic investments in health and monitoring the progress they have made towards meeting their various commitments, such as the 2001 Abuja declaration when African leaders agreed to spend 15 % of their budgets on health. Although governments have increased domestic health spending, there is evidence that in countries that receive significant DAH, health aid may be partially replacing domestic spending.

With the focus on results, donors have shifted from funding inputs to performance based funding and innovative financing mechanisms. Performance based funding directly links on-going payments to demonstrated progress in attaining pre-agreed performance measures and results. These new funding mechanisms aim to improve the performance of the service delivery system, improve efficiency, accountability, change the incentive structure, and invest in system-level changes to achieve better health outcomes. The reproductive health community is equally concerned with results and has an opportunity to adapt to these new approaches, notwithstanding some of the challenges to implementing them (e.g., where setting targets may be counter to the voluntary use of family planning). In addition, less measurable program objectives may be equally important to improving equity and quality of services, including where reproductive health outcomes may need multiple interactions.

During my tenure at the World Bank and work in Nigeria and India, I became aware of the importance of multi-sectoral approaches and how capturing the intersectoral synergies can have multiplier effects for outcomes. Enormous multiplier effects may result from extending female education and economic empowerment with reproductive health, as well as between maternal health and transport, between maternal and child health and nutrition, and between child health and water and sanitation. However, planning and implementing multi-sectoral approaches is extremely difficult because of how government ministries are organized, how planning, implementation and accountability take place at national levels, how budgets are allocated, how NGOs are funded, and how integration is monitored and evaluated. Weak capacity and incentive structures may not support effective inter-sectoral implementation. Similarly, although service integration between different components of reproductive health (e.g. family planning, HIV/AIDS and maternal health) has been supported, it has proved difficult to implement and there have been many missed opportunities. Bangladesh, Malawi and Egypt are good examples of using a

---

[19] A sector-wide approach is an approach to international aid that coordinates governments, donors and other stakeholders in any sector to operate under a set of principles rather than a specific package of policies or activities.

multisectoral approach, through door step delivery of information and services while simultaneously investing in girls' education and other relevant sectors. Given the changes in disease burden, financing, and workforce shortages, integration is imperative when it is appropriate, and more evaluations and studies would be useful to show when it works and when it does not.

At the global level, much has been accomplished since Cairo but much more remains to be done in this changing environment and competing priorities. As I look at what more needs to be done in Uganda and elsewhere, I see many opportunities for bolder action despite the politics and controversies of the field. Effective advocacy requires investing more in rigorous research and evaluations, so that we have solid evidence to make a stronger business case for investing in reproductive health and in girls and women, and to embrace multi-sectoral approaches. We need to think out of the box regarding how we integrate with the new financing approaches, new instruments, services, and other sectors. A more targeted approach and focus on countries where progress is lagging may get us faster progress. Beyond strengthening health systems, we can focus on service delivery performance, governance and accountability, as well as on integrating equity, social justice and individual human rights approaches. Finally, we can take advantage of innovation, new technologies and social media. These efforts will require more cohesion in the movement and effective partnerships with the private sector and civil society. Finally, my dream is to see a global, dynamic youth movement that embraces, owns and energizes this agenda, since their own reproductive health choices will determine their potential and shape the future of our planet.

Conflict of Interest The opinions expressed in this contribution reflect the views of the author and should not be attributed to the World Bank, its executive directors or any of its member countries.

Part III
Strengthening Service and Program Capacity

Chapter 12
Fostering Change in Medical Settings: A Holistic Programming Approach to "Revitalizing" IUD Use in Kenya

Roy Jacobstein

12.1 Introduction

The intrauterine device (IUD) is a highly effective, safe, long-acting, and quickly reversible contraceptive method that is suitable for most women who wish to delay a first birth, or space or limit subsequent births (Kaneshiro and Arby 2010; Thonneau and Almont 2008; WHO 2010a). Globally, the IUD is the most widely used temporary contraceptive method, relied upon by over 150 million women (14.3 %) worldwide (Salem 2006; UN 2011). However, despite excellent method characteristics and high prevalence rates in some countries and regions, the IUD is often difficult to access. On the African continent, prevalence varies from as low as 0.5 % in Eastern Africa and much of sub-Saharan Africa, to as high as 22.3 % in Northern Africa (UN 2011). Provider and client myths and misunderstandings about the IUD abound, and there are numerous other access barriers as well. In the fragile, resource-strapped countries of sub-Saharan Africa (Jacobstein et al. 2009), even those with relatively stronger family planning (FP) programs and higher levels of IUD use, such as Kenya, have experienced declines in IUD prevalence overall, and as a proportion of modern contraceptive use (see Fig. 12.1).

Efforts are being undertaken to "revitalize family planning" (Speidel et al. 2009) and to make "underutilized" contraceptive methods such as the IUD more widely available and accessible. To better inform such efforts, this chapter presents a case study of the experience of one capacity-building agency in providing technical assistance for "IUD revitalization" to the Ministry of Health (MOH) in Kisii District, Kenya. Project design and implementation were informed by the latest scientific evidence and international guidance about IUDs; by considerations of how to foster change in medical settings; and by a holistic programming model for FP service

R. Jacobstein, M.D., MPH (✉)
EngenderHealth, New York, NY, USA
e-mail: Rjacobstein@engenderhealth.org

A. Kulczycki (ed.), *Critical Issues in Reproductive Health*, The Springer Series on Demographic Methods and Population Analysis 33, DOI 10.1007/978-94-007-6722-5_12,
© Springer Science+Business Media Dordrecht 2014

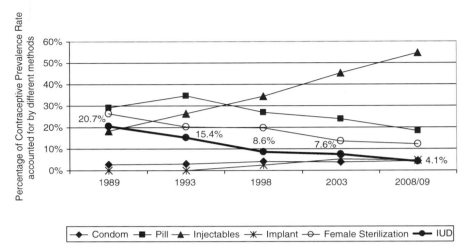

Data Source: Kenyan Demographic and Health Surveys, various years, www.measuredhs.com.
Secondary Analysis by the RESPOND Project. (About the RESPOND Project, see note 13)

Fig. 12.1 Time trends for use of IUDs and other contraceptives as a share of modern contraceptive method mix in Kenya, 1989–2003, among married women of reproductive age (MWRA)

delivery. Although the project was modest in scale and in temporal and geographic scope, it generated substantial increases in IUD use and these higher levels of use were sustained for at least 30 months after project activities ceased. Following brief consideration in Sects. 12.2, 12.3, and 12.4 of the IUD's characteristics and service delivery challenges, the dynamics of successful change, and the nature of medical settings, the Kisii IUD project is presented in detail in Sects. 12.5 and 12.6.

12.2 The IUD: Characteristics, Challenges, New Evidence, and Guidance

The IUD is one of the most effective modern contraceptive methods available, with an annual failure rate of 0.8 % per 100 women in the first year of use (UNDP et al. 1997), comparable to that of female sterilization (Trussell 2007). The IUD is also the most cost-effective of all modern methods, with the lowest service costs per couple year of protection (Tumlinson et al. 2011). It can be provided by a number of health cadres and enjoys a high continuation rate, with an estimated 88 % of women still using the method after 1 year; however, its availability is restricted by commodity stock-outs, limited human resources, competing demands on health providers, and sub-optimal organization and management of work, as well as by widespread misperceptions, myths, and biases (Townsend and Jacobstein 2007; Alnakash 2008). Reproductive health programs have to work hard to address these barriers.

Clients and providers alike often hold erroneous beliefs and perceptions about the IUD's safety and mechanism of action. For example, they often think that the IUD works as an abortifacient by preventing implantation, although it works predominantly by preventing sperm from reaching the fallopian tubes (where fertilization occurs) and/or by altering the egg (Mishell 1998; Sivin 1989). Providers sometimes also fear that the IUD may cause or worsen anemia or increase the risk of ectopic pregnancy. However, while some users of copper-bearing IUDs report increased menstrual bleeding, no significant changes in hemoglobin levels have been found[1] (Milsom et al. 1995). Because IUDs are so effective at preventing pregnancy, women using an IUD have a >90 % lower risk of ectopic pregnancy compared to sexually-active noncontraceptors (Mishell 1998; Sivin 1991).

Provider concern is often centered on the nexus of sexually-transmitted infection (STI), pelvic inflammatory disease (PID), and infertility. Providers often fear that insertion of the IUD—or its ongoing presence in a woman at risk of STI—will increase the risk of PID and in turn lead to infertility. They also often have concerns that the IUD may be unsuitable for HIV-infected women (Jacobstein 2007). The latest scientific evidence on these matters is reassuring. While there is slightly increased risk of clinical PID in the first 20 days after insertion, these rates are much lower than providers typically imagine, and after the first 20 days of IUD use, PID rates are comparable to those in non-users.[2] In addition, any possible link between IUD use and infertility is now considered to be "immeasurable" and "not of public health significance" (Skjeldestad 2008; Hubacher et al. 2001).[3] Even in settings of high STI prevalence, risk of clinical PID due to the IUD is very low, with estimates ranging from 0.075 to 0.15 % in sub-Saharan Africa (Stanback and Shelton 2008). Studies of IUD use among women with HIV/AIDS (conducted mainly in Kenya) have found that IUD complication rates are low comparable to non-HIV-infected women (Sinei et al. 1998; Morrison et al. 2001). The IUD is not associated with increased cervical shedding of HIV, which would be a proxy for increased risk of infecting an uninfected male partner (Richardson et al. 1999). Moreover, multiple studies have found that IUD use does not increase the risk of HIV acquisition (WHO 2010b; Morrison et al. 2001).

Reflecting this latest evidence, the World Health Organization's *Medical Eligibility Criteria* (MEC), which gives guidance on contraceptive safety and

---

[1] Significantly increased vaginal bleeding sometimes occurred with the older, inert IUDs like the Lippes Loop. However, copper-bearing IUDs can generally be used by women with iron deficiency anemia (WHO 2010a).

[2] The rate of clinical PID the first 20 days post-insertion is 7 cases per 1,000 women-years of use (Farley et al. 1992; Mishell 1998); that is, 993 of 1,000 women having an IUD inserted would *not* get PID in the immediate post-insertion period. Rates of clinical PID after the first 20 days of IUD use range between 0.6 and 1.6 cases/1,000 woman-years of IUD use. These findings are the basis for WHO's recommendation that only one *routine* follow-up visit is needed, 3–6 weeks after insertion (WHO 2004).

[3] Tubal infertility was not associated with IUD use per se, or with duration of use, reasons for removal, or gynecologic symptoms during use; rather, it was associated with presence of antibodies to chlamydia.

appropriate use, indicates that most women are eligible to use an IUD. This includes women who: are postabortion, immediately postpartum, or at farther intervals from childbirth (4 weeks postpartum and beyond); want to delay, space, or limit births; are breastfeeding; are HIV-infected (including those with AIDS on treatment); are anemic; or are of any age and parity, including younger women and those who have not yet had any children (WHO 2010a).[4] This guidance informs national service and training policies, guidelines, and standards, and influences provider practice (Peterson 2006).

12.3 The Dynamics of Change

Like any other aspect of reproductive health (or development more generally), those undertaking programmatic efforts to improve knowledge, provider provision, client access, and service quality with respect to the IUD are acting as change agents, and trying to induce others to change their behavior. Yet, change is unsettling to most people.[5] Furthermore, "good changes" are not necessarily adopted—indeed, "knowledge-to-practice" or "research-to-practice" is not only not automatic but is often difficult to achieve. Furthermore, perceptions often differ between programmatic change agents and their intended beneficiaries.[6] The intended recipients of an intervention (e.g., IUD providers or potential clients) have their own "truths" that influence their perceptions and understandings of innovations: they are not simply "empty vessels" waiting to be "filled up" with scientific truth or knowledge of "best

---

[4]The MEC has four classification categories: Category 1, "no restriction: use method in any circumstances"; Category 2, "generally use: benefits outweigh risks"; Category 3, "generally do not use: risks outweigh benefits"; and Category 4, "method not to be used". The MEC schema also distinguishes between providers *with* clinical judgment and providers with *limited* clinical judgment. For the latter group of providers, Categories 1 and 2 are compressed to "Yes" and Categories 3 and 4 to "No." The MEC largely classifies the IUD in Category 1 or Category 2. Women living in high STI- and HIV-prevalence settings or who are HIV-infected now belong to Category 2 with respect to IUD use, whereas on theoretical grounds these conditions had previously been Category 3. Women with high *individual* risk of STI, which can be determined with a checklist in low-resource settings, are in Category 3. Women with AIDS who are not yet on antiretroviral therapy (ART) are also in Category 3, but women with AIDS who are being treated and are clinically well are in Category 2 and thus good candidates for an IUD if they desire one.

[5]"The art of progress is to preserve order amid change and to preserve change amid order," philosopher and mathematician Alfred North Whitehead reminds us (Whitehead 1929); in other words, although change may be inevitable, and indeed its pace may be accelerating, people incline towards homeostasis.

[6]Beauty is indeed in the eye of the beholder: often what the development change agent sees as a "beautiful" new way of doing things is perceived as unattractive by the "changee". In this sense, the type of perspective about change being presented in this chapter can induce a sense of empathy and lead to "bottom-up" programming. As a wise Kenyan midwife/IUD service provider once told the author, "We must walk in their shoes, or we will fail."

practices."[7] Behavior change theory can help implementers of FP programs achieve better program outcomes; yet experience shows that proven principles and dynamics of fostering and maintaining behavior change are often not fully factored into program design and implementation. As a result, access barriers are not fully addressed, and little changes.

The Kisii project for improving IUD services, described below, was influenced by the Diffusion of Innovations theory of how, why, and at what rate new ideas and technologies spread (Rogers 2003). This theory posits that three broad dimensions most influence the speed and extent of the change process associated with the adoption of an innovation: (1) the qualities of the innovation or new practice itself (i.e., the "what," such as a client choosing an IUD for her contraceptive method, a provider providing an IUD, or a program making it more widely available); (2) the characteristics of potential adopters (the "who"); and, (3) contextual factors (the "how," referring to how adoption may be facilitated or impeded by such factors as a health system's structures and policies, human and financial resources, and leadership and management). It is also helpful to consider "where" the IUD is to be provided (typically in medical settings) and "when" (since the timing of IUD provision carries different clinical and programmatic implications for work organization and structure).

The category of "what" comprises both the *objective* (scientific) characteristics of the IUD and, critically, its subjective characteristics, i.e., how the IUD is perceived by potential adopters and providers. Five characteristics of an innovation are identified as most likely to determine its rate and extent of adoption: these are its *perceived* (1) benefit; (2) compatibility; (3) simplicity; (4) observability; and (5) "trialability" (Rogers 2003). The single most important determinant of behavior change is the innovation's perceived benefit, which includes consideration of its *relative* or *comparative advantage* to intended recipients. Perceived benefits may include savings of time or effort, economic gain, or better health, including avoiding unwanted pregnancy and its consequences. Thus when new scientific or programmatic information is conveyed, it is often couched in terms of benefit (e.g., that wider use of the IUD will lead to less aggregate burden on providers, or that it is more convenient, effective, and safe for the client). Providing an IUD or choosing to use one is also more likely to occur if it is perceived as compatible with existing norms, behaviors, and culture (of both the community at large and the medical setting), and if it is perceived as "easy to do." While contraceptive use in general and IUD use in particular are not highly "observable" at the level of individual provision and receipt of the method, FP programs are generally better served by making their activities visible to opinion leaders, decision makers, and communities (as was done in the Kisii project described below).

The adoption process is also influenced by an individual's personality characteristics and openness to change. Diffusion theory identifies five categories of

---

[7]Typically, if these "truths" are scientifically or factually wrong, the public health professional labels them "myths" or "misconceptions."

potential adopters: "Innovators," "Early Adopters," the "Early Majority," the "Late Majority," and "Laggards" and holds that they have discrete, identifiable behavioral and personal characteristics (Rogers 2003). Potential adopters (who may be individual health facilities within a health system, as well as individual FP clients, service providers, program managers and leaders, or community members), layer out in a normal distribution across a population in terms of receptivity to change, time to adoption of new behavior, and likelihood that changed/newly-adopted behaviors will be sustained. Once the innovation is embraced by Innovators and Early Adopters, who typically represent about 15–20 % of the population, the adopter curve arrives at the "tipping point." Then those who adopt later follow as they become progressively more comfortable with the change. The Late Majority adopters (or "skeptics") adopt an innovation only when it has become the standard of practice. In the Kisii project and program context, these are health professionals who require local proof, not trusting outside sources of "evidence."

These categories and characteristics have important implications for program design, the type and nature of program activities, market segmentation, target audiences, and plans for scale-up. For example, an FP program seeking to revitalize IUD use would do well to consider who might choose, provide, support, or impede IUD use, and on what basis. Diffusion theory reminds us that most providers and clients do not adopt new practices because of scientific studies; rather, they are influenced by their "near-peers" who have already adopted the new behavior. Thus, Early Adopters (as distinct from Innovators) are programmatically key: they are the highly-respected and well-networked opinion leaders in a given community (including the community of the medical setting) whose activities are the most closely watched by others, which is crucial to the spread of new practices. They are not only more receptive to change, but they also have the resources, risk tolerance, and willingness to try new things. On the other hand, later adopters of an innovation not only adopt later, but are more likely to discontinue (Rogers 2003).[8]

12.4 Medical Settings and IUD Use

The provision of IUDs largely occurs in medical settings such as clinics, health posts, and hospital outpatient departments. Access to IUDs is thus dependent on the nature and dynamics of medical settings, which are typically hierarchical and conservative, with well-established policies, routine practices, and providers acting as "gatekeepers" to services. There is often little perceived need to change service

---

[8]This gives rise to what Rogers terms "the Innovativeness-Needs Paradox": individuals (or units in a system) who most need the benefits of a new idea, e.g., the less-educated or the poor are generally the last to adopt an innovation, and thus one consequence of technological innovation can be to *widen* socioeconomic disparities in social systems.

policies and practices, and thus resistance to proposed changes that an internal change agent or an external technical assistance agency might try to introduce (Berwick 2003; Jacobstein 2009). Furthermore, busy providers, especially in limited-resource settings, often have difficulty accessing the latest scientific knowledge, and may be unaware of the latest findings and recommendations about the benefits and risks of the IUD and other contraceptive methods, as encapsulated in WHO's MEC and other international guidance.

Another germane dynamic in medical settings is that in following the fundamental medical principle of "do no harm" and avoiding iatrogenic (doctor-caused) disease, inadequate attention is generally paid to "the harm of *not* doing," i.e., to the negative consequences of withholding interventions. The substantial risks a woman faces in (unwanted) pregnancy and childbirth are thus not fully considered, while the relative risk of providing methods like the IUD (or hormonal contraception) is erroneously perceived to be high (Jacobstein 2009; Shelton 2000). Similarly, providers often withhold contraceptives from non-menstruating women seeking FP services (Stanback et al. 1997), even though an unwanted pregnancy may pose far larger risk to their health. Yet in contrast to the aforementioned low rates of IUD-associated PID and infertility, a sub-Saharan African woman faces a one in 31 lifetime risk of maternal death. Of the estimated 358,000 maternal deaths worldwide in 2008, nearly 3/5ths of the total (204,000) occurred in Sub-Saharan Africa, which had the world's highest maternal mortality ratio (MMR) of 640 maternal deaths per 100,000 live births (WHO et al. 2010). Further, for every instance of mortality there may be 20 instances of injury, infection, disability, or disease (Nanda et al. 2005).[9]

A range of cognitive, economic, sociocultural, political, geographic, and health system barriers to quality, access and use are common with respect to IUDs. Some barriers to FP that are manifested in medical settings have been grouped as *medical barriers*: well-intentioned but inappropriate policies or practices based at least partially on a medical rationale which impede or prevent clients from receiving contraception (Shelton et al. 1992). Among the most common and difficult medical barriers to IUD availability, access and use are: provider bias; inappropriate eligibility restrictions on who can receive an IUD (e.g., by age, parity, or marital status); mistaken application of "contraindications" (inconsistent with the WHO MEC); "process hurdles" (e.g., unnecessary lab tests or mandatory return visits); and unjustified restrictions on which health system cadres can provide a method (Bertrand et al. 1995; Stanback and Twum-Baah 2001; Shelton et al. 1992). Poor side effects counseling and/or management are also barriers that arise in the medical setting and limit adoption and continuation of the IUD (RamaRao 2003; Bertrand et al. 1995). All of these barriers are more prevalent with "provider-dependent" clinical methods like the IUD, and thus an understanding of how to change provider behavior is helpful.

---

[9]In striking contrast, there are only 14 maternal deaths per 100,000 live births in industrialized countries (WHO et al. 2010).

12.5   The Kisii Project: Holistic Programming in Action

12.5.1   Background

At the turn of the century, many FP programs in sub-Saharan Africa were considered "fragile," as reflected in low contraceptive prevalence rates or stalled progress (Jacobstein et al. 2009; Westoff and Cross 2006). In Kenya, FP program performance measures improved steadily between 1972 and 1989 before tapering off in the 1990s (Ross and Smith 2010). Modern method use rose from 18 % of currently married women in 1989 to 27 % in 1993, then more slowly to 31.5 % in 1998, and remained unchanged in 2003. As seen in Fig. 12.1, the same period saw declines in the IUD's share of the method mix. (The IUD predominantly used in Kenya, as in most countries with donor-supported national FP programs, is the Copper T 380A). Among currently married women, 3.7 % used the IUD in 1989, accounting for one in five (20.7 %) married users of modern contraceptive methods. By 2003, IUD prevalence fell to 2.4 %, representing less than one in 13 married women (7.6 %) who were using modern contraception. At the same time, 25 % of married women reported having an unmet need for contraception (CBS 2004), and long-acting and permanent methods including the IUD were underutilized (ACQUIRE Project 2006).

In addition, secondary analysis of 2003 Kenya DHS (KDHS) data conducted by the RESPOND Project (see Figs. 12.2 and 12.3), which gives the context just preceding the Kisii project's period of operation (January 2005 to January 2007), suggests that at the aggregate level there is a 'sub-optimal fit' between method use and reproductive intentions among both "spacers" (who want to space a next birth or delay a first birth at least 2 years) and "limiters" (who wish to limit further childbearing altogether).[10] While there is no "ideal" method mix, as individual and program circumstances vary—and it is of paramount importance that FP programs provide informed and non-coerced choice from a full range of methods to the clients that they serve—an aggregate "goodness of fit" with reproductive intentions and with access (or lack thereof) can be inferred by comparing the method mix in countries such as Kenya (and most of sub-Saharan Africa) with the method mix in countries that provide complete access to a full range of contraceptive methods via universal health coverage. In the United Kingdom, for example, where there is full access to a wide range of methods, the modern contraceptive prevalence rate is 84 %, with 40 % of all women using a highly effective clinical method,[11] including 10 % who use the IUD (UN 2011). By contrast,

---

[10] This pattern of high unmet need, limited method availability, and suboptimal fit of methods used with reproductive intentions (as well as, in consequence, excess fertility and high maternal mortality) persisted in Kenya in 2008 (KNBS 2010), and is a typical pattern for sub-Saharan African family planning programs.

[11] Data is not generally available that is stratified by reproductive intention (i.e., for limiters and spacers), thus the use of highly effective clinical methods among limiters is likely to be higher than 40 %, as there is a "dilution" effect when all women comprise the denominator.

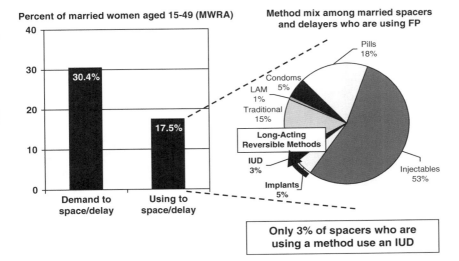

Percent of married women aged 15-49 (MWRA)

Method mix among married spacers and delayers who are using FP

Pills 18%
Condoms 5%
LAM 1%
Traditional 15%
Long-Acting Reversible Methods
IUD 3%
Implants 5%
Injectables 53%

Only 3% of spacers who are using a method use an IUD

Data source: MEASURE/DHS, Kenya DHS Survey, 2003; UN (2011).
Secondary analysis by The RESPOND Project (About the RESPOND Project, see note 13)

Fig. 12.2 Reproductive intentions, FP use, and method mix, among married spacers, Kenya, 2003

as seen in Fig. 12.2, among spacers and delayers in Kenya (30.4 % of married women), only 3 % of those actually using a method were using an IUD,[12] whereas 15 % of spacers and delayers using a method were using traditional methods. An additional 12.9 % of all married spacers and delayers (i.e., those not using a method at all) had unmet need.

The situation was similar with limiters, as seen in Fig. 12.3. One in eight limiters (12.7 %) used no method at all (i.e., had an unmet need), and of limiters actually using a method, only 1 in 25 used an IUD (and only one in four used *any* of the four clinical methods), whereas among women using a method to limit, one in eight was using a traditional method. Again, this is in notable contrast to the levels and patterns of contraceptive use found in the United Kingdom and other countries that provide complete access to a wide range of methods, and thereby women have little unmet need and a better fit of method characteristics with their reproductive intentions.

---

[12]The low IUD use in Kenya (and elsewhere in sub-Saharan Africa) occurs for many reasons, as discussed in Section IV of this chapter. One additional reason for low IUD use among delayers has been the prevailing practice (the received "wisdom") in medical settings that "IUDs are not indicated for women who have not yet had a child." Also, some FP providers and programs are reluctant to provide methods with long duration of action (e.g., 12 or more years with the copper-T 380A) to women who indicate that they might want another child, albeit after 2–3 years of spacing. That is, "long-acting" is conflated with "long-term" and thus the intrinsic method characteristic is confused with how long a woman might choose to use the method.

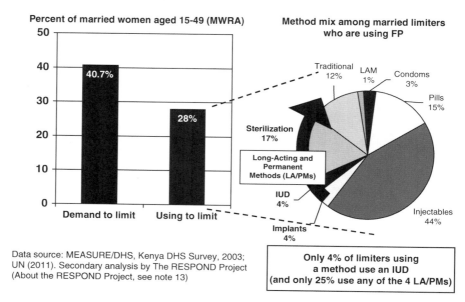

Data source: MEASURE/DHS, Kenya DHS Survey, 2003;
UN (2011). Secondary analysis by The RESPOND Project
(About the RESPOND Project, see note 13)

Fig. 12.3 Reproductive intentions, FP use, and method mix, among married limiters in Kenya, 2003

12.5.2 Chronology and Overview of Project Interventions

The "plateauing" of contraceptive use, coupled with persisting high unmet need, prompted the Kenyan MOH to launch a national initiative in 2003 to "revitalize" FP, with a focus on "underutilized" methods such as the IUD (Fischer 2005). In 2004, Kenya's IUD Task Force, led by the MOH, launched an IUD revitalization initiative in seven districts. The initiative involved national-level advocacy, as well as community outreach and building of capacity to provide IUD services. Among the seven districts that the IUD Task Force identified for programmatic intervention was Kisii District of Nyanza Province in southwestern Kenya, near Lake Victoria and Uganda. Nyanza Province is the third most populous of Kenya's eight provinces, and Kisii the eighth most populous of its 47 districts, with a population of 1.15 million (among Kenya's overall population of 38.6 million) (KNBS 2009). In Kisii, IUD prevalence was even lower than the national average (0.5 % vs. 2.4 %) and unmet need was even higher (35 % vs. 25 %) (CBS et al. 2004).

In late 2004, the ACQUIRE Project,[13] led by EngenderHealth, was asked to provide IUD-related technical assistance to Kisii District. The project began doing so

---

[13] ACQUIRE is an acronym for Access, Quality and Use in Reproductive Health. The ACQUIRE Project was funded by USAID's Office of Population and Reproductive Health to focus on facility-based services and clinical contraception, especially long-acting and permanent methods of contraception (LA/PMs). The ACQUIRE Project was a partnership among several agencies that worked from 2003 to 2008. In 2008 it was succeeded by the RESPOND Project, with a similar mandate and also led by EngenderHealth. Within the LA/PMs, IUDs and hormonal implants are grouped as "long-acting reversible methods," and female sterilization and vasectomy as "permanent methods". "Long-acting" is preferred to "long-term," for reasons discussed in endnote 12.

from January 2005 to January 2007, working with District-level MOH leadership and staff to establish sustainable systems and services for IUD provision (ACQUIRE Project 2006; CBS 2004). In May 2005, after an initial stakeholder meeting, a "performance needs assessment" (PNA) was conducted to identify areas of greatest programmatic need. A formal, data-driven process that compares desired to actual performance and analyzes the nature of "performance gaps" (EngenderHealth 2006; Kisii District MOH 2005), the PNA was conducted by managers and service providers from the Kisii District MOH and Kisii District Hospital in collaboration with ACQUIRE Project staff. Using data from facility audits of each of the project's 13 service sites, interviews with providers and clients, and focus group sessions with women and men in the project's catchment area, the PNA identified barriers to IUD access, quality, and use in Kisii, their root causes, related systems challenges, and possible solutions.

IUD-specific findings from the PNA included that: the IUD was only being provided at the hospital level in Kisii (whereas it is easily and quite appropriately provided in clinic and even community settings via "mobile services"); costs of supplies, equipment, and provider time for counseling, insertion, and removal were limiting health system capacity; providers lacked motivation to provide the IUD; supervision was not aimed at improving provider performance; and myths and misconceptions about the IUD were widespread at both the provider and client levels (Kisii District Ministry of Health 2005). These problems were addressed through closely-linked activities aimed at improving supply, demand, and service policies and practices. The activities were undertaken and coordinated in accord with a model of holistic programming for service delivery. Bimonthly service results were monitored and correlated with key program inputs, as well as with major external events that disrupted services, such as stock-outs, serious political unrest, transfer of staff trained in IUD service provision to other duties and locations, and health system restructuring. Results were further tracked for 30 months after project implementation ended, thus affording a sense of the longer-lasting change that arose.

12.5.3 *The Holistic Programming Approach Followed in Kisii*

A holistic model for FP programming (see Fig. 12.4) served as a conceptual framework for the design and implementation of the IUD-related activities in Kisii District. The Supply–demand-Advocacy (SDA) Program Model[14] reflects EngenderHealth's four decades of experience in providing technical assistance for FP service delivery in clinical settings (ACQUIRE Project 2007). Central to the SDA Program Model is the service interaction that ideally takes place between a knowledgeable, empowered client and a skilled, motivated, well-supported FP service provider at a suitable site.

---

[14]The SDA Program Model for FP/RH Service Delivery was subsequently elaborated upon to accommodate other health sector activities besides FP, and to expand beyond service delivery activities per se. In the process, the SDA Program Model became the Supply-Enabling Environment-Demand (SEED) Programming Model for Sexual and Reproductive Health. The basic elements of both the SDA Model and the SEED Model are similar.

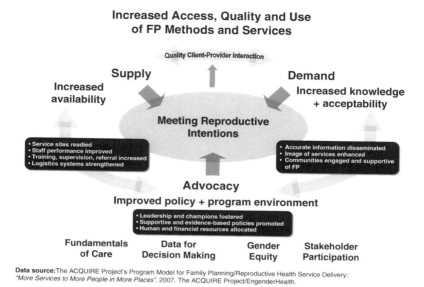

Fig. 12.4 The ACQUIRE Project's program model for FP/RH service delivery

The purpose of these interactions is for women and men to be able to realize their reproductive intentions throughout their reproductive life cycle; in the aggregate, this also helps FP programs achieve their goals of increasing access, quality, and use of FP/RH methods and services on a sustainable basis. Good ("quality") client-provider interactions are enabled by well-functioning supply-side and demand-side program elements that are operating within a supportive (i.e., enabling) policy and program environment. The SDA Model envisions potential synergy among program elements which can be fostered via a coordinated package of mutually reinforcing interventions. The next section gives a sense of how the individual elements of the model helped guide program activities in Kisii.

12.5.4 Key Activities and Outcomes, by Program Model Component

Supply-Side Interventions

On the supply-side, the PNA revealed insufficient provider capacity and service infrastructure in Kisii District, as well as substandard IUD service practices. These included widespread biases against the IUD, outdated training, and insufficient equipment and supplies. To address these deficiencies, a number of activities were undertaken. Knowledge updates that focused on the "fundamentals of care"[15]—safety, quality assurance and improvement, and informed choice—conveyed the latest scientific findings and proven programming practices. Ways to change provider perceptions and practices that impeded client access to IUDs were identified for implementation by the stakeholders. Providers were trained in IUD insertion and removal, FP counseling, and infection prevention, and supervisors were trained in facilitative supervision. Gaps in needed equipment (e.g., IUD kits and sterilization equipment for infection prevention) were addressed at all 13 service sites, which were otherwise readied to provide IUDs. Logistics systems for procuring and distributing IUDs, related equipment (e.g., uterine sounds) and expendable supplies were strengthened, and links between service sites and the community were enhanced. Periodic monitoring visits were also conducted in tandem with MOH staff, with regular reports drawing attention to service system factors and outputs.

Overall, 555 providers were trained at 34 training "events" (e.g., knowledge updates, counseling workshops), and 28 service providers received IUD insertion and removal skills updates. In addition, 72 female and male peer educators from faith-based organizations, women's organizations, and youth groups, and 388 community-based distribution (CBD) agents and their supervisors received basic or comprehensive FP counseling training. These peer educators and CBD agents subsequently served as an important information source in their communities and as a key link between women in the community and the newly-strengthened FP- and IUD-service sites (ACQUIRE Project 2008a).

The Enabling Programmatic Environment

During the project period, significant policy and advocacy efforts were undertaken in Kisii to further enable an environment conducive to FP service delivery in general, as well as to the IUD in particular (as an underutilized method). Sensitization workshops were conducted, IUD advocacy briefs were disseminated, and national FP service guidelines were updated according to the latest WHO guidance. This involved cultivating stakeholder buy-in, participation, and support; identifying, mobilizing, and "nurturing" IUD champions at the district and community levels; and promoting district-level implementation of Kenya's updated, WHO-informed, national FP/RH policies, guidelines, and protocols.

---

[15]Ensuring the "Fundamentals of Care" is one of the SDA Model's four "cross-cutting imperatives." The others are to: use relevant evidence for decision-making in program strategy, design, implementation, and evaluation; promote gender equity, as gender norms and power dynamics often constrain women from accessing methods and services they want and need (Doyal 2000); and ensure widespread stakeholder engagement and "ownership." Important stakeholders whose championship of FP is needed include political, religious and other opinion leaders; program leaders and managers, at national, regional, and district levels the medical community; clinic managers and FP service providers; advocacy groups; community organizations; and individual FP clients. Also implicit in the Model is the need to use the dynamics of change to design and implement program interventions that lead to greater service quality, access, and sustainability. As can be seen in this chapter, all of these aspects were addressed in the IUD-related work in Kisii.

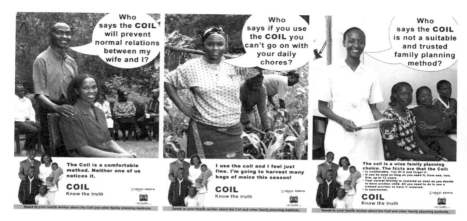

Fig. 12.5 Demand-side programming intervention: IUD-related posters, Kisii Project: "Now You Know the Truth!" (Note: These posters were developed by the ACQUIRE Project/EngenderHealth as part of the Kisii Project to revitalize IUD use in Kenya)

Demand-Side Interventions

The demand-side effort in Kisii was robust, and structured in accord with how best to change behavior and attitudes, as well as to increase knowledge. Much of the overall effort centered on IUD-specific demand-side interventions that integrated marketing and community mobilization and was directed at: (1) improving accurate knowledge among clients, potential clients, providers, and communities by addressing the benefits of FP and IUDs, and by directly counteracting myths, misunderstandings, and misperceptions about the method; (2) improving the IUD's image; and, (3) informing the public where quality IUD and other FP services could be accessed. Mass media and community outreach interventions using satisfied users and IUD champions were sequenced with supply-side interventions and paced with increases in supply-side (service) capacity.

A demand creation campaign was formally launched in July 2006 and conducted for 6 months. This centered on the pretested slogan aimed at combating myths: "Now you know the truth." The campaign used local, regional, and national radio and was supported by 10,000 leaflets, 6,000 brochures, and 1,200 posters. Positive images (see Fig. 12.5) conveyed concepts such as: the IUD's convenience, effectiveness, and safety; the stamina and well-being of IUD users; male involvement and a satisfied couple's happy and mutually supportive relationship; and (your provider will be) a friendly, motivated (female) IUD provider who is "standing up" to challenge the myths and negative perceptions about IUDs (that may be) held by her peers. Advertisements were broadcast in local languages during peak listening periods, and a weekly talk show was mounted featuring IUD advocates (e.g., doctors, peer educators, and satisfied IUD clients and their husbands), which offered listeners an opportunity to phone in and ask questions to local and national medical experts.

Community outreach and mobilization were conducted with women's and men's clubs, youth and religious groups, peer and health educators, and CBD agents. Community leaders (elders, religious leaders, and opinion and other community leaders), CBD agents, and peer educators were also educated and/or trained in FP/IUD basics. Constructive male engagement was promoted in recognition of the crucial role men play in supporting or impeding their partner's access to FP, in furtherance of project survey findings that 70 % of men believed that they shared FP responsibility equally with their partner and would be willing to consider their partner's use of an IUD if they had information about the method. Additionally, gender norms inhibiting access to FP services were challenged. All messaging ended with a call to action, encouraging women and their partners to visit their health care provider together.

The multifaceted communications effort delivered approximately 250,000 exposures to IUD-related messages among the people living in Kisii District, 45 % of whom reported hearing or seeing such a message. Approximately 50,000 people in the communities served, including 21,000 men, were informed about the IUD by female and male peer educators from faith-based organizations, women's organizations, and youth groups at 2,700 community "events" (e.g., "street theatre" performances at community fora and marketplaces). A number of male champions emerged and actively promoted FP within the community at large. Interviews with numerous providers, community volunteers, and survey respondents indicated that the project led to men talking about FP much more, seeking more information on particular contraceptive methods, and even visiting health care sites to talk about FP with providers, which generally did not happen prior to the initiative (Republic of Kenya 2008).

Additionally, CBD agents from the MOH served as referral links between women, communities, and the newly strengthened FP service sites. Nearly one in five residents of Kisii District reported having attended a community session focused on the IUD. The cumulative evidence suggests that such demand-side activities facilitated a closer working relationship between the community and clinic staff. These activities also increased the depth and accuracy of client and community knowledge; improved the acceptability and image of FP; informed clients and communities about when, where, and how services could be obtained; engaged them in defining their FP/RH needs and asserting their rights, and encouraged users to serve as supportive advocates for higher-quality, more-accessible FP/RH and other health services. The consideration of modern contraception, if not its actual use, increasingly became both a community norm and an informed individual choice (ACQUIRE Project 2008a).

Overall, the Project's demand-side, supply-side, and enabling-environment interventions, relied on salient considerations of the dynamics of change (as discussed in Sect. 12.3) and the nature of medical settings (as discussed in Sect. 12.4). On the demand-side, the entire arc of mass media, community-level, and individual-level behavior change communications followed diffusion theory principles. For example, messages and images alike were not only mutually reinforcing, but they focused on known (project-determined and/or project-verified) perceptions of benefit, sociocultural appropriateness, and feasibility (simplicity), at the levels of the individual provider, individual client, contracepting couple, community, and medical setting. Also, the demand creation campaign spanned enough time to allow pulsed repetition of effective images and messages, and thus greater impact in terms of generating positive behavior and attitude change among clients, potential clients, supportive partners, and sympathetic providers alike. On the supply-side, already active and locally influential providers who were Early Adopter IUD champions were used as trainers/change agents and experts available to the public, and organized into an informal network. The trainers as well as the trainees themselves identified the cognitive, structural and practice barriers to be addressed in their own medical settings. Furthermore, they were engaged over the life of the project, since "change takes time" and one-off training (or policy-advocacy) events alone often yield very little in terms of changed provider or program practices. The use of champions in both the supply enhancement and demand creation efforts—both providers and clients, on posters, in mass media, and as experts available to the public—enabled project implementers to "walk the talk."

12.6   Achievements: Sustained IUD Service Utilization and Other Positive Programmatic Changes

The Kisii project was a modestly-funded pilot project of relatively short duration, entailing technical assistance to the district-level public sector for an underutilized and often-misunderstood clinical contraceptive method. IUDs were provided in the context of free and informed choice from among a wide range of available modern contraceptive methods. The project followed a holistic programming model, paying attention to both supply-side elements (e.g., knowledge transfer and skills training) and demand-side elements (e.g., mass media, community-level engagement, and interpersonal communication). Interventions were sequenced and coordinated, with demand-side activities only undertaken once the facilities were equipped and the providers and community workers were trained, so that the increased demand that was created could be met. As can be seen in Fig. 12.6, which plots quarterly IUD insertion totals against project inputs, IUD utilization spiked after each set of interventions, most notably during the robust demand creation campaign from July to December 2006.

Overall, the Kisii project achieved considerable success with respect to improving knowledge, attitudes, and practices. Almost half of the residents of Kisii District reported hearing or seeing an IUD-related mass media message, and 50,000 people were informed about the IUD at community-level events. Knowledge of the IUD increased and a positive attitude toward the method was fostered. For example, a representative household survey conducted in 2006 by a Kenyan market research firm found that 93 % of married women and 85 % of married men in Kisii had knowledge of the IUD, compared to overall national knowledge levels of 75 % for married women and 62 % for married men; in addition, three out of five female

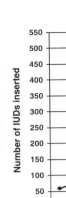
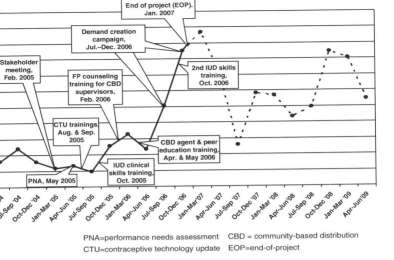

PNA=performance needs assessment   CBD = community-based distribution
CTU=contraceptive technology update   EOP=end-of-project

Fig. 12.6 IUDs inserted in Kisii Project, by quarter and key programmatic inputs (Jan 2005–Aug 2009)

Table 12.1 IUDs inserted in Kisii, before, during, and after Kisii Project (2005–2009), Kisii District, Kenya

Year	Description	Annual total	Monthly average
2004	Baseline, year before project	338	28
2005	First project year	300	25
2006	Second project year	959	80
2007	First year post-project	1,260	105
2008	Second year post-project	1,172	98
2009	Third year post-project (first 8 months only)	787 (8-month total)	98

Data source: Kisii District Service Statistics, 2004–2009

respondents and one of two male respondents agreed that the IUD is a "trusted method of FP" (ACQUIRE Project 2008b).

From the standpoint of changed and improved practices in medical settings, IUD provision and use more than tripled compared to baseline levels, and these gains continued on a sustained basis for more than 30 months after project activities ceased in January 2007, as reflected in Table 12.1's summary of annual insertions and monthly averages, as well as in Fig. 12.6. The annual number and monthly average number of IUD insertions at project sites almost tripled during the second (and final) project year, rising from 338 annual insertions in the baseline year of 2004 to 959 in 2006 (during the second half of which the mass media demand creation campaign was conducted). Annual use rose further still in 2007 and 2008, after formal project activities ceased. Average use peaked at 105 IUD insertions per month in

2007, and then remained at 98 IUD insertions per month for the following 20 months through August 2009 (the last data collection point), a greater than threefold increase compared to the baseline averaged level of 28 monthly IUD insertions.

In addition, positive changes in service quality and access extended beyond the IUD. Specifically, visible improvements were made in the supervision system; linkages between the community and the project sites increased; male engagement in FP increased; and project sites reported having served 33 % more new FP clients (for all contraceptive methods) in the first quarter of 2008 compared to the same period in 2007; (ACQUIRE Project 2008a).

It is also noteworthy that these improvements took place and have been sustained in a difficult (and unfortunately typical) milieu. The usual programming vicissitudes in public health systems such as commodity stockouts and other resource shortages, staff transfers, and competing health service demands from diseases such as HIV/AIDS and malaria, were compounded by jolts from district restructuring and political unrest and strife. That the increases nonetheless occurred, and continued, underscores both the high degree of unmet need for FP in Kenya and the great interest among women and men in accessing effective, safe, and convenient contraception that helps them meet their reproductive intentions to space births for at least several years, or to limit further childbearing.

12.7 Lessons Learned

The results presented in this chapter suggest that meaningful increases in IUD provision and uptake, and other positive service changes, can be fostered and sustained in medical settings initially likely to be resistant to such change, especially if the changes can be conveyed in such a way that their benefits and appropriateness can be readily and widely perceived. Furthermore, these positive changes can be fostered even in—and by—the resource-strapped public sector, and notwithstanding many myths and misperceptions being widespread among both providers and clients. The results also suggest that in order to increase access for provider-dependent clinical methods like the IUD, it is helpful (and feasible) to follow a holistic and sequenced systems approach that addresses barriers in each domain (e.g., the medical setting and its intrinsic resistance to change; and the community, with its gender-based barriers). This entails the coordinated programming of mutually reinforcing supply-side and demand-side activities in accord with evidence-informed principles of the dynamics of successful behavior change.

Efficacious aspects of following this holistic programming approach that is grounded in the realities of the medical setting as well as the dynamics of behavior change include: (1) robust attention to demand-side elements; (2) forging stronger links between communities and facilities; (3) equipping facilities, training staff, and addressing unwarranted service policy restrictions (e.g., which skilled cadre can provide a given FP method); (4) working to address provider-level factors such as their knowledge base, belief systems, structure of work, and rewards; and

(5) engaging men as supportive partners and FP champions. Doing so can create a better image of FP methods and services, increase demand for, and use of, modern contraception, as well as increase system capacity. The holistic programming approach embodied in the SDA model and Kisii project has thus not only been further refined and widely adopted within EngenderHealth's various SRH programs and internal strategic plans (see endnotes 14 and 15), but such an approach is also at the heart of recent FP/RH service delivery projects designed by donors such as USAID (the U.S. Agency for International Development), the UK's Department for International Development (DFID), and the Bill and Melinda Gates Foundation. Furthermore, it is inherent in newer paradigms that relate to working in complex systems such as health systems (and their medical settings) (Pourbohloul and Kieny 2011).

Not unlike many donor-funded FP/RH projects, the "IUD revitalization" project in Kisii was of a more modest size and limited scope and duration than would have been ideal. The project was anticipated to become part of a larger set of activities when it was planned and implemented. While it was not called a "pilot project" or "demonstration project" per se, this is in effect what the Kisii project was. Yet project implementers had quite limited ability to convene and involve—let alone subsequently to fund and assist—those potential stakeholders from other districts and regions who might "view" the Kisii project, be involved in it, and subsequently adopt and adapt it as a high impact practice elsewhere, as part of a larger program of scale-up.

In addition, while the results support the utility of a holistic approach to service delivery programming that is informed by evidence of what variables most contribute to behavior change (by providers, clients, and communities), implementing such an approach is often difficult for FP programs. Indeed, the World Bank has recently identified the lack of integration and coordination of supply and demand interventions as typically deficient in country social sector programs (Peters et al. 2009).[16] Such programming not only entails advocacy and "demonstration" by donors and technical assistance agencies, but ongoing commitment of scarce human and financial resources for FP program subsystems (e.g., supervision, training, and logistics) by the resource-strapped public sector (whether or not the services themselves are provided in a public, private, or NGO setting). The need for these systems that ensure safety, choice, and quality is particularly strong for the longer-acting and/or permanent (clinical) methods of FP like the IUD.

Finally, it is important to note that the increase in IUD use in the Kisii project occurred in a context of strong government and donor support to "revitalizing FP," which undoubtedly contributed in important ways to improving the enabling environment. One reflection of this increased governmental and donor attention to FP has been the resumption in rising contraceptive prevalence seen in the 2008–2009 DHS (KNBS 2010). In this latest DHS, which spans the time period during which

---

[16]"All case studies show demand-side interventions and demand creation to be largely neglected—an omission bound to influence implementation" (Peters et al. 2009).

the Kisii project was operative, modern method CPR is 39.4 %, up from 2003's stalled level of 31.5 % (unchanged from 1998). That is, the Kisii project was operating during a time of generally increasing contraceptive uptake in Kenya. On the other hand, both IUD prevalence and the IUD's share of overall contraceptive use continued their more than 20-year decline in Kenya (see Fig. 12.1). IUD use among married women fell to 1.6 % in 2008–2009, which represents 4.1 % of modern method contraceptive use.[17]

Acknowledgements Many staff from both the Kisii District Ministry of Health, the ACQUIRE Project, the RESPOND Project, and EngenderHealth worked on the IUD revitalization effort in Kisii. Too numerous to acknowledge individually, they contributed the knowledge and expertise of a number of professional disciplines including medicine, midwifery, nursing, communication, marketing, and project management and evaluation. Appreciation is also given to the many community leaders and volunteers who worked to increase access, quality, and use of FP among women and men in Kisii. The continuing encouragement and commitment of Patricia MacDonald and Carolyn Curtis of USAID was indispensible in allowing this project to proceed and succeed.

References

ACQUIRE Project. (2006). *Revitalizing the IUD in Kenya* (Acquiring knowledge no. 2). New York: EngenderHealth/The ACQUIRE Project.

ACQUIRE Project. (2007). *The ACQUIRE Project's program model for FP/RH service delivery.* New York: EngenderHealth/The ACQUIRE Project. http://www.acquireproject.org/archive/files/1.0_introduction/3_ACQUIRE_Program_Model.pdf. Accessed 30 Jan 2011.

ACQUIRE Project. (2008a). Programming for IUD services: Experience and lessons learned in field implementation and global leadership (Acquiring knowledge no. 14). New York: EngenderHealth/The ACQUIRE Project.

ACQUIRE Project. (2008b). *Revitalizing underutilized family planning methods: using communications and community engagement to stimulate demand for the IUD in Kenya* (Acquiring knowledge no. 7). New York: EngenderHealth/The ACQUIRE Project.

Alnakash, A. H. (2008). Influence of IUD perceptions on method discontinuation. *Contraception, 78*(4), 290–293.

Bertrand, J. T., Hardee, K., Magnani, R. J., & Angle, M. A. (1995). Access, quality of care and medical barriers in family planning programs. *International Family Planning Perspectives, 21*(2), 64–74.

Berwick, D. M. (2003). Disseminating innovations in health care. *Journal of the American Medical Association, 289*(15), 1969–1975.

Central Bureau of Statistics (CBS) [Kenya], Ministry of Health (MOH) [Kenya], & ORC Macro. (2004). *Kenya demographic and health survey 2003.* Calverton: CBS, MOH, & ORC Macro.

Doyal, L. (2000). Gender equity in health: Debates and dilemmas. *Social Science & Medicine, 51*(6), 931–939.

EngenderHealth. (2006). *Performance needs assessment: Lessons learned from EngenderHealth/The ACQUIRE Project.* Unpublished report prepared for EngenderHealth/The ACQUIRE Project, New York.

---

[17]For the first time, the prevalence of hormonal implants (1.9 %) surpassed that of IUDs, a trend that may well continue, given increasing donor, program and client interest in implants, and the availability in Kenya of a much less expensive implant (KNBS 2010).

Farley, T. M., Rosenberg, M. J., Rowe, P. J., Chen, J. H., & Meirik, O. (1992). Intrauterine devices and pelvic inflammatory disease: An international perspective. *The Lancet, 339*(8796), 785–788.

Fischer, S. (2005). *Translating research into practice: Reintroducing the IUD in Kenya.* Research Triangle Park: Family Health International.

Hubacher, D., Lara-Ricalde, R., Taylor, D. J., Guerra-Infante, F., & Guzmán-Rodríguez, R. (2001). Use of copper intrauterine devices and the risk of tubal infertility among nulligravid women. *The New England Journal of Medicine, 345*(8), 561–567.

Jacobstein, R. (2007). Long-acting and permanent contraception: An international development, service delivery perspective. *Journal of Midwifery & Women's Health, 52*(4), 361–367.

Jacobstein, R. (2009). Fostering change in medical settings: Some considerations for family planning programs. *International Planned Parenthood Federation (IPPF) Medical Bulletin, 43*(3), 3–4.

Jacobstein, R., Bakamjian, L., Pile, J. M., & Wickstrom, J. (2009). Fragile, threatened, and still urgently needed: Family planning programs in sub-Saharan Africa. *Studies in Family Planning, 40*(2), 147–154.

Kaneshiro, B., & Arby, T. (2010). Long-term safety, efficacy, and patient acceptability of the intrauterine Copper T-380A contraceptive device. *International Journal of Women's Health, 9*(2), 211–220.

Kenya National Bureau of Statistics (KNBS) (2009). *Kenya 2009 population and housing census highlights.* Available at: http://www.knbs.or.ke/Census%20Results/KNBS%20Brochure.pdf. Accessed 3 Apr 2011.

Kenya National Bureau of Statistics (KNBS) & ICF Macro. (2010). *Kenya demographic and health survey 2008–09.* Calverton: KNBS & ICF Macro.

Kisii District Ministry of Health (MOH). 2005. *Report on a performance needs assessment on revitalization of family planning and the IUCD, Kisii, Kenya.* Unpublished report prepared for USAID/The ACQUIRE Project, New York.

Milsom, I., Andersson, K., Jonasson, K., Lindstedt, G., & Rybo, G. (1995). The influence of the gyne-T 380S IUD on menstrual blood loss and iron status. *Contraception, 52*(3), 175–179.

Mishell, D. R. (1998). Intrauterine devices: Mechanisms of action, safety, and efficacy. *Contraception, 58*(3), 45S–53S.

Morrison, C. S., Sekadde-Kigondu, C., Sinei, S., Weiner, D., Kwok, C., & Kokonya, D. (2001). Is the intrauterine device appropriate contraception for HIV-1-infected women? *British Journal of Obstetric Gynecology, 108*(8), 784–790.

Nanda, G., Switlick, K., & Lule, E. (2005). *Accelerating progress towards achieving the MDG to improve maternal health: A collection of promising approaches.* Washington, DC: World Bank.

Peters, D. H., El-Saharty, S., Siadat, B., Janovsky, K., & Vujicic, M. (Eds.). (2009). *Improving health service delivery in developing countries: From evidence to action.* Washington, DC: World Bank.

Peterson, H. B., & Curtis, K. M. (2006). The World Health Organization's global guidance for family planning: An achievement to celebrate. *Contraception, 73*(2), 113–114.

Pourbohloul, B., & Kieny, M.-P. (2011). Complex systems analysis: Towards holistic approaches to health systems planning and policy. *Bulletin of the World Health Organization, 89*, 242.

RamaRao, S., Lacuesta, M., Costello, M., Pangolibay, B., & Jones, H. (2003). The link between quality of care and contraceptive use. *International Family Planning Perspectives, 29*(2), 76–83.

Republic of Kenya, Ministry of Public Health and Sanitation, Division of Reproductive Health. (2008). *Kenya comparative assessment of long-acting and permanent methods activities, final report.* Nairobi: Government of Kenya.

Richardson, B. A., Morrison, C. S., Sekadde-Kigondu, C., Sinei, S. K., Overbaugh, J., Panteleeff, D. D., Weiner, D. H., & Kreiss, J. K. (1999). Effect of intrauterine device use on cervical shedding of HIV-1 DNA. *AIDS, 13*(15), 2091–2097.

Rogers, E. (2003). *Diffusion of innovations* (5th ed.). New York: The Free Press.

Ross, J., and Smith, E. (2010). *The family planning effort index: 1999, 2004, and 2009.* Washington, DC: Futures Group, Health Policy Initiative, Task Order 1.

Salem, R. (2006). *New attention to the IUD: Expanding women's contraceptive options to meet their need* (Population reports, series B, no. 7). Baltimore: INFO Project, Johns Hopkins Bloomberg School of Public Health.

Shelton, J. D. (2000). The harm of "first, do no harm". *Journal of the American Medical Association, 284*(21), 2687–2688.

Shelton, J., Angle, M., & Jacobstein, R. (1992). Medical barriers to access to family planning. *The Lancet, 340*(8831), 1334–1335.

Sinei, S. K., Morrison, C. S., Sekadde-Kigondu, C., Allen, M., & Kokonya, D. (1998). Complications of use of intrauterine devices among HIV-1-infected women. *The Lancet, 351*(9111), 1238–1241.

Sivin, I. (1989). IUDs are contraceptives, not abortifacients: A comment on research and belief. *Studies in Family Planning, 20*(6), 357–359.

Sivin, I. (1991). Dose- and age-dependent ectopic pregnancy risks with intrauterine contraception. *Obstetrics and Gynecology, 78*(2), 291–298.

Skjeldestad, F. E. (2008). The impact of intrauterine devices on subsequent fertility. *Current Opinion in Obstetrics and Gynecology, 20*(3), 275–280.

Speidel, J. J., Sinding, S., Gillespie, D., Maguire, E., & Neuse, M. (2009). *Making the case for U.S. International family planning assistance.* Baltimore: The Bill & Melinda Gates Institute for Population and Reproductive Health.

Stanback, J., & Shelton, J. D. (2008). Pelvic inflammatory disease attributable to the IUD: Modeling risk in West Africa. *Contraception, 77*(4), 227–229.

Stanback, J., & Twum-Baah, K. A. (2001). Why do family planning providers restrict access to services? An examination in Ghana. *International Family Planning Perspectives, 27*(1), 37–41.

Stanback, J., Thompson, A., Hardee, K., & Janowitz, B. (1997). Menstruation requirements: A significant barrier to contraceptive access in developing countries. *Studies in Family Planning, 28*(3), 245–250.

Thonneau, P. F., & Almont, T. (2008). Contraceptive efficacy of intrauterine devices. *American Journal of Obstetrics and Gynecology, 198*(3), 248–253.

Townsend, J. W., & Jacobstein, R. (2007). The changing position of IUDs in reproductive health services in developing countries: Opportunities and challenges. *Contraception, 75*(Suppl), S35–S40.

Trussell J. (2007). Contraceptive efficacy. In R. A. Hatcher, et al. (Eds.), *Contraceptive technology* (19th Rev. ed.). New York: Ardent Media.

Tumlinson, K., Steiner, M., Rademacher, K., Olawo, A., Solomon, M., & Bratt, J. (2011). The promise of affordable implants: Is cost recovery possible in Kenya? *Contraception, 83*(1), 88–93.

United Nations (UN). (2011). *World contraceptive use 2010.* New York: United Nations, Department of Economic and Social Affairs, Population Division.

United Nations Development Programme (UNDP), United Nations Population Fund (UNFPA), World Health Organization (WHO), & World Bank. (1997). Long-term reversible contraception: Twelve years of experience with the TCu380A and TCu220C. *Contraception, 56*(6), 341–352.

Westoff, C. F., & Cross, A. R. (2006). *The stall in the fertility transition in Kenya* (DHS analytical studies 9). Calverton: ORC Macro.

Whitehead, A. N. (1929). *Process and reality: An essay in cosmology.* New York: The Free Press.

WHO. (2010a). *Medical eligibility criteria for contraceptive use* (4th ed.). Geneva: Department of Reproductive Health and Research, WHO.

WHO. (2010b). *Review of priorities in research: Hormonal contraception and IUDs and HIV infection.* Report of a technical meeting, Geneva 13–15 Mar 2007.

WHO, UNICEF, UNFPA, & World Bank. (2010). *Trends in maternal mortality: 1990–2008. Estimates developed by WHO, UNICEF, UNFPA and The World Bank.* Geneva: WHO.

World Health Organization (WHO). (2004). *Selected practice recommendations for contraceptive use* (2nd ed.). Geneva: Department of Reproductive Health and Research, WHO.

Chapter 13
Radical Common Sense: Community Provision of Injectable Contraception in Africa

John Stanback and Reid Miller

13.1 Introduction and Background

Sub-Saharan Africa lags far behind the rest of the world in the use of family planning. Myriad factors contribute to low contraceptive prevalence in the region, but clearly, existing demand is not being met, and governments, donors and non-governmental organizations (NGOs) have failed to ensure access to a range of contraceptive options for Africa's people. Rural areas are particularly neglected: clinics are few and far between, and typically offer few family planning choices. This chapter describes a recent innovation in sub-Saharan Africa that began to diffuse when four determining factors came into play simultaneously: (1) high unmet need for contraception, (2) strong preference for injectable family planning methods, (3) a critical shortage of clinical health workers, and (4) the existence of under-utilized, community-based family planning programs. The result of the innovation was logical, but radical: the provision of the continent's favorite contraceptive by its lowest level health workers.

This chapter first briefly clarifies how these four conditions spurred the introduction of community-based distribution (CBD) of injectables in sub-Saharan Africa, and reviews the history of this practice in other regions. Next, it describes how CBD provision of injectables began and spread in Africa, anticipates what is next on the horizon, and concludes with a discussion of why CBD of injectables is becoming a standard of practice rather than a "radical" innovation.

J. Stanback, Ph.D. (✉)
PROGRESS Project, FHI 360, Durham, NC, USA
e-mail: jstanback@fhi360.org

R. Miller, MPH
Department of Reproductive Health and Research, WHO, Geneva, Switzerland

A. Kulczycki (ed.), *Critical Issues in Reproductive Health*, The Springer Series on Demographic Methods and Population Analysis 33, DOI 10.1007/978-94-007-6722-5_13, © Springer Science+Business Media Dordrecht 2014

13.1.1   Factor 1: Unmet Need for Family Planning Services

Sub-Saharan Africa faces a huge unmet need for contraception. Approximately 25 % of women of reproductive age want to delay or limit future childbearing, but do not use a modern family planning method (United Nations 2011). This gap has important implications for the well-being of the region and its people. At the macro level, governments struggle to feed, house, and educate citizens, but fall further behind in these efforts as populations continue to grow rapidly in size. An extreme example is Niger, an impoverished country in West Africa's Sahel region, whose population is doubling every 20 years (Ibid). At the micro level, bluntly stated, pregnancy is a dangerous business. Rates of maternal mortality and morbidity are up to a hundred times higher than in more developed countries. On average, women in sub-Saharan Africa run a 1 in 31 lifetime risk of dying of pregnancy-related causes, and the risk in Guinea Bissau, Somalia, and Chad, is greater than 1 in 20 (WHO et al. 2010).

Unmet need for contraception reflects gaps in both demand for and supply of contraceptive services. Most African women know about contraception, but the practice remains controversial among large swathes of the population. Fertility is highly-valued, while contraception is widely viewed with suspicion and sometimes associated with promiscuity. Pronatalist societal norms, combined with gender inequities and widespread mistrust of contraception, keep use low in many areas, even where family planning services are available. Prevalence of modern contraceptive methods in the region is only 19 % (compared to 62 % in more developed regions), while in some Sahelian countries, such as Mali, Benin, and Niger, prevalence remains in the single digits (Population Reference Bureau 2011). Women who *do* want to control their fertility face an uphill battle as well. Services are non-existent in many rural areas, and where clinics do exist, they are often understaffed, crippled by chronic commodity shortages, or both.

13.1.2   Factor 2: Preference for Injectable Contraception

In contrast to the rest of the world, where the most popular contraceptive methods are sterilization, IUDs, and the pill, women in sub-Saharan Africa largely prefer progestin-only injectable hormonal contraceptives, usually Depo Provera (DMPA, depo-medroxy progesterone acetate) or, less commonly, NET-EN (Noristerat, or norethindrone enanthate). "Injectables" are used by nearly half of African women using modern contraception (Population Reference Bureau 2008), in part, because they are highly effective, simple to administer and, relatively speaking, widely available. However, injectables are also popular with users because they require no daily or coitally-dependent regimen, only a simple injection every 3 months (every 2 months for NET-EN). This simple regimen is important for many women because it enables the method to be used discreetly—many women in the region want to use contraception without the knowledge of their partners or family.

13.1.3   Factor 3: Shortage of Clinically-Trained Health Workers

A crippling shortage of health workers exacerbates the difficulties of providing effective contraceptive services in sub-Saharan Africa. The World Health Organization (WHO) estimates that poor countries will require 2.5 health workers per 1,000 population to achieve their Millennium Development Goals (MDGs). However, of the 57 countries in the world that fall below this threshold of having a critical shortage of medical personnel, 36 are located in Sub-Saharan Africa, which has only 4 % of the world's health workers, but 25 % of its burden of disease (WHO 2006). Trained health workers have always been in short supply on the continent, especially in rural areas, because health workers are typically concentrated in urban areas. But, in recent years, the AIDS epidemic and the "brain-drain" of qualified doctors and nurses to higher paying jobs in industrialized countries has dealt a double-blow to the numbers of qualified health workers available to provide family planning to the rapidly growing population in the region. Coupled with outdated or insufficient contraceptive training curricula in medical, nursing, and midwifery schools, and a dire unmet need for curative services, it is not surprising that family planning is widely neglected on the continent.

13.1.4   Factor 4: Reliance on Community-Based Distribution Programs to Reach Rural Populations

Faced with shortages of clinically-trained health workers, many poor countries have relied for decades on community health workers (CHWs). The process of delegating certain tasks, where appropriate, to less specialized health workers is called "task shifting" (WHO 2007). In Africa, the practice of task shifting in health has increased in recent years to meet the needs of millions infected with HIV. Today, countries hard-hit by HIV/AIDS, particularly in Southern and Eastern Africa, rely on both paid and volunteer CHWs to provide not only condoms and counseling, but also testing services and even anti-retroviral treatment.

Interestingly, long before the term "task shifting" (or its newer incarnation, "task sharing" (Janowitz et al. 2012)) came into vogue, family planning programs made use of the concept, usually under the name "community-based distribution" or "CBD." Since the 1970s, CBD agents have been a fixture of family planning programs around the world, usually providing pills and condoms, but sometimes even injectable contraceptives in a few Asian and Latin American countries. Research suggests that community-based family planning programs not only go beyond improving the *supply* of contraception, but also increase *demand* as well. This is particularly true for regions with low contraceptive prevalence rates, such as Sub-Saharan Africa. By promoting family planning at the community level and increasing local knowledge of contraceptive methods, CBD agents can create new demand for these services (Phillips et al. 1999).

In Africa, funding for CBD has been sporadic, and programs come and go. But, by and large, CBD programs have been an important mechanism for reaching vulnerable women in rural areas with life-saving contraceptive services.

13.2 A Radical Solution—Community-Based Distribution of Injectable Contraceptives

The four conditions reviewed above have led to the introduction of CBD of injectables in sub-Saharan Africa. The end result was logical, and perhaps even inevitable. But it was also radical. Why should this be so? After all, the practice is not uncommon in Asia and Latin America.

The answer lies, in part, with exaggerated fears about hormonal contraceptives, even among those in the medical community. The dangers of hormonal contraception are over-stated in outdated curricula still in use in many medical, nursing, and midwifery schools in Africa, particularly in the former French colonies, where antiquated pronatalist laws outlawing contraception remained on the books until recently (Huston 1992).

But fears of hormonal methods pale in comparison to the reluctance, among some clinicians, to allow paramedical workers—however well-trained—to give injections of any kind. Such fears are sometimes justified: Africa has a widespread problem of informal and untrained healthcare providers who give unsafe injections. Clinicians fear, naturally enough, that CHWs trained to provide DMPA may be tempted to give other, less safe, less necessary injections.[1] But the reluctance also arises from "turf" issues; the injection of any medicine is considered by many a skilled medical act reserved for clinically trained providers. For this reason, professional associations of physicians, nurses, and midwives at the national level have opposed CBD of injectables on the grounds that it is unsafe or can take jobs away from more clinically trained health workers. These groups have long been opposed to CHWs taking on a larger share of the work in HIV prevention, care and treatment (McPake and Mensah 2008).

It is also worth noting that giving injections is often well-remunerated. Of the nearly two billion injections given every year in sub-Saharan Africa (Hutin et al. 2003), a large number are provided by the private health sector (which includes the many public sector health workers who provide private services during evenings, weekends, and even during the workday). Many clinicians thus equate CBD of injectables with threats to their livelihood from what amounts to low-cost competition.

---

[1] One review has estimated that, in many parts of the developing world, most injections are both unsafe and unnecessary (Simonsen et al. 1999). Another by the same authors estimated that, each year, unsafe injections are responsible for tens (or hundreds) of thousands of cases of HIV, and millions of cases of hepatitis (Kane et al. 1999).

No wonder community-based access to injectables was—and still is—considered radical in many quarters. The fear and distrust of CBD of injectables explains in large part why this common-sense practice did not spread to Africa until very recently, despite the co-existence, for more than a decade, of the four factors which should have jump-started community-based provision of injectables. In the rest of this chapter, we review the history of community-based provision of injectables in other regions, describe how the practice began and diffused in Africa, look ahead to the future of the practice, and conclude with a discussion of why CBD of injectables is becoming a standard of practice rather than a "radical" innovation.

13.3 A Brief History of CBD of Injectables in Asia and Latin America

Community-based distribution of DMPA began nearly four decades ago. In 1975, the government of Bangladesh, in collaboration with the International Centre for Diarrhoeal Disease Research, Bangladesh, introduced community-based distribution of condoms and oral contraceptives to 150 villages in the Matlab subdistrict, where contraceptive use was only 1 %. Soon thereafter, six of the villages incorporated DMPA into the method mix to assess its effect on the program. The results were impressive enough that, in 1977, DMPA was expanded to all participating villages with improvements made to the training and supervision of local providers. This service expansion led, in turn, to substantial increases in contraceptive acceptance and nearly doubled the 1-year contraceptive continuation rate. By early 1979, DMPA had replaced oral contraceptives as the most popular method in Matlab, accounting for roughly half of all contraceptive use (Ashraf et al. 1997; Huber and Khan 1979).

Beyond Bangladesh, four projects in the 1990s expanded the concept of CBD of injectable contraception in Latin America. Beginning in 1992, 180 randomly assigned CHWs affiliated with Peru's Ministry of Health (MOH) were trained to begin providing DMPA. Although this operations research project was never scaled up nationally, it was credited with jump-starting the popularity of DMPA, now Peru's most widely used method (Leon 2000).

In 1995 the Guatemalan affiliate of the International Planned Parenthood Federation (IPPF), Asociación Pro-Bienestar de la Familia de Guatemala (APROFAM), in partnership with the Population Council, conducted operations research comparing acceptance and continuation rates between clinic provision and community-based provision of DMPA. The study found that most women sought services from CBDs, and that 65 % had never used a family planning method before, suggesting that CBD provision increased contraceptive uptake. Furthermore, at 15 months, DMPA continuation rates for CBD provision were high and nearly identical to those for clinic provision: about 90 %. Because of the success of this program, APROFAM expanded community-based distribution of DMPA throughout the country (Fernandez et al. 1997). A small study in

Bolvia in 1998, and a second study in Guatemala a few years later confirmed the popularity of this service delivery mechanism in those countries, as well as CHWs' ability to use screening checklists and safely provide injectables (McCarraher 2000; Ramirez 2008).

Finally, in Mexico, a large introductory study of the monthly combined injectable contraceptive Cyclofem included community-based provision to women in rural areas. CBD workers actually achieved a higher continuation rate than MOH staff: 37 % of the 640 rural women served by CBD workers were still using Cyclofem after 1 year, compared with 24 % of the 2,817 urban and suburban women who visited health centers (Garza-Flores et al. 1998).

It is notable that the experiences in Bangladesh and Latin America were all conducted as part of research projects. High quality data from these pilot studies documented that community workers could screen and counsel clients, and safely provide DMPA injections. As important, the data showed that clients were satisfied with the services and that the CHWs were proud of the contributions they were making to their communities. Finally, the data showed that CHWs could success-fully reach women in a variety of cultural and geographic contexts (Malarcher et al. 2011). These findings have created a solid evidence base for initiating CBD of DMPA in settings with diverse cultures, environments, and health systems, but which all shared high levels of unmet need for contraception, particularly for rural populations.

13.4   Uganda: Africa's Pilot for CBD of Injectables

At century's end, CHWs still could not provide injectable contraceptives in Africa. Change was coming, however. In the late 1990s, the influential Navrongo Community Health and Family Planning Project in northern Ghana began offering DMPA door-to-door by community nurses. The project was not specifically designed to assess the effect of introducing community access to injectables, but the overwhelming majority of clients (92 %) chose DMPA from the range of methods offered by nurses during home visits. Community access to injectables also had a substantial impact on fertility levels. In 3 years, births per woman declined by16 % compared with fertility levels in similar communities served by standard MOH services (Asuru et al. 2002).

The Navrongo Project set the stage for real CBD of injectables, but it took several more years to achieve even a pilot version. A safety and feasibility study was proposed in 2000 but, due to the controversial nature of the topic in Africa, languished for 4 years while researchers looked for a country willing to host the research. Finally, in 2004, with a change in leadership in Uganda's MOH Family Planning Commission, plans were made to conduct research in Nakasongola, an impoverished rural district north of Kampala. The study, a collaboration between Uganda's Ministry of Health, the NGO Save the Children-USA, and Family Health

Table 13.1 Key results[a] from community-based distribution of injectables pilot study in Nakasongola District, Uganda, 2007

	CHW clients % (n = 449)	Clinic clients % (n = 328)
Client received second injection	88	85
Client 'Satisfied' or 'highly satisfied' with:		
Provider care	95	93
DMPA as contraceptive method	93	90
Quality indicators; client reported that provider:		
Discussed side effects	85	86
Gave written appointment slip	87	91
Discussed STI/HIV/AIDS	69	71
Offered condoms	36	34
Explained that DMPA does not protect against HIV	80	81
Infections/abscesses reported	0.0	0.0

Source: Stanback et al. (2007)
[a]Comparison of proportions of CHW clients and clinic-based clients with selected characteristics

International (FHI 360), trained Save's cadre of local CHWs to provide DMPA in addition to the condoms and pills they normally distributed. The CHWs' clients were invited to enroll in the study when they accepted the DMPA, and were followed up approximately 14 weeks later, as was a control group of DMPA clients receiving their method from local government clinics. More than 700 women were enrolled in the study, and researchers determined that the safety, acceptability, and quality of service delivery by the CHWs was comparable to that of clinic-based services (Stanback et al. 2007). Table 13.1 summarizes key findings from this research study on the first pilot of provision of injectables by CHWs in Africa.

The results of the study were widely disseminated and engendered interest both within and beyond Uganda. The stage was now set for widespread introduction of community provision of injectables in Africa.

13.5   Diffusion Within Uganda

In 2007, after the success of the pilot in Nakasongola District, CBD of DMPA began to spread within Uganda. At the time, the private, non-profit sector was more willing to innovate than the MOH, so the "early adopters" of the practice in Uganda were Save the Children, which scaled up its Nakasongola pilot to two additional districts, and also two other NGOs, Conservation Through Public Health and WellShare International. The former implemented community-based access to DMPA in the far-west Kanungu District as part of their work to mitigate human population pressures on rare mountain gorillas. WellShare implemented the project in Mubende District in south-central Uganda. Results of this expansion in the NGO sector provided more evidence of the effectiveness of the practice and also allowed for refinements prior to consideration of national scale-up (Akol et al. 2009).

While these NGO pilots were ongoing, FHI launched an advocacy campaign to create awareness of the benefits of the practice in Uganda's public sector health programs. The campaign made use of "champions," influential advocates tasked with mobilizing key district and national level stakeholders. At the national level, a high-level government official from the Ugandan MoH's Division of Reproductive Health was identified as a national-level champion. He had served as a co-principal investigator on the original pilot study and used his insider's position to maintain momentum for the project. At the district level, local champions used radio and community meetings to disseminate locally tailored messages about the importance of family planning and the use of CBD of DMPA to provide access to these services.

The success of the early adopters and the impact of the champions led the Ministry of Health to request in 2007 that the project be tested in the public sector. Local health officials who wished to replicate the project in their own districts were encouraged to apply for technical support. Little by little, Ugandan districts began adding DMPA to their existing CBD programs, and in March 2011, Uganda's MoH officially changed the national health policies to enable CHWs to provide injectable contraception. While this policy-change process was slow in comparison to several of the countries described in the following section, it showed that not every country follows the same policy path, and that diffusion of the innovation can occur even in the absence of policy change. Today, although overall contraceptive prevalence and Depo Provera use (26 % and 14 %, respectively, in 2011) remain low nationally, Uganda continues to scale up CBD of Depo Provera, and is once again taking the lead in Africa by experimenting with ways to safely provide injectable contraceptives in that country's ubiquitous private drug shops (ICF Macro 2011). Such a strategy, though controversial, makes good sense; drug shops have access to low-cost, socially marketed injectables in many countries, and drug shop operators are often far more qualified to be trained as family planning providers than typical CHWs (Stanback et al. 2011).

13.6   Diffusion in Africa

After the pilot in Uganda had demonstrated that CHWs could safely and effectively distribute DMPA, the potential for this practice was not lost on some other sub-Saharan African countries with similar health care worker shortages and limited ability to meet the contraceptive needs of women in rural areas. Nor was it lost on donors, such as USAID, who not only used their considerable influence to advocate for the practice, but also rushed to fund pilot projects. This set the stage for several countries to initiate their own programs and begin the process of policy change.

Fortunately for these countries, community provision of injectable contraception shares many of the characteristics of innovations that, according to "Diffusion of Innovation" theory, predispose an innovation to successful diffusion (Rogers 1962).

Key factors that influence the decision to accept or reject an innovation include trialability (the ease with which an individual can adopt the innovation) and observability (the extent to which the results of the innovation are visible).[2] As described above, community provision of injectables fits both of these criteria. Additional factors include the relative advantage of the innovation compared to existing practices, the simplicity of adoption, and the compatibility of the innovation with accepted values. Community provision fits these criteria as well: local needs for task shifting and benefits of CDB of contraception point to the relative advantage of community provision of injectables; pilot studies to date have demonstrated the relative ease of adoption; and, lastly, CBD programs have been active and well-accepted in Africa for decades, thus demonstrating compatibility with norms and values.

To date, however, diffusion of this innovation in Africa has been anything but uniform. There are as many models for the introduction of CBD of Depo in Africa as there are countries where it is now being piloted and scaled up. However, they all share a few common steps as they move from concept to pilot to scale up. Specifically, six such steps have been well-described by Krueger et al. (2011) with regard to how they occurred in Uganda: (1) advocacy for policy, program, and community support; (2) choice of setting for introduction; (3) commitment of resources; (4) training; (5) commodity management; and (6) process and outcome documentation.

Each of these steps implies its own set of challenges. Most of the dozen or so countries now implementing this practice are dealing with all of these challenges, and nearly all have required significant donor-funded technical assistance to move ahead.[3] Another set of issues, often unique to a given country, better illustrates the uneven diffusion of this innovation thus far. Below, short country case studies are presented that highlight idiosyncratic factors or events that have inhibited or accelerated the introduction of CBD of Depo in each case. Figure 13.1 summarizes the recent history of use of injectables in each of these countries.

13.6.1 Madagascar: "An Early Adopter"

Shortly after the Ugandan pilot ended, Madagascar's MOH approved a pilot project and subsequently scaled up its CBD of Depo program more quickly and broadly than Uganda did. Several factors contributed to Madagascar's early adoption and

---

[2]In his 1962 book "Diffusion of Innovations," Everett Rogers synthesized existing diffusion studies to popularize a theory for the adoption of innovative ideas and technologies through cultures. His theory defined five key characteristics of innovations that influence an individual's decision to adopt or reject an innovation, which include its trialability and observability (see Rogers 1962; and Chap. 12 by Jacobstein in this book for more information).

[3]The fact that these programs are donor-funded implies no criticism whatsoever of their value or usefulness. Nearly all family planning programs in sub-Saharan Africa rely partially or totally on donor funding. Community-based family planning programs are, if anything, particularly dependent, since they usually operate in remote areas and target the poorest of the poor.

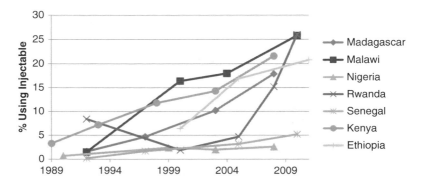

Fig. 13.1 Changing use of injectable contraceptives among married women, selected African countries, c. 1990–2011 (Source: National DHS survey data from seven sub-Saharan African countries (ICF Macro 2011))

scale-up of this innovative practice. First, the MOH's open-minded leadership was looking for results rather than focused on obstacles. These officials had heard results of Uganda's pilot from trusted advisors before publication and promptly embraced the potential of CBD of Depo as a means to reach vulnerable women in Madagascar's remote areas (Hoke et al. 2012). Since then, Madagascar, although not typically thought of as an exemplar in Africa, has served admirably in the role of innovator. Teams of policy makers and program managers from several African countries have visited Madagascar on study tours and themselves become early adopters of this practice.

13.6.2 Malawi: "Using Paid, MOH-Employed CHWs to Provide Depo Provera"

Malawi has a paid cadre of trained CHWs who provide most primary health care services to the largely rural population. In spite of the country's rapid population growth and high unmet need for family planning, these health surveillance assistants (HSAs) were, until recently, associated largely with provision of services related to HIV/AIDS, tuberculosis, and malaria. Community-level family planning was an obvious gap, filled incompletely by volunteer community-based distribution agents who were allowed to provide condoms and pills. In 2008, after Malawian family planning stakeholders participated in a learning tour to Madagascar, the MOH changed its policy and allowed HSAs to begin providing injectable contraceptives in nine pilot districts. A recent evaluation of the pilot concluded that "HSA provision of DMPA is acceptable, is safe, and expands access to family planning" (Katz et al. 2010) and has become the basis of a plan to scale up services to the rest of the country. The likely outcome is true national scale-up because HSAs are a pre-existing, paid cadre of workers.

13.6.3   Nigeria: "Stalled Introduction After Pilot"

Nigeria's successful 2008 pilot of community-based provision of injectables was one of the first completed in Africa. Like its predecessors in Uganda and Madagascar, it showed that CHW provision of DMPA was safe, feasible and popular (Abdul-hadi 2013). However, following the small pilot, the practice was not scaled up within the country or even the state where the pilot took place. Several factors explain why: first, the sponsor of the pilot (FHI 360) had neither an ongoing family planning program in Nigeria, nor local staff dedicated to moving the project forward after data collection ended. Second, Nigeria is de-centralized enough to make it very difficult to translate state-level activities into federal policies, much less successfully implement them in other states.

The potential for scale-up remains. Because the pilot was conducted in the conservative northern Nigerian state of Gombe, known for its extremely low contraceptive prevalence and antipathy towards family planning, it is hoped that less conservative states will be more quick to adopt the practice if a concerted effort is made to scale up. To that end, a national working group meeting was recently held to discuss scale-up, and funds have been allocated for both advocacy efforts and necessary training. As of this writing, Nigeria is well-positioned for provision of DMPA by its large cadre of Community Health Education Workers, which may allow the practice to finally reach a "tipping point."

13.6.4   Rwanda: "Policy Constraints That Limit the Effectiveness of CBD of Injectables"

Rwanda is a true success story for family planning in Africa. In 2010, 45 % of married women aged 15–45 used a modern method of contraception, up from only 10 % in 2005 (ICF Macro 2011). However, among the early adopters in Africa of community-based provision of injectables, Rwanda is the first to embrace a practice that has long been a feature of some CBD programs offering oral contraceptive pills: allowing CHWs to re-supply, *but not initiate*, the method. Some experts consider this a significant barrier to access, because CHWs exist exactly because some people do not have good access to clinical services. Rwanda is currently expanding community-based provision of DMPA, and already has many more trained providers than early-adopting countries such as Uganda, Zambia, and Nigeria. It remains to be seen, however, whether the improved access to family planning will be offset in any way by this policy constraint.

13.6.5   Senegal: "Outsized Influence of a Champion"

In his recent tenure as Director of the Senegalese MOH's Division of Reproductive Health, Dr. Bocar Daff has reversed decades of restrictive policy on family planning in this influential francophone West African country. He has made enemies of some conservative *médecins* along the way, but Senegal is becoming a favorite of family planning donors, and Dr. Daff shares their commitment to improved access to life-saving family planning services.

The changes in Senegal during Dr. Daff's tenure are striking. Although Senegal has only just begun community-based provision of *pills*—20 years after most African countries—the country is now piloting contraceptive injections by its extensive system of "matrones" who operate from small health huts or "cas de santé" throughout rural Senegal. Senegal was also chosen as one of only two sites in the world to study the acceptability of contraceptive injections by CHWs using subcutaneous Depo Provera in the Uniject device (see below). Host in 2011 to the second International Conference on Family Planning, Senegal is already influencing the rest of Francophone Africa to liberalize their rigid family planning policies and allow long-overdue "task sharing" between the *ancien régime* of conservative-minded clinicians and a more dynamic new cadre of community-based workers.

13.6.6 Kenya: "Slow Adoption in an Otherwise Successful Family Planning Program"

In comparison with other countries in East Africa, Kenya is relatively affluent and has high modern method contraceptive prevalence (39 % in 2008–2009). However, because of strong opposition from professional bodies as well as senior officials in the Ministry of Public Health, efforts aimed at official acceptance of CBD of injectables have been unsuccessful to date, exacerbated by the erosion of Kenya's formerly extensive system of community-based family planning. Some observers are hopeful, however, citing results of a successful local pilot (Olawo et al. 2011) and the recognition of a new, largely theoretical, cadre of trained MOH CHWs.

13.6.7 Ethiopia: "Ambitious Programs Going Beyond CBD of Injectables"

Even among early adopting countries of CBD of injectables, Ethiopia stands out. While Uganda, Madagascar and other countries were training their first cohorts of community workers to provide DMPA, Ethiopia was planning to roll out a national system of 30,000 Health Extension Workers trained not only to give Depo injections, but also to insert the single-rod contraceptive implant Implanon. These workers have more training and skills than most CHWs in Africa, but the audacity of the program is still striking on a continent that remains resolutely conservative about family planning. As of this writing, about half of the Ethiopian Health Extension Workers have been trained in implant insertion and are providing local women with what most other sub-Saharan African countries lack: access to long-acting contraception, even for women in remote rural areas.

While the pace and method of introduction has varied greatly across these seven countries, there is reasonable agreement on optimal strategies required for CBD programs to deliver family planning services in a sustainable manner. Phillips et al.'s (1999) thorough analysis of CBD programs identified overarching lessons in program management that are also relevant to the challenge of adding injectables to CHWs' workload. These should include (1) political support; (2) the involvement of communities in the selection of the CBD agents; (3) community involvement in information dissemination and outreach; (4) initial investments in quality training programs; (5) compensation of CBD agents; (5) supportive (rather than directive) supervision of CBD workers; and (6) sufficient attention given by information systems to the quality-of-care information needs of CBD agents.

Phillips et al. (1999) also provide recipes for CBD program failure. These include perceptions by planners that CHWs are simple and self-sustaining; preoccupation by programs with a single commodity or service, premature program focus on sustainability, and the failure to address quality-of-care requirements and social barriers to family planning. Since this 1999 review, community health programs in Africa have gradually shed some of these weaknesses and adopted many of Phillips' suggestions for strengthening programs. Well-trained, public sector CHWs are far from ubiquitous, but are now a goal in many countries.

13.7 Diffusion of Injectable Contraceptive CBD Programs Beyond Africa

With a foothold in Africa, CBD of injectable contraception may also make a much-needed comeback in Asia and Latin America, both in countries where it was introduced and has since languished, and in new countries as well. A good example of the latter is Afghanistan, where the practice was never attempted in decades past, but recently has had demonstrable success in the face of widespread skepticism about the acceptability of community-based provision of family planning. In the three areas of Afghanistan selected for the 2005–2006 "Accelerating Contraceptive Use" project, contraceptive prevalence—led by injectables—increased by 24–27 % in only 8 months (Fig. 13.2, Huber et al. 2010). Since then, Afghanistan has trained more than 9,000 CHWs, leading to a 5 % per year increase in contraceptive prevalence (Mushfiq et al. 2011). CBD of injectables presents a wonderful opportunity to expand family planning in countries, like Afghanistan and others, where poverty, rugged terrain, and sparsely populated rural areas make clinic-based services untenable. Pakistan, home to nearly 100,000 lady health workers, is another country making strides with community-based access to injectables. Until recently, Pakistan's lady health workers only allowed to re-supply injectables, but policies were changed recently and these community providers can now screen new clients and initiate the method, allowing women who live far from clinics to access injectables.

India also holds huge potential for CBD of injectables, along with a well-organized system of community health workers. However, because of past abuses

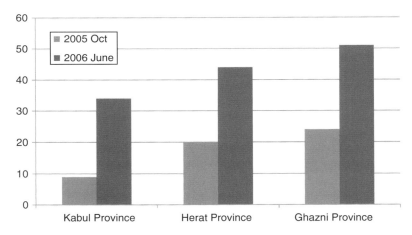

Fig. 13.2 Contraceptive prevalence rates in the accelerating contraceptive use project, Afghanistan (Source: Huber et al. 2010)

by the Indian government's family planning program (Gwatkin 1979), along with exaggerated fears of DMPA's side effects, a small but vocal minority of women's groups have prevented provision of Depo Provera by government health programs (Hirve 2005). Even in the private sector, current regulations allow only physicians to prescribe and give the first injection of DMPA. Efforts are now underway to convince the Indian Government to change these restrictive policies. If policy change does succeed, the impact could be significant in large, poor states such as Uttar Pradesh where contraceptive prevalence lags far behind other parts of India.

Community-based provision of injectables will also continue to spread in Africa. A particular challenge lies ahead in the francophone countries of West Africa, which, in the past, have often harbored a deeper mistrust of contraception than their anglophone counterparts. But even in the Sahel, a region long associated with conservative beliefs about family planning, the tide is turning, due in part to progressive changes in Senegal. As of this writing, Togo has initiated CBD of injectables, and countries such as Niger and Burkina Faso have agreed in principle to begin pilots.

13.8 Two Potential Accelerators of Diffusion

Two recent developments will likely accelerate the spread of community-based provision of injectables. These include the guidance from two WHO Technical Consultations related to the subject and the approval by European regulatory authorities of a new formulation of DMPA pre-packaged in a novel, simple-to-use injection device called Uniject®.

13.8.1   Technical Consultation on Community-Based Provision of Injectables

In an effort to inform policies and programs related to community based provision of injectables, WHO, USAID, and FHI convened a Technical Consultation on "Expanding Access to Injectable Contraception" in Geneva, 2009. Thirty technical and program experts found that community-based provision of progestin-only injectable contraceptives by appropriately trained CHWs is safe, effective, and acceptable. They concluded that evidence supports the introduction, continuation, and scale-up of community-based provision of progestin-only injectable contraceptives, provided as part of a family planning program offering a range of contraceptive methods. In 2010, a number of large international organizations added their endorsements to this brief. They included the International Confederation of Midwives, International Council of Nurses, and International Federation of Gynecology and Obstetrics (FIGO); and the IPPF, Marie Stopes International, United Nations Population Fund (UNFPA), and the World Bank.

More recently, WHO (2012) published new guidelines on task shifting for key maternal and newborn health interventions, including family planning. Through a rigorous process of systematic reviews and expert opinion, WHO concluded that lay health workers such as CHWs can provide injectable contraceptives "with targeted monitoring and evaluation."

13.8.2   Depo subQ 104 in Uniject

Advances in technology will also speed the diffusion of community-based provision of injectables. In particular, Pfizer Pharmaceuticals has developed a new formulation of DMPA that is injected subcutaneously—with a markedly shorter needle—rather than the deep intramuscular injection used for standard DMPA. This new DMPA, with a hormone dose a third lower than regular Depo Provera, comes in a simple-to-use, pre-filled injection device called Uniject® developed by PATH (see Fig. 13.3). Depo subQ 104 in Uniject, also called "Sayana Press®," is compact, non-reusable, and may change the face of family planning in Africa and in other countries where injectables are popular. The new product is more simple for CHWs to administer, and, because the injecting device looks nothing like a standard syringe, countries that have previously balked at allowing community workers to give injections may be more likely to change their policies. Depo subQ 104 in Uniject will also open up the possibility of self-injection of DMPA (Keith 2011). In the past, contraceptive self-injection was studied in a few limited trials, but was never scaled up, due in part to the intimidating nature of injecting oneself with the long needle required for deep intramuscular injection.

As of this writing, Sayana Press is not yet widely available, but three studies have recently been completed to study the acceptability of self-injection with the same subcutaneously-injected formulation of DMPA in a prefilled glass syringe

Fig. 13.3 Depo subQ 104
in Uniject® (Photo credit:
PATH/Patrick McKern)

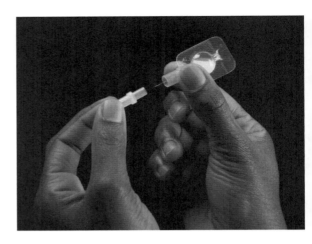

(Cameron et al. 2012; Prabhakaran and Sweet 2012; Beasley et al. 2011). Hopes are
high that, once a woman is taught to self-inject by a qualified provider, she could
buy the product, perhaps in a socially-marketed format, when needed, or keep a small
stock at home for future use. The latter could be particularly important for women
who live far from services or are seasonally cut off from services due to weather.

13.9   Are We Betting on the Wrong Method?

This chapter has highlighted the growing popularity of injectables in Africa. They
are indeed popular, but their real and perceived benefits are counter-balanced by a
number of disadvantages. Although DMPA and NET-EN do not contain estrogen
and thus are free of some of the risks of combined hormonal contraception, use of
progestin-only injectable contraceptives nearly always results in menstrual irregularities such as sporadic or prolonged bleeding and, eventually, amenorrhea. Less
common side effects include headaches, dizziness and weight gain. Long-term use
has also been associated with loss of bone density, a risk serious enough that, in
2004, the U.S. FDA added a so-called "Black-Box" warning to DMPA's labeling
requirements.[4] There are also literal costs to use of injectables, for which governments and donors spend from $0.60 to $1.12 a dose, making them one of the most
expensive family planning methods per woman-year of use (Reproductive Health
Supplies Coalition 2011).

Another potential disadvantage of DMPA is its possible association with
HIV acquisition and transmission. While no research has proven that injectable

---

[4]However, several studies have shown that the lost bone mass is usually recouped after the method
is discontinued (Kaunitz et al. 2008) and, more recently, calls to remove the black box warning
have appeared (Kaunitz and Grimes 2011).

contraceptives influence HIV risk, some studies have suggested such a link with HIV infection, while others have not. The most recent major study, by Heffron et al. (2012), suggested that, among sero-discordant couples, HIV negative women had a two-fold risk of acquiring HIV if they used progestin-only injectables. All of these studies, the Heffron study included, were observational in design, so may be biased by self-selection or some other unexplained variables. In addition, DMPA users may differ in important ways from non-users, for example, by having higher coital frequency or lower condom use. Thus, these types of studies are usually not considered conclusive. As of this writing, WHO's position reflects the conclusions of a technical consultation held in January 2012, which upheld earlier guidance that the balance of evidence suggests no association between HIV infection or progression and the use of progesterone-only contraceptive use. However, the new Technical Statement also adds that, "because of the inconclusive nature of the body of evidence on possible increased risk of HIV acquisition, women using progestogen-only injectable contraception should be strongly advised to also always use condoms, male or female, and other HIV preventive measures (WHO 2012)."

Finally, it is worth noting that the typical family planning clinic in sub-Saharan Africa offers only pills, condoms, and DMPA. Thus, the popularity of injectables in Africa is due in part to the lack of access of other acceptable methods, particularly long-acting and permanent contraceptives such as implants, IUDs and sterilization. For example, in the study of Uganda's pilot experience with CBD of injectables, 27 % of new clients seeking DMPA from CHWs wanted no more children (Stanback et al. 2007). These women likely had zero access to long-acting or permanent contraceptives, so it is reasonable to assume they would have preferred a method more appropriate to their situation. In the future, rural women in Africa may have better access to a broad range of methods, rendering injectables the top choice for only a small niche population, as is now the case in many industrialized countries. For now, however, injectables remain the available method of choice for many rural African women.

13.10   Conclusion

Community-based provision of injectable contraception is still a radical notion in most African countries, its common-sense unrecognized. Powerful groups, such as professional nurses' associations, argue vehemently against the practice, while poor women, who stand to gain the most from this innovation, have no voice in the matter.

However, a growing number of countries do recognize the good sense of task sharing. They are now training cadres of community workers to provide routine health services, and thereby freeing the time of doctors, nurses, and midwives to make best use of their specialized clinical skills. As these CHWs provide more—and more specialized—care for those suffering from HIV/AIDS, malaria, tuberculosis, and other ailments, it should become obvious to even the most entrenched interests that providing healthy women with safe contraceptive methods is a good idea.

As the practice spreads to more and more countries, a tipping point will be reached and community-based provision of injectables will take its rightful place as a new standard of practice.

References

Abdul-hadi, R. A., Abass, M. M., Aiyenigba, B. O., Oseni, L. O., Odafe, S., Chabikuli, O. N., Ibrahim, M. D., Hamelmann, C., & Ladipo, O. A. (2013). The effectiveness of community based distribution of injectable contraceptives using community health extension workers in Gombe State, Northern Nigeria. *African Journal of Reproductive Health, 17*(2), 80–88.

Akol, A., et al. (2009). *Scaling up community-based access to injectables in Uganda: Lessons learned from private- and public-sector implementation.* Research Triangle Park: Family Health International.

Ashraf, A., Ahmed, S., & Phillips, J. F. (1997). The example of doorstep injectables. In Barkat-e-Khuda, T. T. Kane, J. F. Phillips (Eds), *Improving the Bangladesh health and family planning programme. Lessons learned through operations research. Monograph No. 5.* Dhaka: International Centre for Diarrhoeal Disease Research.

Asuru, R., Phillips, J. F., Akumah I., et al. (2002, November 9–13). *The success and failure of alternative strategies for community-based distribution of contraception in the Navrongo Project.* American Public Health Association 130th Annual Meeting, Philadelphia.

Beasley, A., White, K. O., & Westhoff, C. (2011). *Self versus clinic administration of depot medroxyprogesterone acetate: A randomized controlled trial.* Poster presented at the 59th Annual Clinical Meeting of American College of Obstetricians and Gynecologists, Washington, DC.

Cameron, S. T., Glasier, A., & Johnstone, A. (2012). Pilot study of home self-administration of subcutaneous depo-medroxyprogesterone acetate for contraception. *Contraception, 85*(5), 458–464.

Fernandez, V. H., Montúfar, E., Ottolenghi, E., et al. (1997). *Injectable contraceptive service delivery provided by volunteer community promoters.* Unpublished paper. New York: Population Council.

Garza-Flores, J., Del Olmo, A. M., Fuziwara, J. L., et al. (1998). Introduction of cyclofem once-a-month injectable contraceptive in Mexico. *Contraception, 58*(1), 7–12.

Gwatkin, D. R. (1979). Political will and family planning. *Population and Development Review, 5*(1), 29–59.

Heffron, R., Donnell, D., Rees, H., et al. (2012). Use of hormonal contraceptives and risk of HIV-1 transmission: A prospective cohort study. *The Lancet Infectious Diseases, 12,* 19–26.

Hirve, S. (2005). Injectables as a choice – Evidence-based lesson. *Indian Journal of Medical Ethics, 11*(1), 12–13.

Hoke, T. H., Wheeler, S. B., Lynd, K., Green, M. S., Razafindravony, B. H., Rasamihajamanana, E., & Blumenthal, P. D. (2012). Community-based provision of injectable contraceptives in Madagascar: 'Task shifting' to expand access to injectable contraceptives. *Health Policy and Planning, 27*(1), 52–59.

Huber, D. H., & Khan, A. R. (1979). Contraceptive distribution in Bangladesh villages: The initial impact. *Studies in Family Planning, 10,* 246–253.

Huber, D. H., Saeedi, N., & Samadi, A. K. (2010). Achieving success with family planning in rural Afghanistan. *Bulletin of the World Health Organization, 88*(3), 227–231.

Huston, P. (1992). *Motherhood by choice: Pioneers in women's health and family planning* (p. 161). New York: International Planned Parenthood Federation.

Hutin, Y. J., Hauri, A. M., & Armstrong, G. L. (2003). Use of injections in healthcare settings worldwide, 2000: Literature review and regional estimates. *British Medical Journal, 327*(7423), 1075.

ICF Macro. (2011). *MEASURE DHS STATcompiler*. Available at: http://www.statcompiler.com. Accessed 10 June 2012.

Janowitz, B., Stanback, J., & Boyer, B. (2012). Task sharing in family planning. *Studies in Family Planning, 43*(1), 57–62.

Kane, A., Lloyd, J., Zaffran, M., Simonsen, L., & Kane, M. (1999). Transmission of hepatitis B, hepatitis C and human immuno-deficiency viruses through unsafe injections in the developing world: Model-based regional estimates. *Bulletin of the World Health Organization, 77*, 801–807.

Katz, K., Ngalande, R., Jackson, E., Kachale, F., & Mhango, C. (2010). *Evaluation of community-based distribution of DMPA by Health Surveillance Assistants in Malawi*. Final report. FHI 360. Research Triangle Park.

Kaunitz, A. M., & Grimes, D. A. (2011). Removing the black box warning for depot medroxy-progesterone acetate. *Contraception, 84*, 212–213.

Kaunitz, A. M., Arias, R., & McClung, M. (2008). Bone density recovery after depot medroxy-progesterone acetate injectable contraception use. *Contraception, 77*(2), 67.

Keith, B. M. (2011). *Home-based administration of depo-subQ provera 104™ in the Uniject™ injection system: A literature review*. Seattle: PATH.

Krueger, K., Akol, A., Wamala, P., & Brunie, A. (2011). Scaling up community provision of inject-ables through the public sector in Uganda. *Studies in Family Planning, 42*(2), 117–124.

Leon, F. (2000). *Utilization of DMPA and other operations research solutions in Peru*. Lima: Population Council.

Malarcher, S., Meirik, O., Lebetkin, E., Shah, I., Spieler, J., & Stanback, J. (2011). Provision of DMPA by community health workers: What the evidence shows. *Contraception, 83*, 495–503.

McCarraher, D. (2000). *Informe final. Administracion de Depo Provera a traves de asistentes voluntaries y personal del Centro de Salud CIES – El Alto*. Unpublished project report. Family Health International, Durham, NC, USA.

McPake, B., & Mensah, K. (2008). Task shifting in health care in resource-poor countries. *The Lancet, 372*(9642), 870–871.

Mushfiq, H., & Aitken, I. (2011). *Scaling up community health worker provision of Depo-Provera as part of a broader birth spacing program*. Presentation at 2011 International Conference on Family Planning, Dakar, Senegal.

Olawo, A. A., Washika, E., Gitonga, J., Malonza, I., & Manyonyi, K. (2011). *Task sharing in reproductive health: Community-based distribution of depot medroxyprogesteroine acetate in Kenya: Findings from a pilot project in Tharaka District*. Presentation at 2011 International Conference on Family Planning, Dakar, Senegal.

Phillips, J. F., Greene, W., & Jackson, E. (1999). *Lessons from community-based distribution of family planning in Africa*. New York: Population Council.

Population Reference Bureau. (2008). *Family planning worldwide data sheet*. Washington, DC: Population Reference Bureau.

Population Reference Bureau. (2011). *World population data sheet*. Washington, DC: Population Reference Bureau.

Prabhakaran, S., & Sweet, A. (2012). Self-administration of subcutaneous depot medroxyproges-terone acetate for contraception: Feasibility and acceptability. *Contraception, 85*(5), 453–457.

Ramirez, L. (2008). *Introduction of a training program for the delivery of Depo-Provera® by community-based providers from the Ministry of Public Health in Guatemala*. Unpublished project report 2008. Final Report. Guatemala City, Guatemala: Centro de Investigación Epidemiológica en Salud Sexual y Reproductiva.

Reproductive Health Supplies Coalition. (2011). *RH interchange*. Available from: http://rhi.rhsup-plies.org. Accessed 18 Dec 2011.

Rogers, E. M. (1962). *Diffusion of innovations*. Glencoe: Free Press.

Simonsen, L., Kane, A., Lloyd, J., Zaffran, M., & Kane, M. (1999). Unsafe injections in the devel-oping world and transmission of blood-borne pathogens: A review. *Bulletin of the World Health Organization, 77*(10), 789–800.

Stanback, J., Otterness, C., Bekiita, M., Nakayiza, O., & Mbonye, A. K. (2011). Injected with controversy: Sales and administration of injectable contraceptives in drug shops in Uganda. *International Perspectives on Sexual and Reproductive Health, 37*(1), 24–29.

Stanback, J., Mbonye, A., & Bekiita, M. (2007). Contraceptive injections by community health workers in Uganda: A non-randomized trial. *Bulletin of the World Health Organization, 85,* 768–773.

United Nations. (2011). *The millennium development goals report 2011.* New York: Department of Economic and Social Affairs.

WHO, Department of Reproductive Health and Research. (2012). *Hormonal contraception and HIV: Technical statement.* http://whqlibdoc.who.int/hq/2012/WHO_RHR_12.08_eng.pdf

World Health Organization. (2007). *Task shifting to tackle health worker shortages.* Geneva: World Health Organization.

World Health Organization. (2010). *Medical eligibility criteria for contraceptive use* (4th ed., p. 51). Geneva: World Health Organization.

World Health Organization (WHO). (2006). *The world health report 2006: Working together for health.* Geneva: World Health Organization.

World Health Organization (WHO), UNICEF, UNFPA, World Bank. (2010). *Trends in maternal mortality: 1990 to 2008: Estimates.* Geneva: World Health Organization.

World Health Organization. (2012). *WHO recommendations: Optimizing health worker roles to improve access to key maternal and newborn health interventions through task shifting.* Geneva: WHO.

Chapter 14
Global Introduction of a Low-Cost Contraceptive Implant

Kate H. Rademacher, Heather L. Vahdat, Laneta Dorflinger,
Derek H. Owen, and Markus J. Steiner

The best way is the implant. A person like me is always forgetful. I cannot lie as I'm talking about myself. If I say that I want to take the pill…I will not. I will use [implants] because I will definitely forget to take the pills. ~ Kenyan woman, focus group participant

The [implant] is a good method, but unaffordable. The health clinic should stock it and reduce its price. ~ Kenyan woman, focus group participant[1]

Hormone-releasing subdermal implants are a safe, highly effective, and reversible form of contraception that provides continuous pregnancy protection for 3–5 years depending on the type of implant. Implants are among the most effective forms of contraception available; efficacy is comparable to other long-acting and permanent methods including the intrauterine device (IUD) and sterilization, with annual pregnancy rates less than 1 % for women using these methods (Mansour et al. 2010). However, unlike the IUD or female sterilization which requires a gynecological procedure, implants are inserted under the skin of a woman's upper arm. Because no regular action is required by the user and no routine resupply or clinical follow-up is needed, implants are widely seen as an ideal method for women with limited

---

[1]Quotations are from unpublished interview transcripts recorded in a 2008 study of female sex workers in Kenya, from which some results have been published in Sutherland et al. (2011).

K.H. Rademacher, MHA (✉)
Program Sciences, FHI 360, Durham, NC, USA
e-mail: krademacher@fhi360.org

H.L. Vahdat, MPH
Social and Behavioral Health Sciences, FHI 360, Durham, NC, USA

L. Dorflinger, Ph.D.
Global Health, Population and Nutrition, FHI 360, Durham, NC, USA

D.H. Owen, Ph.D. • M.J. Steiner, Ph.D., MSPH
Clinical Sciences, FHI 360, Durham, NC, USA

A. Kulczycki (ed.), *Critical Issues in Reproductive Health*, The Springer Series on
Demographic Methods and Population Analysis 33, DOI 10.1007/978-94-007-6722-5_14,
© Springer Science+Business Media Dordrecht 2014

access to health services, particularly women in developing countries (Frost and Reich 2008). However, despite the advantages of this method, worldwide use of implants is low: whereas 56 % of married women between the ages of 15 and 49 around the globe use a modern method of contraception, less than 1 % use implants (United Nations 2011).

A key barrier to uptake of contraceptive implants has been their high cost. While implants are cost-effective compared to other methods (Mavranezouli 2009), the high upfront commodity cost of implants can be prohibitive for governments and donors who tend to invest in less expensive, shorter-acting methods such as oral contraceptives or injectables (Hubacher et al. 2007). The global introduction of Sino-implant (II), a two-rod implant which is manufactured in China that cost less than half of the cost of other implants on the market as of mid-2012, has the potential to increase access to a popular family planning method and increase contraceptive security in resource-constrained settings (Tumlinson et al. 2011).

This chapter reviews efforts to facilitate the introduction of Sino-implant (II) in Sub-Saharan Africa, Latin America and Asia starting in 2007. The manufacturer of Sino-implant (II), Shanghai Dahua Pharmaceutical Company, Ltd. (subsequently referred to as "Dahua"), has sold the product in China since 1996 and in Indonesia since 2003. However, Dahua had very limited international reach at the start of the global initiative, which is coordinated by Family Health International (FHI 360), a global development organization, and funded by the Bill & Melinda Gates Foundation. This chapter outlines and analyzes the strategy that has been used by Dahua, FHI 360, distributors, and other organizations to seek regulatory approval of Sino-implant (II) at the national level while simultaneously pursuing prequalification from the World Health Organization (WHO) for the product. The WHO prequalification process is described in detail later in the chapter, and organizations involved in the Sino-implant (II) initiative and related activities are listed in Table 14.1.

The experience with the introduction of Sino-implant (II) highlights the upfront investment that is required to help manufacturers from developing countries reach a global market. Whereas the international introduction of drugs that have been approved by a strict regulatory authority (SRA), such as the U.S. Food and Drug Administration (USFDA) or the European Medicines Agency (EMA), may assume a more linear path, the Sino-implant (II) initiative has involved an iterative, multi-stage process. This model may provide a roadmap for other non-SRA approved products that are manufactured and distributed in developing countries.

14.1   History of Implants

The first contraceptive implant, Norplant, was developed by the Population Council, a non-governmental organization (NGO) based in New York. Consisting of six rods each containing 36 mg of levonorgestrel, a progestin hormone, Norplant was first

Table 14.1 Organizations involved in Sino-implant (II) initiative and related activities

Organization or entity	Role in the global introduction of Sino-implant (II)
Bill & Melinda Gates Foundation	Provides the primary funding for the global Sino-implant (II) initiative. The goal of the initiative is to increase access to affordable contraceptive implants in resource-constrained settings.
DKT	Distributor for Sino-implant (II) in Ethiopia under the trade name "Trust."
EngenderHealth	Works in developing countries to increase access to long-acting and permanent methods, including implants. Involved in a pre-marketing study of Sino-implant (II) in Bangladesh.
Family Health International (FHI 360)	Coordinates independent quality testing activities for Sino-implant (II); negotiates public sector price ceilings; supports national registrations; leads post-marketing studies; and provides technical assistance for additional introduction activities.
Marie Stopes International (MSI)	Distributes Sino-implant (II) in Africa and Asia under the trade name "Femplant," and is a lead service-delivery group providing contraceptive implants.
Ministries of Health	Approve introduction of Sino-implant (II) after registration, and support scale up.
National Population and Family Planning Commission (NPFPC)	Helped lead the development of Sino-implant (II) and currently supports provider trainings in China.
Pharm Access Africa, Ltd. (PAAL)	Distributes Sino-implant (II) in Africa under the trade name "Zarin."
The Population Council	Led the development of first- and second-generation implants.
Progyne	Distributor for Sino-implant (II) in Columbia.
PSI	Conducted an audit of Dahua early in the initiative and approved procurement for its international programs.
Shanghai Dahua Pharmaceutical Company, Ltd. (referred to as "Dahua")	Manufactures the two-rod implant, Sino-implant (II).
United Nations Population Fund (UNFPA)	Serves as a major donor of contraceptive implants globally. In 2011, UNFPA established an interim approval mechanism for contraceptives that have begun the WHO prequalification process.
United States Agency for International Development (USAID)	Serves as a major donor of contraceptive implants globally. USAID's policy that only allowed procurement of US-manufactured, SRA-approved drugs was changed in 2011 to allow more flexibility. USAID funds post-marketing studies of Sino-implant (II) in two countries.
WomanCare Global	Distributor for Sino-implant (II) in Nepal, Russia and several Latin American countries under the trade name "Simplant."
World Health Organization (WHO)	Leads the Prequalification Programme for medicinal products including reproductive health commodities.

licensed in Finland in 1983. International pre-introduction trials began in the early 1980s (Sivin et al. 2002). Numerous clinical, pre-introduction, post-marketing and acceptability studies in over 44 countries demonstrated the safety and acceptability of the new method. However, Norplant faced challenges when introduced at scale in multiple countries. Problems included limited access to removal services; public perception that as a provider-controlled method, implants might be pushed upon vulnerable populations without their full consent or understanding; and a high commodity cost which reduced access among poor women. In addition, in the mid-1990s, a class action lawsuit in the United States was brought against Wyeth-Ayerst, the private sector manufacturer of Norplant, by women who complained about scarring and substantial pain upon removal, and about side effects that they had not been informed about prior to insertion. Demand for the product declined, and after the suits were either settled or dismissed, Norplant was taken off the US market in 2002 (Frost and Reich 2008).

Around the world, however, an estimated six million women had used Norplant by 2003 and the product was registered in over 58 countries. In acceptability trials in developing countries, women reported that they were very satisfied with the method (Frost and Reich 2008). Continuation rates among Norplant users were high; studies in developing countries showed that after 2 years of use, 91 % of women were still using Norplant (Power et al. 2007). Studies also showed that women who received pre-insertion counseling about side-effects and other aspects of the method were more likely to be satisfied (Coukell and Balfour 1998).

By the late-1980s, the Population Council developed a new two-rod implant named Jadelle. The intention was to make insertion and removal easier. Each of Jadelle's two rods has 75 mg levonorgestrel (for a total of 150 mg), and the product is registered for 5 years of continuous use. Jadelle was approved in 1996 by the USFDA, although it was never marketed in the US, and is currently licensed for global distribution by Bayer HealthCare (Hohmann and Creinin 2007). Subsequently, Implanon, a single-rod implant, was introduced by Schering-Plough, now Merck/MSD. Implanon contains 68 mg of etonorgestrel, is registered for 3 years of use, and was approved by the USFDA in 2006 (Adams and Beal 2009). Contraceptive efficacy of these second generation implants is comparable to Norplant, with annual pregnancy rates of less than 1 %. As with Norplant, continuation rates for Jadelle and Implanon are high, particularly in developing countries (Power et al. 2007).

Studies and field experience demonstrated that compared to Norplant, one- and two-rod implants are easier and quicker to insert and remove. This advantage led to the replacement of Norplant by Jadelle and Implanon in health programs around the world; in 2008, global production of Norplant was discontinued (Ramchandran and Upadhyay 2007).

However, the high cost of both Jadelle and Implanon has remained a barrier to wider scale availability. The RHInterchange database (maintained by UNFPA, the United Nations Population Fund) indicates that in 2010, Jadelle was available at an average cost of $22 per unit and Implanon at $20 per unit (RHInterchange 2011). Procurement of implants by most donor agencies and governments has remained low, and stockouts of implants have been common in developing countries.

While the true demand for implants is not known due to shortage of supplies, evidence suggests that many more women would choose implants in resource-constrained settings if they were reliably available (Hubacher et al. 2007; Neukom et al. 2011).

14.2   Development of Sino-implant (II) in China

Sino-implant (II) is a two-rod implant with the same active ingredient, delivery system and mechanism of action as Jadelle. The development of Sino-implant (II) was initiated and led by the China State Family Planning Commission (now named the National Population and Family Planning Commission or NPFPC) between 1986 and 1996. The research process was led by Chinese research institutions affiliated with NPFPC, with some limited technical assistance provided by WHO.

Although not a member of the initial research team, Dahua bought the rights from the research institutions for the production technology for Sino-implant (II) in 1991. In 1994, the core research and development team along with Dahua obtained approval for pilot production of Sino-implant (II) from the China Ministry of Health Drug Bureau (now named the State Food and Drug Administration or SFDA), and approval was granted to Dahua for commercial production in 1996.

Sino-implant (II) is approved as a 4-year product in China. A review of four randomized clinical trials conducted in China with over 15,000 women indicated that the cumulative pregnancy rate for Sino-implant (II) at the end of 4 years was 0.9–1.06 % and side-effects were comparable to other implants (Steiner et al. 2010).

Despite the availability and proven effectiveness of Sino-implant (II), uptake of implants has been relatively low in China. While the contraceptive prevalence rate is 85 % in China, only 0.3 % of women of reproductive age use implants (United Nations 2011). Female sterilization and IUDs are the dominant methods that became firmly entrenched due to the one-child policy in China that was established in 1979. The government has favored both methods because of their low cost (d'Arcangues 2007; Sullivan et al. 2006; Bertrand et al. 2000). According to Dahua, almost 300,000 units of Sino-implant (II) were sold in China in 2010 in more than 20 provinces, primarily in central and western China. Customer surveys have shown a high level of satisfaction with the method. Provider trainings are offered by NPFPC; recently, NPFPC has committed to increasing utilization of implants through implementation of a national training program for providers in China and in Tibet (Zhou 2011).

In 2002, Sino-implant (II) was registered in Indonesia and then introduced in 2003. Rates of implant use in Indonesia are somewhat higher than other countries; 2.8 % of women ages 15–49 use implants (United Nations 2011). According to Dahua, in 2010, over 300,000 units of Sino-implant (II) were sold in Indonesia (Zhou 2011).

Figure 14.1 illustrates the cost advantages of Sino-implant (II). Average direct service delivery costs—including commodity costs and staff time for resupply or insertion and removal—were calculated over 3 years of continuous use based on mid-2012 prices. The results show that Sino-implant (II)'s average direct service

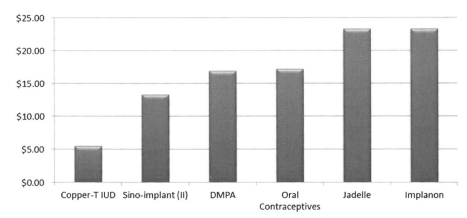

Fig. 14.1 Average direct service delivery costs for 3 years of protection from various contraceptive methods across 12 countries based on mid-2012 commodity prices* (Sources: Cost data from RHInterchange (http://rhi.rhsupplies.org) and personal correspondence with USAID 2012. Data on labor and supply costs from UNFPA's RH costing model, 2008 v. 3; received through personal correspondence, 2012 (see http://www.unfpa.org/public/home/supplies/pid/3595). Average direct service delivery costs based on labor costs from UNFPA model from 12 countries: Democratic Republic of Congo, Ethiopia, Haiti, Kenya, Madagascar, Malawi, Nigeria, Pakistan, Rwanda, Tanzania, Uganda, and Zambia)

Note: This figure includes commodity costs plus staff time for resupply or insertion and removal assuming a unit price of $8 for Sino-implant (II) and $18 for Jadelle and Implanon.

*As noted in the postscript, as this publication was going to press, Bayer HealthCare and Merck/MSD announced price reductions of Jadelle and Implanon respectively to under $9 per unit (Bayer HealthCare 2012; MSD 2013).

delivery costs were lower than that of most other reversible methods over a 3-year period including oral contraceptives, injectables and other implants in 2012, making it second only to the Copper-T IUD.[2]

14.3   Global Introduction: Overview of the Sino-implant (II) Initiative

In 2006, FHI 360 learned that a low cost implant was being manufactured in China by Dahua. FHI 360 staff visited Dahua to assess the facility and to discuss Dahua's interest and capacity to become a global manufacturer of contraceptive implants. Subsequently, a team at FHI 360 submitted a proposal to the Bill & Melinda Gates

---

[2] Costs include commodities, supplies and labor.

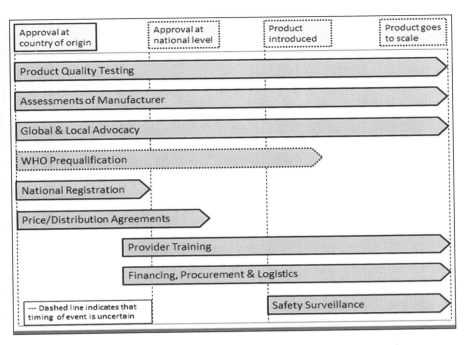

Fig. 14.2 Key milestones in introduction of new contraceptive method. Although some countries require WHO prequalification prior to national registration, under the Sino-implant (II) initiative, registration and introduction has moved forward in a number of countries while WHO prequalification is pending

Foundation to support a 1-year effort to initiate quality testing and assistance with product registration activities. Funding for this initial phase was awarded in 2007 followed by a second grant in 2008 to expand these efforts for an additional 5 years (2009–2013). The primary objective of the grant is to develop a global business model between public and private organizations to ensure access to affordable, high quality contraceptive implants in resource-constrained settings.

Key activities of the initiative include (1) establishing processes and procedures to monitor the quality of Sino-implant (II) through independent product testing; (2) coordinating on-going evaluations of the manufacturing facility through audits and inspections; (3) negotiating public sector price-ceiling agreements with distributors; (4) providing technical assistance to distributors for their applications for regulatory approval at the national level with an emphasis on designated focus countries; (5) supporting a dossier submission to the WHO's prequalification program; (6) conducting post-marketing surveillance activities in select countries; and (7) providing technical assistance for introduction activities at the country level. The remainder of this chapter describes the progress that has been made in these areas. Figure 14.2 depicts key milestones in the process to introduce a new contraceptive product at the country-level, including the activities that Dahua, FHI 360, distributors and other groups engaged in through the Sino-implant (II) initiative. Two case studies of country-level experiences with product introduction are presented from Sierra Leone and Kenya.

14.4 Quality Evaluation

Because procurement of contraceptive products by donor organizations is generally tied to a product being SRA-approved or being WHO prequalified, lack of these approvals significantly impacts the availability of a product. However, securing these approvals can be a lengthy process. In the absence of these approvals, assuring quality of non-SRA-approved pharmaceutical products manufactured in emerging markets and distributed outside the countries of origin can be challenging.

This challenge can be further exacerbated by incidents that highlight deficiencies in the quality of other products manufactured in the same country of origin. This was the case as Dahua moved forward with registration efforts for Sino-implant (II) in Sub-Saharan Africa in late 2007. Registration activities were initiated on the heels of high profile scandals of other Chinese exports, including pet food containing melamine and toys containing lead-based paint, and continued through the melamine infant milk scandal of 2008 (USFDA 2010; Story 2007; Macartney 2008). Such events deepen consumer mistrust of all products coming from emerging markets, and China specifically, thus placing additional onus on manufacturers, procurement organizations, and health agencies to provide reassurance of product quality.

14.4.1 Quality Testing Program

Dahua's manufacturing facility is assessed through various Good Manufacturing Practice (GMP) inspections and audits.[3] In addition, a key component of FHI 360's work under the Sino-implant (II) initiative has been the development of a quality testing program designed to help resource-poor countries make informed registration and procurement decisions. The Sino-implant (II) initiative established a process that includes independent lot release testing of each shipment distributed to countries supported under the project coupled with more extensive annual quality testing of the active pharmaceutical ingredient (API), the final product, and the packaging.

Product testing activities are conducted using samples of the final implant product provided by Dahua. Samples of levonorgestrel (LNG), the API, are obtained

---

[3] These GMP inspections were conducted by the Chinese SFDA; NQA, an international assessment group based in the UK; national drug regulatory authorities as part of the product registration process; and international NGOs and procurement organizations such as PSI.

Table 14.2 Summary of product evaluation activities: 2008–2011

Test	Number of lots 2008	2009	2010	2011	Results
Quality monitoring activities					
Verification that each lot of Sino-implant (II) meets the requirements specified by the regulatory authority.	10	3	4	9	Met requirements
Annual quality evaluation					
Specifications for levonorgestrel content	3	3	3	3	Met requirements
Evaluation of residuals remaining after the sterilization process	3	3	3	3	Met requirements
Evaluation of levels of metal elements	3	3	3	3	Met requirements
Evaluation of residual levels of solvents utilized during the manufacturing process	3	3	3	3	Met requirements
Tests to identify the presence of possible bacterial components	3	3	3	3	Met requirements
Tests to predict how the body will react to product contact	3	3	3	3	Met requirements
Tests to ensure that the package is sealed appropriately	3	3	3	3	Met requirements
Tests to show that the package can be used in contact with the product	1	1	2	3	Met requirements

Sources: FHI 360. Sino-implant (II) Initiative: Quality Assurance Evaluation. Durham, NC. Final reports (unpublished) for the years 2008–2011.

from both Dahua and directly from the API manufacturer. Test methods used in the lot release testing[4] are approved by the Chinese SFDA, while those used in annual product testing are based on accepted international standards.[5] Table 14.2 summarizes the findings from the quality testing program from 2008 to 2011. The conclusion from the first 4 years of the quality evaluation was that Dahua demonstrated the ability to consistently produce a contraceptive implant that meets international standards.

In addition, assessments of data from Sino-implant (II) lots manufactured between 2004 and 2011 evaluating three test parameters (dissolution, content and tube thickness) showed that Dahua's manufacturing process is stable and well-controlled based on Process Capability Analysis techniques (FHI 360 2009 and 2012). In addition, in 2010, an analysis was conducted of the LNG release rate for Sino-implant (II) explants (i.e. implants removed from users at various time points);

---

[4]Lot release testing refers to the conduct of a series of contingency tests of representative samples from a single manufacturing run of product. Based on the results of these tests, the product is either cleared for distribution or rejected. For additional information on lot release testing, see Table 14.2.

[5]These include the United States Pharmacopoeia, British Pharmacopoeia, International Organization for Standardization, and ASTM (formerly the American Society for Testing and Materials).

results were then compared to publicly available release rate data for Jadelle. Although the analysis was limited due to the timespan for which public data were available for Jadelle, the results indicated that "LNG release rates *in-vivo* are consistent with the hypothesis that Sino-implant (II) and Jadelle are bioequivalent up through 3 years of use" which was the time period that was studied (Jenkins et al. 2010).

Additionally, in partnership with Ministries of Health, distributors and service delivery organizations, FHI 360 initiated several post-marketing activities. Prospective cohort studies funded by United States Agency for International Development (USAID) and the Bill & Melinda Gates Foundation in Madagascar, Kenya, Pakistan and Bangladesh followed Sino-implant (II) users for at least 12 months to assess safety, effectiveness and acceptability. Meanwhile, pharmacovigilance for the Africa region, which involves voluntary reporting from service delivery groups, is coordinated by distributors.

No quality testing program is capable of providing an absolute guarantee of quality. However, in the absence of SRA approval or WHO prequalification, the Sino-implant (II) initiative's independent product testing program was designed to allow key decision-makers in government, regulatory, procurement, and service delivery sectors to make informed decisions regarding the introduction of Sino-implant (II) into their family planning programs.

14.5 Setting Price Ceilings and Seeking National Regulatory Approvals

Another important objective of the Sino-implant (II) initiative was to help ensure that the product remains affordable for programs in developing countries. To that end, FHI 360 has entered into an agreement with Dahua that allows FHI 360 to negotiate public sector price ceilings with Sino-implant (II) distributors in exchange for the provision of technical assistance supporting their product registration applications. Early in the initiative, Pharm Access Africa Ltd. (PAAL), a company founded in 2001 and based in Nairobi with the mission to increase access to health services and products in sub-Saharan Africa, became Dahua's exclusive distributor of Sino-implant (II) in a number of African countries. Marie Stopes International (MSI), a leading international NGO with a long history of delivering family planning services, also signed on as a distributor in several African, Asian and Latin American countries. DKT, an NGO that promotes family planning through social marketing, became the exclusive distributor in Ethiopia. WomanCare Global signed on later as the distributor in Nepal, Russia, and a number of Latin American countries, and Progyne as the distributor in Columbia. These groups were granted freedom to set private sector prices for Sino-implant (II), but agreed to keep public sector prices low in focus countries under the project. Sino-implant (II) is registered under the trade name "Zarin" in countries where PAAL is the distributor, as "Femplant" where MSI is the distributor, as "Trust" in Ethiopia by DKT, and as "Simplant" in countries where WomanCare Global is the distributor.

Once distribution agreements were in place, distributors initiated dossier preparation and submissions with national drug regulatory authorities, with technical assistance from FHI 360. Dossier preparation involved gathering and translating highly technical reports from Chinese into English, French and Spanish; understanding the specific requirements for each country; and determining how existing documentation, some of which was many years old, could be used to meet those requirements. The process illustrated that registration requirements vary across countries, and that even within countries, some guidelines are not entirely clear and require interpretation. Also, there were challenges involved with registering a product that was developed over 20 years ago because many available documents date back from a period when regulatory standards were different from today (Luo 2011).

A number of countries—including Kenya, Madagascar, Malawi, Uganda, Ghana, Nepal, Tanzania, and Ethiopia— have conducted GMP inspections as part of the national registration processes for Sino-implant (II). Despite the involvement of translators, language barriers still presented challenges during some of the inspection visits. In addition, GMP guidelines are open to interpretation such that inspection findings were not always consistent across inspectors. Occasionally, recommendations contradicted one another. For example, one country wanted the Standard Operation Procedures mounted on the wall in the production room. Another country said that posting such documents would collect dust and cause contamination problems (Luo 2011). This experience highlights that interpretation of GMP is subjective; currently there is a global movement towards harmonization of standards.[6]

Despite the challenges, national registrations of Sino-implant (II) have moved forward. By the beginning of 2012, over 20 countries had registered the product in Africa, Asia, and Latin America under the initiative,[7] and the dossier was under review in over ten additional countries.

14.6 World Health Organization Prequalification Programme

A priority of the Sino-implant (II) initiative has been to pursue WHO prequalification, while simultaneously seeking approval at the national level. Because some developing countries lack the capacity to rigorously evaluate and monitor pharmaceutical

---

[6]To this end, the Chinese government is in the process of updating their current GMP guidelines; the latest draft was issued in early 2011. The revised version incorporates key concepts from the ICH GMP guidance as well as EU and US GMP regulations, thus strengthening the international credibility of future Chinese inspections.

[7]By May 2012, Sino-implant (II) had been registered in Burkina Faso, Cambodia, Chile, Ethiopia, Fiji, Ghana, Jamaica, Kenya, Madagascar, Mali, Malawi, Mongolia, Mozambique, Nepal, Nigeria, Pakistan, Sierra Leone, Uganda, Zambia, and Zanzibar, as well as China and Indonesia.

drugs (Milistein et al. 2009; Hall et al. 2007) and because SRA-approval is out of reach for most manufacturers based in developing countries, the WHO Prequalification Programme was established in 2001 to provide an international mechanism to assess the quality, safety and effectiveness of both generic and patented drugs used for the treatment of HIV/AIDS, tuberculosis, and malaria. In 2006, the Prequalification Programme was expanded to cover reproductive health essential medicines (WHO 2010). Although not a regulatory authority, the Prequalification Programme requires manufacturers to meet GMP criteria and uses "internationally harmonized standards for evaluating information on product quality and bio-equivalence, inspecting manufacturing sites, and undertaking quality control of pharmaceutical production" (Gross 2006).

A benefit of WHO prequalification is that countries and donor organizations can be more confident about the quality and effectiveness of the drugs, without having to verify safety independently (Gross 2006). Increasingly, decision-makers—including Ministry of Health officials and procurement groups—desire WHO prequalification before importing certain drugs, including family planning methods, into a country. According to Dr. Bashir Issak, Head of the Division of Reproductive Health in the Kenyan Ministry of Health, "WHO prequalification is a recognized standard. Countries in Sub-Saharan Africa rely on WHO for guidance and reliable technical information. Generally once you have WHO prequalification, you have sufficient backing that a product is safe and acceptable" (Issak 2011).

However, securing WHO prequalification has been challenging for suppliers of contraceptives from the developing world (Hall et al. 2007).[8] By early 2012, 11 contraceptive methods had been WHO prequalified (WHO 2012). However, all of these products except two had already been SRA-approved. In addition, the WHO prequalification process is often lengthy; an assessment showed that for antiretroviral (ARV) drugs submitted to both the USFDA and WHO, WHO prequalification took 2.5 times longer than USFDA approval (Clinton Health Access Initiative 2011).

In 2011, UNFPA and WHO created interim approval processes for manufacturers of hormonal contraceptives, allowing UNFPA to purchase products for country programs while the WHO prequalification review was ongoing. Interim approval would be granted for a limited time period after a successful review of the product dossier and a GMP inspection of the facility, as long as sufficient evidence was available that a manufacturer continued to pursue WHO Prequalification (UNFPA 2011). The process has been used successfully with non-contraceptive drugs; in the case of ARV drugs, the Clinton Health Access Initiative's assessment found that this type of interim approval process "served a useful role in speeding access to new products" (Clinton Health Access Initiative 2011).

---

[8] At the outset of the process, Dahua did not have any English speakers on staff. FHI 360 helped navigate the application process, assisted with development of a Common Technical Document dossier, and engaged consultants to conduct mock GMP audits and advise Dahua on preparations. The Common Technical Document was submitted to WHO and accepted for official review in the fall of 2010.

14.7   Case Studies: Country-Level Introduction in Sierra Leone and Kenya

Because Sino-implant (II) has had a successful track record in China since 1996 and clinical evidence demonstrated its clinical efficacy (Steiner et al. 2010), a strategic decision was made to pursue country-level introduction in parallel to seeking WHO prequalification. Experiences with product introduction in Sierra Leone and Kenya provide insight into some of the successes and challenges encountered at the country level.

14.7.1   Sierra Leone

In Sierra Leone, where a decade-long civil war devastated public health infrastructure and extreme poverty persists, only 8 % of women use a modern method of contraception. Family planning options are generally limited to short-acting methods including condoms, pills and injectables. In 2008, less than 1 % of women used a long-acting method (Statistics Sierra Leone and ICF Macro 2009). In this context, Marie Stopes Sierra Leone (MSSL) partnered with the Ministry of Health starting in 2008 to expand access to contraceptive services throughout the country. A priority of this initiative was to introduce contraceptive implants in Sierra Leone for the first time.

PAAL, the distributor in Sierra Leone, worked with MSSL as a leading service delivery group to develop and submit a dossier for product registration under the trade name Zarin. According to MSSL, after dossier submission, "keeping in constant contact with the Pharmacy Regulation Board to ensure that the implant did not fall off the agenda was fundamental. MSSL's liaison officers kept in touch regularly to monitor the progress of the application" (MSI 2010). As part of the application, a country-specific pharmacovigilance plan was developed and submitted to the Pharmacy Regulation Board which outlined steps for voluntary reporting of any serious adverse events by providers and managers. In late 2008, Zarin was approved as the first contraceptive implant to be made available in Sierra Leone (FHI 2010).

Once approval was secured, MSSL organized trainings with private sector providers and MSSL clinicians. Training was provided on informed decision-making and counseling skills, infection prevention, insertion and removal techniques, and management of side effects. Members of the medical development team travelled to other countries to learn the clinical skills for implant service delivery, and expert trainers were brought to Sierra Leone from neighboring countries to conduct trainings (Brett 2011).

Zarin was first introduced through MSSL's social franchise network of private providers, Blue Star, and then more broadly within MSSL clinics. In private clinics, the implants were initially offered for free to increase demand, and then the price was subsidized. According to Tracey Brett, Associate Director of Procurement and Logistics of MSI, cost was an important factor. "With Zarin, we could afford the subsidy. With Jadelle, we could not have afforded it" (Brett 2011). Demand creation activities at the community level included distribution of educational materials, radio advertising, and public health talks (MSI 2010). A national product launch meeting was sponsored by the Ministry of Health, MSSL and PAAL, with technical assistance from FHI 360. Stakeholders were informed about the benefits of implants, the potential cost-savings that could be realized from investing in Zarin, and the results of the quality testing program.

Initial procurement of Zarin was led by MSI. In 2009, in response to a request from the Ministry of Health, UNFPA purchased 5,000 units of Zarin for use in Sierra Leone. By the middle of 2011, over 51,000 units of Zarin had been procured and shipped to Sierra Leone, primarily purchased by MSI.

When reflecting on the initial successes of Zarin introduction in Sierra Leone, MSSL representatives concluded that "establishing a broad advocacy coalition with government, development partners, civil society, and the private sector was key to the rapid registration and roll-out of Zarin. At every step…a range of partners were involved." (MSI 2010). According to Ms. Brett, "we've really seen the benefits of Zarin in Sierra Leone. For women who don't want an IUD and need to travel very far, we've been able to bring a new method and offer women more choice. However, the next hurdle is to encourage the Ministry of Health to purchase Zarin for the public sector." Ms. Brett acknowledges that the up-front expense of procuring Zarin can be prohibitive. As Fig. 14.1 illustrates, "Compared to the IUD, Zarin is still expensive" (Brett 2011).

14.7.2 Kenya

In 2009, Kenya was the first country outside of Asia to register Sino-implant (II) under the trade name Zarin. Kenya's experience with Zarin reflects similar successes with product introduction in Sierra Leone through MSI clinics. However, significant challenges with public sector procurement have limited large scale access to the product.

Contraceptive use among married women in Kenya rose considerably from 7 % in the late 1970s to 46 % by 2008–2009, after stalling in the late 1990s. However, only 8.3 % of married women had chosen sterilization, implants or IUDs by 2008–09 (Kenya National Bureau of Statistics and ICF Macro 2010), despite the government's efforts to promote longer-acting methods (Engenderhealth 2009). Norplant was first introduced through the national family planning program in 1992. A decade later, nurses and clinical officers were given authority to insert and remove implants and approximately 95,000 Kenyan women were using the method. In 2004, Kenya made the transition to the second generation implants, Jadelle and Implanon (Hubacher et al. 2007). Only 1.9 % of married women used implants in 2008–09, although among non-users who intended to use family planning in the future, 8 % said that their preferred method would be implants (Kenya National Bureau of Statistics and ICF Macro 2010) and key informants indicated somewhat higher demand for implants (Hubacher et al. 2007).

However, service delivery constraints in Kenya impact the availability of implants. In 2006, approximately 1,000 providers in over 1,200 health facilities were trained on insertion and removal of implants (Hubacher et al. 2007), but with over 6,000 health facilities in Kenya, there still are not sufficient numbers of trained providers, particularly in rural and poorer areas. To increase access and uptake, the Ministry of Health wants to expand training to all cadres of health care providers (Issak 2011).

The cost of implants has been another barrier to wide scale availability and commodity stock-outs have also impeded access. In 2004, only a third of facilities that had the service delivery capacity to provide implants had stocks of Jadelle or Implanon available (Hubacher et al. 2007). According to Dr. Issak of the Kenya Ministry of Health, high commodity costs contribute to these stock-outs; while demand drives forecasts for procurement needs, actual procurement must be based on funds available (Issak 2011). A recent study revealed that clients in both public and private service delivery settings reported a willingness to pay out-of-pocket fees for implants that would cover 100 % of the direct costs of providing Zarin. In addition, private sector clients currently pay a price for implant insertion that is greater than the direct cost of Zarin delivery. Thus, wide scale introduction of Zarin provides an opportunity to reduce reliance on donor money and, in turn, to improve commodity security (Tumlinson et al. 2011).

By the end of 2010, MSI had procured over 16,000 units of Zarin and introduced them into Marie Stopes Kenya clinics. To monitor and identify any possible problems with Zarin, two activities were initiated. PAAL established a passive pharmacovigilance plan whereby providers of Zarin were asked to file reports on adverse medical events. Second, an existing phone hotline for contraceptive users added Zarin so that clients can report problems or ask questions; Zarin clients receive a card with the hotline telephone number. During the first 2 years, no service delivery problems or serious adverse events were reported by these mechanisms. Additionally, FHI 360 initiated a post-marketing study in public sector clinics to provide stakeholders with evidence of acceptability, safety and effectiveness in MOH clinics.[9]

Despite the initial introduction of Zarin in the NGO sector in Kenya, large-scale procurement for the public sector has not yet occurred. PAAL's outreach efforts with the MOH have included advocacy for public sector introduction of Zarin. However, the Kenya Medical Supplies Agency, which oversees logistics of medical supplies nationally, has chosen not to procure Sino-implant (II) to date for the public sector, despite the potential cost advantage, indicating that WHO prequalification is a critical milestone to achieve.

---

[9]The study followed 600 women over a period of 12 months. Results are expected by the end of 2013.

14.8 Discussion

With WHO prequalification pending, the Sino-implant (II) initiative has implemented an independent quality testing program for Sino-implant (II) while simultaneously pursuing regulatory approval at the national level. However, as the country case studies illustrate, without WHO prequalification or SRA approval, expanding public sector procurement will continue to be challenging in some countries.

In particular, because of persistent mistrust of Chinese products, internationally recognized quality assurance mechanisms will remain important in coming years. Sino-implant (II) is not unique in this respect. With over 80 % of APIs in products sold in the US produced in other countries—mostly in China or India—issues of quality assurance loom large for both the regulatory and public health communities. A report released by the USFDA, entitled "Pathway to Global Product Safety and Quality," acknowledges the enormity of the task of monitoring quality of pharmaceutical products coming out of developing countries (Harris 2011).

In addition, other factors present potential challenges to the success of the Sino-implant (II) initiative, several of which were recently highlighted in an FHI 360 evaluation of the project (Adamchak 2010):

1. Some stakeholders have incorrectly assumed that Sino-implant (II) is an FHI 360 product. One goal of the Sino-implant (II) initiative is to provide information to relevant stakeholders about who the distributors are and to clarify the roles and responsibilities of various organizations involved in the project.
2. It is unlikely that Sino-implant (II) would have gained traction globally without technical assistance from the organizations involved in the initiative. For example, Dahua would likely not have had the capacity to apply for WHO prequalification or to work with distributors to prepare dossiers for national registration in Sub-Saharan Africa without substantial support. Despite the importance of FHI 360's role as coordinator in the initiative, a fundamental objective of the project is sustainability. To that end, a priority of the project is the phase out of FHI 360's role over time and the assumption of full responsibility by the manufacturer, logistics export agent, distributors and service delivery groups for Sino-implant (II) distribution, delivery, and pharmacovigilance.
3. The value proposition of Sino-implant (II) as a low-cost alternative is not entirely guaranteed in the future. It is uncertain whether price ceiling agreements with distributors will continue once they expire. In addition, if capital investments in the manufacturing process are required for expansion, Dahau may need to increase the price to offset higher production costs. Also, data from the RHInterchange shows that the prices of Jadelle and Implanon dropped by 13 and 37 % respectively between 2005 and 2009 (Tumlinson et al. 2011). Additional price reductions of these other implants may make the cost advantage of Sino-implant (II) less significant (see postscript).

Despite these issues, significant successes have already been achieved. By early 2012, over 700,000 units of Sino-implant (II) had been procured in countries under

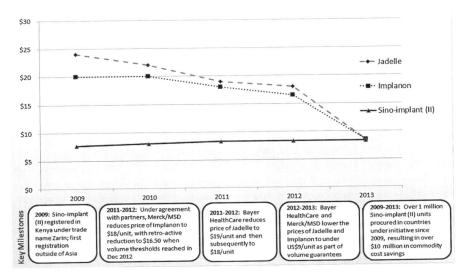

Fig. 14.3 Changes in contraceptive implant prices since global introduction of Sino-implant (II) and key milestones, 2009–2013. Sources: 2009–2010 prices based on weighted averages from RH Interchange in Kenya, Ethiopia and Sierra Leone. 2011–2013 prices for Jadelle and Implanon based on information from the Reproductive Health Supplies Coalition and from press releases issued by international donors and the manufacturers (BMGF 2013; Bayer HealthCare 2012; RHSC 2012b).

the initiative.[10] This represents a total savings of almost US $8.4 million in commodity costs.[11] In addition, according to the MSI Impact calculator, these units of Sino-implant (II) translate into over 2.4 million couple-years of protection from pregnancy, and can lead to the prevention of over 660,000 unintended pregnancies, 2,600 maternal deaths, and 126,000 abortions (MSI 2012).

The introduction of Sino-implant (II) may have begun to put market pressure on other implant manufacturers to continue to lower their prices. As of mid-2012, both Bayer HealthCare and Merck/MSD had each announced price reductions of Jadelle and Implanon respectively to $18 per unit for both products. Merck/MSD has also promised an additional retro-active price drop if procurement volumes reach certain thresholds (RHSC 2011, 2012a) (see postscript and Fig. 14.3). If this trend continues or if Sino-implant (II) gains substantial market share in developing countries, the underlying public health objective will be achieved as access to more affordable contraceptive implants grows.

[10]FHI 360 does not procure or donate commodities under the initiative. Rather, donors, NGOs and Ministries of Health buy units of Sino-implant (II) for country-level programs.

[11]Savings are calculated based on a price of $8 for Sino-implant assuming the alternative is to purchase Jadelle (average unit price for Jadelle was $24 in 2009, $22 in 2010, $19 in 2011 and US$18 in 2012). Prices were calculated using information from the Reproductive Health Supplies Coalition and the RHInterchange: http://rhi.rhsupplies.org/.

14.9 Conclusion

Increasingly, lower cost pharmaceutical products produced in the developing world help meet an urgent need for lifesaving and preventative drugs among underserved populations. Currently, over 200 million women in developing countries want to delay or limit births but are not using contraception (Barot 2008). As a highly effective, long-acting and popular method, implants have the potential to help address this unmet need for family planning and improve contraceptive security, particularly in contexts where short-acting methods that require frequent resupply put pressure on healthcare systems. Yet, the potential impact of implants has been limited due to their high cost. A low-cost implant could help address chronic problems with affordability and accessibility—both through its position in the global market as a less expensive alternative product and by putting pressure on competing manufacturers to lower their prices.

However, the Sino-implant (II) initiative has demonstrated that the road to international acceptance of a Chinese-made contraceptive can be difficult. Obtaining WHO prequalification is essential for wide scale uptake, yet the process is lengthy and costly. While the review of Sino-implant (II) has been underway at WHO, pursuing national registration of the product has been an efficient way to facilitate initial introduction in developing countries. In addition, an independent quality testing program and coordinated efforts among the manufacturer, distributors, and NGOs to set price ceilings and push for procurement has allowed global introduction of the product to move forward.

14.10 Postscript

At the time this publication was going to press, Bayer HealthCare announced a reduction in the price of Jadelle to $8.50 per unit in low-income countries (effective January 2013). A coalition of partners including the Bill & Melinda Gates Foundation, the Clinton Health Access Initiative, the governments of Norway, the United States, the United Kingdom, and Sweden, as well as other groups, negotiated this price based on a volume guarantee to Bayer Healthcare for 27 million units of Jadelle over 6 years (BMGF 2013; USAID 2012; Bayer Healthcare 2012). In addition, after reducing the price of Implanon to $16.50[12], Merck/MSD announced another 50 % price reduction in May 2013 as part of an agreement with the same coalition of partners (MSD 2013). These reductions mean that both Jadelle and Implanon are now available at a price comparable to that of Sino-implant (II).

Under the negotiated agreements, the donors providing the volume guarantees, rather than the manufacturers, will assume the financial risk in the event that the

---

[12] At the end of 2012, the volume thresholds were reached for Implanon sales which triggered an additional retro-active price reduction to $16.50, according to the Reproductive Health Supplies Coalition (RHSC 2012b).

volume targets are not met. Other similar third-party financing negotiations have resulted in reduced prices of critical public health commodities including ARV drugs used to treat HIV infection. It has been well documented that the introduction of generic alternatives also contributed to the lowering of prices of ARVs (Ford et al. 2011; Waning et al. 2009; Wirtz et al. 2009). The increasing availability of Sino-implant (II) may have played a role in helping to lower the price of Jadelle and Implanon. Additional analysis in this area in the future is warranted.

The true demand for contraceptive implants has been difficult to determine in developing countries because supply has been limited and stock-outs common (Hubacher et al. 2007). According to the RH Interchange, a combined two million units of all three implants—Implanon, Jadelle and Sino-implant (II)—were procured in 2011, and 4 million were procured in 2012 (RHInterchange 2013). Even with the dramatic increase in procurement of implants over recent years, questions remain regarding whether and at what pace national markets will be able to absorb the increased influx of Jadelle and Implanon supplies, as well as whether Dahua can maintain its current market share given the changing landscape.

A report from the UN Commission on Life-Saving Commodities for Women and Children which was released at the same time that the Jadelle price drop was announced, identifies implants as one of thirteen priority health commodities. The Commission recognizes that to strengthen quality and ensure accessibility for these products, it is essential that "at least three manufacturers per commodity are manufacturing and marketing quality-certified and affordable products" (United Nations Commission 2012). In order to sustain reduced prices of contraceptive implants, it will be important for multiple implant manufacturers to stay in the market so that competition remains. Having diversity in the market will also help guarantee that there is sufficient supply to meet the potentially growing demand, and to provide choice to countries, procurement groups, and women.

Dahua is not eligible to enter into a volume guarantee similar to the one established with Bayer Healthcare and Merck/MSD until Sino-implant (II) is prequalified by WHO. Therefore, achieving this key regulatory milestone continues to remain a priority. Because the WHO prequalification process is lengthy and can be difficult for manufacturers in developing countries to navigate, it will be important that Dahua continues to receive technical assistance, as needed, in this area from international groups.

If introduction and scale-up of implants continues to increase rapidly and substantially, it will be essential that Ministries of Health, donors and service delivery groups ensure that adequate, affordable implant services are available to women, particularly reliable access to removals. Implant programs will be threatened if women cannot reliably have their implants removed (or if there is a public perception that these services are not available) (Hubacher and Dorflinger 2012; Frost and Reich 2008).

The overall goal of the Sino-implant (II) initiative has been to increase access to high quality, affordable contraceptive implants for women in low-resource settings. Substantial successes have been achieved towards this goal with the increasing availability of lower-cost implants and the growing procurement of implants worldwide.

Acknowledgments The authors appreciate the contribution of John Bratt and Katherine Tumlinson to the analysis of direct service delivery costs for contraceptive methods. The authors also want to thank Timothy Mastro, Charles Morrison, Diane Luo, David Asante and David Hubacher for their review of the chapter.

References

Adamchak, S. (2010). Sino-implant (II): Year 2 monitoring, learning and evaluation experience. *FHI*. Unpublished report.

Adams, K., & Beal, M. W. (2009). Implanon: A review of the literature with recommendations for clinical management. *Journal of Midwifery & Women's Health, 54*(2), 142–149.

Barot, S. (2008). Back to basics: The rationale for increased funds for international family planning. *Guttmacher Policy Review, 11*, 3.

Bayer HealthCare. (2012, September 26). Bayer joins global initiative for better access to safe and effective contraception. Press release. http://press.healthcare.bayer.com/en/press/news-details-page.php/14732/2012-0429. Accessed Sept 2012.

Bertrand, J. T., Rice, J., Sullivan, T. M., & Shelton, J. (2000). *Skewed method mix: A measure of quality in family planning programs*. Chapel Hill: MEASURE Evaluation.

The Bill & Melinda Gates Foundation. (BMGF). (2013). *Innovative partnership reduces cost of Bayer's long-acting reversible contraceptive implant by more than 50 percent*. Press release. February 27, 2013. http://www.gatesfoundation.org/Media-Center/Press-Releases/2013/02/Partnership-Reduces-Cost-Of-Bayers-Reversible-Contraceptive-Implant. Accessed May 2013.

Brett, T. (2011, May 24). Associate Director of Procurement, MSI. Interview.

Clinton Health Access Initiative. (2011). *Regulatory approvals for ARVs: An analysis of review timelines under the US FDA, WHO PQ, and ERP* (Internal report). Received via personal correspondence.

Coukell, A. J., & Balfour, J. A. (1998). Levonorgestrel subdermal implants: A review of contraceptive efficacy and acceptability. *Drugs, 55*(6), 861–887.

d'Arcangues, C. (2007). Worldwide use of intrauterine devices for contraception. *Contraception, 75*, S2–S7.

Engenderhealth. (2009). Respond project. Meeting national goals and people's needs with LA/PMs: Kenya country assessment. http://www.respond-project.org/pages/index.php

FHI. (2010). Zarin launch in Sierra Leone. Fact sheet. Unpublished.

FHI 360 (2009 and 2012). Process capability analysis reports. Unpublished.

Ford, N., Calmy, A., & Mills, E. J. (2011). The first decade of antiretroviral therapy in Africa. *Globalization and Health, 7*, 33.

Frost, L. J., & Reich, M. R. (2008). *Access: How do good health technologies get to poor people in poor countries?* Cambridge: Harvard University Press.

Gross, O. (2006). WHO program for prequalification of antiretroviral, antimalarial and antituberculosis drugs. *Médecine Tropicale, 66*(6), 549–551.

Hall, P., Oehlera, J., Woo, P., et al. (2007). A study of the capability of manufacturers of generic hormonal contraceptives in lower- and middle-income countries. *Contraception, 75*, 311–317.

Harris, G. (2011, June 20). FDA confronts challenge of monitoring imports. Agency head outlines difficulties and risks of food and drug imports. *The New York Times*, B3. http://www.nytimes.com/2011/06/21/health/policy/21food.html

Hohmann, H., & Creinin, M. D. (2007). The contraceptive implant. *Clinical Obstetrics and Gynecology, 50*(4), 907–917.

Hubacher, D., & Dorflinger, L. (2012). Avoiding controversy in international provision of subdermal contraceptive implants. *Contraception, 85*(5), 432–433.

Hubacher, D., Kimani, J., Steiner, M., et al. (2007). Contraceptive implants in Kenya: Current status and future prospects. *Contraception, 75*(6), 468–473.

Issak, B. (2011, May 18). Head of the Division of Reproductive Health, Kenya Ministry of Health. Interview.

Jenkins, D., Taylor, D., Owen, D., & Steiner, M. (2010). *Evaluation of Sino-implant (II) explants* (Final report). Family Health International. Durham, NC, USA

Kenya National Bureau of Statistics (KNBS) and ICF Macro. (2010). *Kenya demographic and health survey 2008–09*. Calverton: KNBS & ICF Macro.

Luo, D. (2011, May 24). Independent regulatory consultant. Interview.

Macartney, J. (2008, September 22). China baby milk scandal spreads as sick toll rises to 13,000. *Times Online*. http://www.timesonline.co.uk/tol/news/world/asia/article4800458.ece

Mansour, D., Inki, P., & Gemzell-Danielsson, K. (2010). Efficacy of contraceptive methods: A review of the literature. *The European Journal of Contraception & Reproductive Health Care, 15*(1), 4–16.

Marie Stopes International. (2012). Impact calculator. www.mariestopes.org

Marie Stopes International (MSI), FHI, Pharm Access Africa, Ltd. (2010). *Introducing the contraceptive Sino-implant (II) (Zarin) in Sierra Leone* (Final report). Available at: http://www.k4health.org/toolkits/implants/country_experiences/sierraleone

Mavranezouli, I. (2009). Health economics of contraception. *Best Practice & Research. Clinical Obstetrics & Gynaecology, 23*(2), 187–198.

Milistein, J., Costa, A., Jadhav, S., & Dhere, R. (2009). Reaching international GMP standards for vaccine production: Challenges for developing countries. *Expert Review of Vaccines, 8*(5), 559–566.

MSD. (2013). *MSD and partners announce agreement to increase access to innovative contraceptive implants Implanon® and Implanon Nxt® in the poorest countries*. Press release. May 2013. http://www.rhsupplies.org/fileadmin/user_upload/Announcements/MERCK_EXTERNAL_STATEMENT_FINAL_May_2013__4_.pdf. Accessed May 2013.

Neukom, J., Chilambwe, J., Mkandawire, J., et al. (2011). Dedicated providers of long-acting reversible contraception: New approach in Zambia. *Contraception, 83*(5), 447–452.

Power, J., French, R., & Cowan, F. (2007). Subdermal implantable contraceptives versus other forms of reversible contraceptives or other implants as effective methods of preventing pregnancy (review). *Cochrane Database of Systematic Reviews, 3*(3), 1–31.

Ramchandran, D., & Upadhyay, U. D. (2007). Implants: The next generation. *Popul Rep Ser K Injectables Implants, 7*, 1–19.

Reproductive Health Supplies Coalition (RHSC). (2011, June 24). Private and public sectors announce commitments to increase access to contraceptives. Press release. http://www.rhsupplies.org/. Accessed 13 July 2011.

Reproductive Health Supplies Coalition (RHSC) (2012a, February). *Supply Insider*. http://www.rhsupplies.org/. Accessed 7 May 2012.

Reproductive Health Supplies Coalition (RHSC) (2012b, November 19). Coalition-supported initiative triggers more than $15 million in savings. Press release. http://www.rhsupplies.org/. Accessed 20 Nov 2012.

RHInterchange. http://rhi.rhsupplies.org/rhi/index.do?locale=en_US. Accessed May 2011 and May 2013.

Sivin, I., Nash, H., & Waldman, S. (2002). *Jadelle levonorgestrel rod implants: A summary of scientific data and lessons learned from programmatic experience*. New York: The Population Council.

Statistics Sierra Leone, & ICF Macro. (2009). *Sierra Leone demographic and health survey 2008*. Calverton: Statistics Sierra Leone (SSL) and ICF Macro. Available at: http://www.measuredhs.com/pubs/pdf/FR225/FR225.pdf

Steiner, M. J., Lopez, L. M., Grimes, D. A., et al. (2010). Sino-implant (II) – A levonorgestrel-releasing two-rod implant: Systematic review of the randomized controlled trials. *Contraception, 81*, 197–201.

Story, L. (2007, August 2). Lead paint prompts mattel to recall 967,000 toys. *The New York Times*. http://www.nytimes.com/2007/08/02/business/02toy.html

Sullivan, T. M., Bertrand, J. T., Rice, J., & Shelton, J. D. (2006). Skewed contraceptive mix: Why it happens, why it matters. *Journal of BiosocialScience, 38*, 501–521.

Sutherland, E. G., Alaii, J., Tsui, S., et al. (2011). Contraceptive needs of female sex workers in Kenya – A cross-sectional study. *The European Journal of Contraception & Reproductive Health Care, 16*(3), 173–182.

Tumlinson, K., Steiner, M., Rademacher, K., et al. (2011). The promise of affordable implants: Is cost recovery possible in Kenya? *Contraception, 83*, 88–93.

U.S. Agency for International Development (2012, September 26). New partnership expands access to contraception for 27 million women and girls in low-income countries. Press release. http://www.usaid.gov/news-information/press-releases/new-partnership-expands-access-contraception-27-million-women-and. Accessed Sept 2012.

United Nations Commission on Life-Saving Commodities for Women and Children (2012, September). Commissioners' report. http://www.everywomaneverychild.org/images/UN_Commission_Report_September_2012_Final.pdf. Accessed Oct 2012.

United Nations, Department of Economic and Social Affairs, Population Division. (2011). *World contraceptive use 2010*. New York: United Nations. http://www.un.org/esa/population/publications/wcu2010/Main.html.

United Nations Population Fund (UNFPA) (2011, April). First invitation to manufacturers of reproductive health medicines to submit an Expression of Interest (EOI) for product evaluation and UNFPA Technical assessment by the Expert Review Panel (ERP) or the Internal Technical Committee. Received through personal correspondence, May 2011.

US FDA. (2007). Melamine pet food recall of 2007. http://www.fda.gov/animalveterinary/safetyhealth/recallswithdrawals/ucm129575.htm

Waning, B., Kaplan, W., King, A. C., et al. (2009). Global strategies to reduce the price of antiretroviral medicines: Evidence from transactional databases. *Bulletin of the World Health Organization, 87*(7), 520–528.

Wirtz, V. J., Forsythe, S., Valencia-Mendoza, A., et al. (2009). Factors influencing global antiretroviral procurement prices. *BMC Public Health, 9*(Suppl 1), S6.

World Health Organization. (2010, August). WHO prequalification. http://www.who.int/mediacentre/factsheets/fs278/en/index.html. Accessed Dec 2010.

World Health Organization. (2012). Prequalification programme. http://apps.who.int/prequal/. Accessed Nov 2012.

Zhou, C. (2011, June 27) Sales Manager, Shanghai Dahua Pharmaceuticals Co., Ltd. Personal correspondence.

Chapter 15
An Integrated Approach to Targeted, Evidence-Based Livelihood and Sexual and Reproductive Health Programs for Vulnerable Young People in Fragile States: The Case of Liberia

Adam Weiner and Andrzej Kulczycki

15.1 Introduction

Liberia has one of Africa's smallest, poorest, and most rapidly growing populations. The 2008 census showed a population growing at a rate of 2.6 % per annum and numbering 3.48 million people (LISGIS 2009), 84 % of whom lived on less than $1.25 per day (World Bank 2010).[1] Young people between the ages of 10 and 24 make up one-third of the total population (LISGIS 2009). They not only face the same issues of identity, relationships and transition to adulthood common to young people everywhere, but today Liberian youth also confront tremendous adversity as a result of the country's 14-year civil conflict (1989–2003) that wreaked havoc on the economy and infrastructure (Ellis 2006).[2] Youth in Liberia have a huge influence

---

[1]Population estimates, total fertility rates and other key demographic data vary by source, underscoring how difficult it is for the staff of agencies working on the projects discussed to obtain sufficient, reliable evidence to support their efforts. For the purposes of this chapter, the 2008 Liberia Population and Housing Census is used whenever possible and UN population estimates are used as a backup where key data are not readily available. The 2007 Demographic and Health Survey (DHS) is the most reliable source for much of the education and reproductive health data presented here.

[2]The civil conflict almost completely stopped all mining activities and severely disrupted rice production, financial services, electricity and water production (Republic of Liberia 2008).

A. Weiner, M.A. (✉)
Adam M Weiner Consulting, San Francisco, CA, USA
e-mail: adam.weiner813@gmail.com

A. Kulczycki, Ph.D.
Associate Professor, Department of Health Care Organization and Policy,
University of Alabama at Birmingham (UAB), Birmingham, AL, USA
e-mail: andrzej@uab.edu

A. Kulczycki (ed.), *Critical Issues in Reproductive Health*, The Springer Series on Demographic Methods and Population Analysis 33, DOI 10.1007/978-94-007-6722-5_15, © Springer Science+Business Media Dordrecht 2014

on which path the country takes due to their large numbers and the role they play in society as future leaders. Liberia's ongoing security and development challenges cannot be addressed without current stabilization policies being better synchronized with developing productive sectors that could be used to secure sustainable livelihoods (Solà-Martín 2011). For the country's development and growth, therefore, it is vital both to protect young people's health and social well-being, as well as to implement interventions that channel them into meaningful and productive employment.

Working in a post-conflict setting presents many challenges specific to the extreme circumstances and traumas a large proportion of society has experienced and is still struggling to overcome. This chapter discusses a project that has attempted to ensure a significant proportion of resources flowing into Liberia address the needs of the most vulnerable young people, adolescent girls in particular. These marginalized groups are critical to development efforts, but despite numerous activities to improve young people's sexual and reproductive health (SRH) and livelihoods,[3] at the time this project commenced, there was no concerted effort to focus such attention in a unified manner (involving non-governmental organizations (NGOs), United Nations (UN) agencies, government ministries, research institutions, and donors) on those being left behind.

A key component of this project has involved the expanded use of data regarding adolescents and young adults to inform decision-making processes at all levels. Quality data are often not disaggregated effectively in order to highlight young people's daily experiences in ways relevant to program officials and policy-makers, the end-users of the data. This is particularly true in post-conflict settings such as Liberia where data files, reports and equipment were destroyed and old sampling frames were rendered invalid by major population displacements.[4] A collaboration between the Population Council and the United Nations Population Fund (UNFPA) has led to the production of numerous analytical reports on the situation of the most vulnerable young people in many resource-poor countries that held a Demographic and Health Survey (DHS) since 2000. These reports highlight the diversity of their youth populations, identify their conditions of vulnerability, and clarify the SRH context of adolescent females.[5] This effort included Liberia and was part of a

---

[3]Livelihood refers to the economic, social, and cultural means of securing the necessities of life. 'Livelihoods' is broadly defined as the skills needed to become economically or financially productive as an important means to increased autonomy and empowerment. A livelihoods approach to programming is one where service providers work to develop these specific skills.

[4]The civil conflict also destroyed earlier census records, survey results, and much of Liberia's statistical infrastructure. This makes it impossible to reconstruct many aspects of the country's demographic and socio-economic situation, including empirical evidence on the large-scale population losses and displacements that occurred during the civil conflict.

[5]*The Adolescent Experience In-depth* series set out to be accessible to a range of audiences, particularly decision-makers from governments, NGOs, and advocacy groups. A complete list of reports is available at: http://www.popcouncil.org/publications/serialsbriefs/AdolExpInDepth.asp.

macro-level set of actions to support in-country efforts to establish holistic, evidence-based programs for vulnerable and marginalized youth.

The Liberian civil conflict had also severely disrupted family and community support systems that care for and guide adolescents through their difficult transitions. The reconstruction and expansion of the health and educational infrastructure is a slow process, one that requires a parallel set of interventions to develop the human and social capital of young people in a way that is sensitive to their life-cycle specific challenges within the Liberian context. This requires an ever-increasing need for accurate, relevant information.

This chapter describes and explains the evolution of an integrated approach to establish targeted, evidence-based livelihoods and SRH programs for vulnerable young people. It presents a detailed, empirically informed framework and its application to marginalized Liberian youth. Beyond Liberian youth, this framework can be more broadly applied and utilized by practitioners, health and social service agencies, donors, researchers, and policymakers in other resource-poor or post-conflict settings. While each of the steps comprising the approach described here is not unique, their integration into a cohesive process sets it apart from other needs assessment activities or situation analyses conducted elsewhere. This process involves data collection and analysis, policy review, capacity building, mentoring, and information sharing to inform the design of more effective, holistic programs for vulnerable young people. Before discussing this process in greater detail, it is first necessary to review the socio-economic and reproductive health situation of Liberia.

15.2   Liberia in the Post-Civil War Period

The ruinous civil conflict killed over 250,000 people and displaced almost half the population. It shattered the job market as well as the education and health sectors, which had earlier suffered from years of neglect. Research conducted for the 2008–2011 Poverty Reduction Strategy (PRS) showed that almost five years after the end of the conflict, approximately 70 % of school buildings were still partially or entirely destroyed (Republic of Liberia 2008). Widespread corruption and a dearth of trained professionals continue to hinder recovery efforts.

The initial influx of humanitarian and development aid brought with it hope for change. A great deal is riding upon the education of the country's youth so they can be adequately prepared to participate in the labor force. However, despite the introduction of compulsory free primary education in government schools, in 2007 only 40 % of primary school-aged children were enrolled in school while the gross attendance ratio was 83 % (LISGIS et al. 2008), meaning that a large number of primary school students were not in the official primary school age group. Many older youth had entered school for the first time after the end of the conflict, increasing pressure on an educational system still in the nascent stages of recon-struction. The vast majority of students are facing challenges that threaten their advancement through primary into secondary education as school leaving disproportionately affects the poor and vulnerable, such as adolescent girls and ethnic minorities. The proportion of adults aged 15–49 who had never attended school was more than twice as high among women than men (42 % vs. 18 %); and the median years of education stood at only 1.6 years for women compared to 5.8 for men and as low as 0 for rural women (LISGIS et al. 2008). Additionally, adult literacy is far lower for women (41 %) than for men (70 %), though there are major geographic and socio-economic variations.

There is a growing literature on the linkages between economic well-being, educational attainment, and reproductive health outcomes in low- and middle-income countries (e.g., Esiet and Whitaker 2002; Lloyd 2006; Population Council 2009a). A healthy transition from school to work and from youth to adulthood depends upon the acquisition of the social and human capital necessary to make decisions that minimize negative outcomes (Knowles and Behrman 2005; Lloyd 2005). Conversely, an unhealthy transition threatens the overall well-being of the individual through exposure to violence, exploitation, or sexually transmitted infections (STIs) including HIV/AIDS, and increases the risk of early marriage and childbearing, particularly for females.

15.3 The Reproductive Health Situation in Liberia

The limited available data indicate a bleak overall reproductive health outlook for Liberia. As in several other West African countries, sexual activity, marriage, and childbearing start early on average and young people of both sexes are typically poorly informed about how to protect themselves from unwanted pregnancies and STIs, including HIV/AIDS. Young females are more vulnerable to many SRH threats due to cultural and gender norms that limit their autonomy. Child marriage occurs when one or both of the spouses are under the age of age 18, suggesting the union may not have been completely consensual. It may be equally or more significant, however, to focus on those marriages occurring before the age of 15 due to the extreme nature and even more potentially devastating consequences of such events.[6]

---

[6]Child marriage has come to be viewed by the international community as unfair and dangerous to children as well as a fundamental violation of human rights. International conventions (notably the Convention on the Rights of the Child adopted by the UN General Assembly in 1989) establish the legal age of consent to marriage as 18 years, but the legal age of marriage may vary across countries because governments can determine at which age a child has reached majority and can therefore be allowed to marry. The definition of child marriage includes boys, but most children who are married are girls, typically to fully-grown men. The effects of child marriage include health problems related to premature pregnancy with increased risks of maternal and infant mortality, stillbirth, and obstetric fistulae. Social consequences may include the denial of further education, constrained decision-making, social isolation, reduced life choices, abuse, and violence. In countries where child marriage remains common, many governments have tended to overlook, or discount, problems that it causes.

Table 15.1 Key reproductive health data, according to sex, Liberia, 2007

Sex and age	Marriage		Sexual initiation	Ever used modern method of contraception		HIV prevalence
	Percent married by age 15	Percent never married	Percent who had sex by age 15	All sexually active (married and unmarried)	Sexually active and unmarried	Percent HIV positive
Females						
15–19	5.8	79.7	18.7	21.9	35.5	1.3
20–24	10.8	38.5	15.8	35.9	56.6	2.0
15–49	14.2[a]	26.1	19.3[a]	32.7	48.3	1.9
Males						
15–19	0.0	96.8	8.6	17.0	39.9	0.4
20–24	0.2	69.6	8.3	55.2	66.3	0.7
15–49	0.3[a]	37.8	6.1[a]	43.0	59.0	1.2

Source: Liberia demographic and health survey 2007 (LISGIS et al. 2008)
[a]Age group is 20–49

Child marriage is still widespread in Liberia as in West Africa.[7] Data from the 2007 Liberia DHS show that among females aged 20–24, over 10 % were married by age 15 and almost 38 % by age 18 (LISGIS et al. 2008). Such early marriage for girls is invariably associated with the cessation of schooling and early onset of childbearing (Esiet and Whitaker 2002), often without any connection to programs that keep them connected to a social support network. Child marriage is almost a non-issue for young males. Table 15.1 shows major differences by sex in this and other key SRH indicators for young people and for the whole childbearing period. Among those aged 15–19, for example, the percentage of females who had initiated sexual relations by age 15 is more than double that for males (18.7 % vs. 8.6 %).

Childbearing begins early in Liberia. The 2007 DHS showed that over one-quarter of females aged 15–19 had already had a child and despite a recent decline, the total fertility rate (TFR) still stood at 5.2 children per woman, with major differentials by region, urban–rural residence, educational attainment, and wealth status. For both married and unmarried people in every age group except those aged 15–19, higher proportions of sexually active males than females reported having ever used a modern method of contraception. This may indicate that females have less bargaining

---

[7]Child marriage has decreased globally but its practice remains prevalent in certain countries, especially in impoverished rural areas, where it is deeply grounded in cultural, social, and economic structures. Child marriage is still widespread in many African and South Asian countries. At the turn of the millennium, over 50 % of females aged 20–24 were married by age 18 in Niger, Chad, Mali, Guinea, Burkina Faso, Central African Republic, Mozambique, Uganda, Cameroon, as well as Bangladesh and Nepal (UNICEF 2005). In West Africa, the practice is also common but the percentage of 20–49 year old women married by age 15 varied greatly across the region: Benin (9.7), Burkina Faso (6.7), Ghana (6.8), Guinea (23.5), Liberia (14.2), Mali (23.6), Mauritania (29.3), Niger (37.4), Nigeria (21.9), Sierra Leone (22.2) (Macro International Inc 2011).

power than males with respect to contraceptive use, although more in-depth research would be required to determine the cause of these differences.

Table 15.1 also shows a high female-to-male ratio of HIV prevalence among youth, a disturbing feature that is common in much of sub-Saharan Africa.[8] The 15–19 year old population in Liberia is characterized by a 3.3 female-to-male ratio of HIV prevalence, which falls somewhat to 2.9 among the 20–24 age-group. Like many other sub-Saharan African nations, Liberia is facing a grave situation where young women are at much greater risk of contracting HIV/AIDS than their male counterparts, an issue that requires significantly more attention.

Access to SRH information and other health and social services is very limited, particularly outside of Monrovia, the capital city. The 2008 census indicated that over half of all households and three-fourths of all rural households were located 40 minutes or more walking distance from a health facility (LISGIS 2009). In Nimba County, which experienced especially high levels of violence and destruction during the war, residents on average lived over 7 km from the closest health facility and had to walk 136 minutes to get there (Kruk et al. 2010). Thus, large numbers of young females are exposed to the dangers of early marriage and childbearing with little access to health care. Poor health and SRH indicators, as well as precarious economic circumstances, are often associated with school-leaving and the inability to work. This leads many young people on a path to a difficult and unhealthy transition to adulthood.

Among 15–19 year old females in Liberia, 58.4 % of those without an education had begun childbearing compared to 31.1 and 16.9 % of females with primary and secondary or higher education, respectively (LISGIS et al. 2008). Also, 45.9 % of those from the lowest wealth quintile had begun childbearing versus 18.2 % of those from the highest wealth quintile (LISGIS et al. 2008). Similarly, among 15–49 year old women with a recent live birth, 35.7 % of women with no education had a birth attended by a skilled provider,[9] compared with 47.4 % of women who had completed primary school and 74.7 % who had attained secondary or higher education (LISGIS et al. 2008).

Approximately 19 % of Liberian youth were neither in school nor in the labor force (Twerefou and Kawar 2008), with limited opportunities to develop critical social capital and job skills; they are highly vulnerable to the adverse impacts of poverty. Overall, 84 % of the population was active in the informal economy (Twerefou and Kawar 2008). Petty trading and precarious economic activities such as the sale of inexpensive merchandise, foodstuff, water, or clothing on the streets and in crowded, often dangerous market areas offer little stability, support, or protection, especially for young girls.

---

[8] Many sub-Saharan countries were experiencing high female-to-male ratios of HIV prevalence among their 15–24 year old populations. For example, ratios of 2.5 or greater are found in Gabon (2.5), Ghana (2.6), Guinea-Bissau (2.5), Lesotho (2.6) and Mozambique (2.8) (UNAIDS 2010).
[9] A skilled provider is defined as a doctor, nurse, midwife, and physician's assistant (LISGIS et al. 2008).

15.4   Targeted, Evidence-Based Policies and Programs

15.4.1   Holistic SRH and Livelihoods Programs

SRH, education, and poverty alleviation programs are unlikely to improve the lives of vulnerable young people if they do not empower their target beneficiaries. This is particularly true for adolescent girls and other subgroups coping with strong asymmetries of power. The integration of a livelihoods approach within SRH programming recognizes that such problems as STIs/HIV, early pregnancy, early marriage, or sexual violence, are linked to circumstances of vulnerability related to poverty, lack of education, and limited understanding of one's rights.[10] It is not uncommon for girls and young women to trade sex for favors or money to obtain the resources needed for their schooling and families' necessities. Nationally representative data on young women's engagement in transactional sex are unavailable due to the sensitive and complex nature of the topic, but surveys show that in some sub-Saharan African settings, this is known to occur frequently (Swidler and Watkins 2007; Wamoyi et al. 2010). Providing women with safe and dignified livelihood opportunities will likely decrease the need for such high-risk behavior, as they will have more tools with which they can support themselves.

In resource-poor or post-conflict settings, young people often suffer multiple disadvantages. A livelihoods program for vulnerable young people that includes SRH and general health information can serve as a bridge to preventive and treatment services for those who need them (Bruce 2007). This chapter presents a new, phased approach to address the needs of the most vulnerable populations of young people, using a process that integrates research evidence into institutional decision-making processes.

15.4.2   The National Policy Climate in Liberia

In early 2008 staff members from the Population Council and UNFPA launched a collaborative effort to engage local partners in Liberia. They sought to ensure policies and programs for young people included evidence-based strategies to reach the most vulnerable and marginalized youth. Although UN agencies, government ministries, and NGOs had been working to deliver the much-needed resources and services, they were not doing so as part of a unified approach that could generate and integrate data into the decision-making process. The national policy environment

---

[10]For example, South African girls and boys aged 14–19 who have experienced nonconsensual sex are less likely to be enrolled in school than those who have not experienced nonconsensual sex (Hallman 2007). Although study data and design issues prevent the attribution of causality, this and other research provides ample evidence of the linkages between sexual abuse or violence and educational attainment.

at the time was quite friendly to a new approach, due in large part to the unequivocal support of President Ellen Johnson Sirleaf, Africa's first democratically elected female head of state and 2011 Nobel Peace Prize winner. She brought with her an acute awareness of the struggles of women and their children, as well as an explicit mandate to improve their lot. Her government sought to ensure more equitable distribution of resources and to eradicate poverty among women, recognizing an important link between the socio-economic status of women and levels of intergenerational poverty. Liberia's 2008–11 PRS included gender equity, children, and youth as crosscutting issues key to achieving the goals of consolidating peace and security, revitalizing the economy, strengthening governance and the rule of law, and rehabilitating infrastructure and basic service delivery (Republic of Liberia 2008). The PRS additionally provided the framework for establishing efforts to target resources at highly vulnerable young people, girls in particular, since it is the country's roadmap to development and growth.

The government's high level of openness to re-targeting resources in this way was quite rare in countries where the Population Council had been working up to that time.[11] However, there were many challenges to implementing a broad-based strategy for employing data more systematically to inform policy and programmatic decision-making for vulnerable young people.

15.4.3   Adapting the Integrated Approach to the Liberian Context

The methodology applied in Liberia adapted an integrated, seven-step approach recently developed to ensure investments in social programs reach the most vulnerable young people (Population Council 2009b). The approach was adapted to the expressed needs of in-country partners who would implement the various activities and participate in extensive capacity-building exercises. In actuality, a more phased approach was adopted that combined several of these steps, with many of the specific activities or projects within the five action areas described below performed with some overlap between activities. The process proved critical to building an evidence base to strengthen institutions and establish locally run programs to address the SRH, livelihood, and educational needs of vulnerable young people, particularly female adolescents and young adults.

Step 1: Making the Case
Both the Population Council and UNFPA understood that the success of the project rested on engaging a strong base of partner institutions and civil society representatives who recognized the importance of pushing the project's agenda. Accordingly,

---

[11] Similar work was undertaken in Ethiopia, Guatemala, and other countries as part of a larger group of actions focused on adolescent girls and supporting their transitions to adulthood. For a full list of references on these projects, see: http://www.popcouncil.org/topics/youth.asp#/Projects.

the Liberian Working Group for Vulnerable Youth was formed to bring together parties interested in establishing the evidence required to make the case for both targeting interventions to subgroups of young people and for generating holistic programming approaches that included SRH, livelihoods, and other areas deemed important. This group was later renamed the Adolescent Girls Working Group (AGWG) after it was determined that girls aged 10–19 received the least policy attention and programmatic assistance, and therefore required significant advocacy to mainstream their needs.

Analysis of the national Millennium Development Goals (MDGs) and the PRS helped build the argument that achievement of the specified goals required channeling resources into innovative programs targeting the vulnerabilities experienced by many young people. The demographic dividend (i.e. the rise in the economic growth rate that may result from an increased share of working age people in the population) cannot be attained without investments targeted to improve the education, health, and SRH outcomes of young people. Evidence was presented to stakeholders from the governmental, non-governmental, and UN sectors that: (1) investments in young people, especially in marginalized subgroups, were critical to achieving development goals; and (2) these investments had to occur early enough in their lives to have significant impacts on a host of interrelated matters. These included alleviating poverty and breaking the cycle of intergenerational poverty; achieving universal primary school enrollment and expanding secondary enrollment; reducing the spread of STIs/HIV and the prevalence of maternal and infant mortality; and fostering gender equity throughout society.

Analysis of the 2007 Liberian DHS revealed that 33 % of males and 34.6 % of females aged 10–14 were not in school (Population Council 2009a). While many AGWG members and other stakeholders were aware of these problems anecdotally, few had been shown the empirical evidence needed to justify programmatic and policy responses. A broader-based analysis of available data was then required to meet the different programmatic needs of the local partners and to build their capacity in utilizing the data to better inform decision-making. As described below, Steps 2 and 3 cover the activities used for generating and disseminating data, Step 4 focuses on working with local partners to use these data in the design of programs for vulnerable youth, and Step 5 outlines the need for more in-depth research to support this process.

Step 2: Using data to identify vulnerable populations of young people
The creative use of cross-tabulations provides a relatively simple analytic approach to locate concentrations of young people with limited access to resources and services; a situation that can lead to poor SRH, education, and other unfavorable outcomes. Population Council staff disaggregated data by indicators of age (in single years or, at a minimum, in 5-year age cohorts), sex, school enrollment and educational attainment status, marital and childbearing status, region, as well as other issues considered relevant to the local context. This helped to highlight the geographic prevalence of factors that allow for more effective targeting of interventions for improving and equalizing access among diverse groups of young people.

Table 15.2 Children's school attendance and household living arrangements, children age 10–14, according to sex, geographic region, and urban–rural residence, Liberia 2007

Region and residence	Percent not in school and not living with either parent		Not attending school		Attending primary school	
	Male	Female	Male	Female	Male	Female
Region						
Monrovia	4.5	7.7	13.3	17.9	75.5	72.0
North Western	7.5	6.3	47.8	34.9	49.1	59.3
South Central	8.4	6.1	40.6	44.5	55.2	51.8
South Eastern A	8.4	5.6	39.0	44.6	59.3	54.3
South Eastern B	7.7	8.9	27.1	31.6	70.1	67.3
North Central	7.9	8.7	46.0	46.7	51.8	52.4
Residence						
Urban	5.1	7.1	17.5	20.4	73.0	71.0
Rural	8.2	8.4	44.4	47.2	53.2	51.4
TOTAL	6.9	7.8	33.0	34.6	61.6	60.6

Source: Population Council (2009a)

A large body of descriptive statistics on the educational, health, social, and SRH lives of young Liberians was prepared as evidence to assist government, UN, and NGO partners on the use of data in decision-making. Tools included easily accessible reports and presentation templates, data tables, charts, and maps of the various indicators of interest. These tools were presented at a variety of dissemination meetings where their programmatic and policy implications were discussed, and hands-on support was provided to local NGOs who wished to use the presentation templates and other data in their work. Thus, the in-country stakeholders had access to simple yet powerful tools to assist their goal setting as well as their advocacy campaigns and fundraising efforts (Table 15.2).

Of particular interest to this project are the young people likely living under severe social isolation: those who are neither in school nor living with their parents (Population Council 2009a).[12] The 2007 DHS showed that in rural Liberia, 8.4 % of boys and 8.2 % of girls were socially isolated with limited or no access to resources to help them develop their social and human capital. Also, 24 % of rural 5–14 year

---

[12] By way of comparison, a 2004 study of 10–19 year olds in the slums of Addis Ababa, Ethiopia, showed that 22.2 % of female domestic workers had never been to school (compared to 8 % of non-domestic workers), 19.8 % lived with at least one parent (compared to 54.4 % of non-domestic workers), 96.3 % migrated from rural areas (compared to 35.1 % of non-domestic workers), and 13.6 % agreed with the statement that they have many friends (compared to 25.2 % of non-domestic workers) (Erulkar et al. 2004a). Many of these same girls reported having faced negative experiences such as physical abuse and pressure to have sex. As a result, not being in school and not living with either parent is used as a proxy for social isolation among adolescents, particularly females aged 10–14. Young people who are not in school and are working may also be isolated because they have little opportunity to socialize or gather with friends.

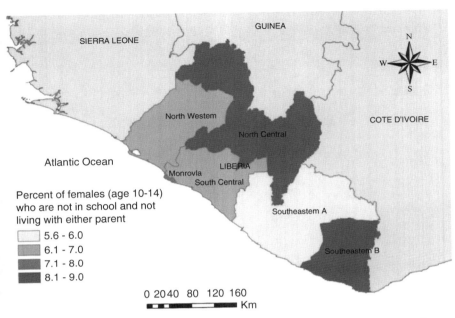

Fig. 15.1 Social isolation among young girls aged 10–14, Liberia, 2007 (Source: Data – Population Council (2009a), Map – ICF Macro (2011))

olds were engaged in some form of child labor (LISGIS et al. 2008). Many of these young people likely had some form of employment in the informal economy, while another large percentage of young people's employment activities go unmeasured due to the complexity of collecting this type of information. Table 15.2 shows sample data on school attendance and living arrangements for young boys and girls aged 10–14. As mentioned earlier, about one-third of all 10–14 year olds were not in school, but this proportion reached 47.8 % for boys in the North Western region and 46.7 % for girls in the North Central region, and was as high as 44.4 and 47.2 % for all rural boys and girls, respectively. Primary school enrollment was as low as 49.1 % for boys in the North Western region and 51.8 % for girls in the South Central region.[13] Schooling and household composition data disaggregated by age, sex, and region underscore the specific circumstances in the lives of young people that lead to disadvantage and increased vulnerability.

Figure 15.1 depicts the same social isolation data presented in Table 15.2. Such maps and figures allow users to easily identify regional variations in different indicators to locate pockets of vulnerability (Weiner 2010). Maps also speak to a wide audience and are easily interpreted by those less comfortable with data tables and charts.

---

[13]The North Western region is comprised of Bomi, Gbarpolu and Grand Cape Mount counties; North Central is comprised of Bong, Lofa and Nimba counties; and South Central is comprised of Grand Bassa, Margibi and Montserrado (excluding Greater Monrovia) counties.

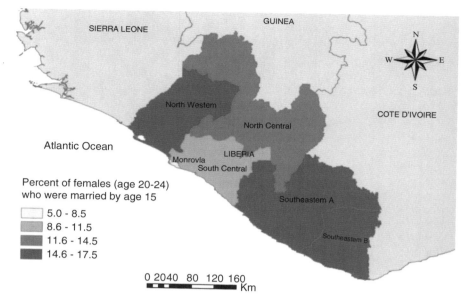

Fig. 15.2 Child marriage rates among women aged 20–24, Liberia, 2007 (Source: Data – Population Council (2009a), Map – ICF Macro (2011))

As stated, the early cessation of schooling and lack of enrollment and attendance are associated with early or child marriage, an issue that is of particular importance to those working to alleviate poverty and improve the SRH conditions of young people. Figure 15.2 shows that rates of child marriage are highest in the South Eastern A region (comprised of Grand Gedeh, River Cess and Sinoe counties) for women aged 20–24. Such data help establish an information base for working with local partners to analyze existing policies and programs, and permit consideration of marginalized young people in geographic areas of higher prevalence. This can help close existing gaps within the regional pockets of vulnerability.

Step 3: Coverage Exercise Study

Steps 1 and 2 set the stage for a coverage exercise study, which can determine if local partner agencies are reaching their target beneficiaries and the types of services being used by particular subgroups of interest (Weiner 2011).[14] A coverage exercise study is a program-monitoring tool that yields data on the demographic characteristics of service clients and is one of a range of possible activities for a larger situation analysis. A simple survey or register is employed on-site to gather

---

[14] A coverage exercise is a situation analysis used to provide data needed to differentiate between the intended and actual beneficiaries of a program (Bruce 2003). The Population Council has conducted coverage exercise studies in Ethiopia, Mauritania, Guinea Bissau, Burkina Faso, Malawi, and Guatemala, each with a slightly different methodology as determined by the local context (Weiner 2011).

information on age, sex, school attendance, educational attainment, household composition, marital and childbearing status, work, distance traveled to reach the program/service, and other pertinent information such as ethnicity or language. A dataset is later created to analyze the profiles of the different subgroups of beneficiaries in order to: (1) gain a clearer understanding regarding how services are distributed by client characteristics; and (2) help identify vulnerable subgroups under-represented at the service delivery sites participating in the study (Weiner 2011). These data can be triangulated with census, DHS, or other survey data to help design future rounds of programming, advocacy campaigns, and policy initiatives aimed at mainstreaming the needs of the vulnerable and marginalized.[15] This yields supply- and demand-side perspectives for broadening access to programs and the scope of programming activities. Coverage exercise data can provide program-monitoring information and be used to illustrate examples or case studies. However, unless the coverage exercise study is designed to be representative at a certain level, data are not fully representative and should not be used to generalize about trends in service provision when disseminated.

In Liberia, 39 youth-serving organizations from all 15 counties participated in the coverage exercise study and collected data over six weeks. Analysis of the descriptive statistics helped build a picture of the subgroups receiving services during this time period and highlighted several significant findings. Firstly, almost 80 % of service beneficiaries were in urban areas despite the 2008 census indicating that over 50 % of the population lived in rural areas (LISGIS 2009; Weiner 2011). This finding suggested a need to expand service provision into rural communities; additional studies would be necessary to make any conclusive recommendations. Secondly, although participating NGOs had reported during the preparatory phase of the coverage exercise that they worked on a wide range of program areas (e.g. education, mentoring, health, SRH, livelihoods, business development, and recreation), the coverage exercise data showed that 59 % of services recorded during the 6 weeks of data collection were for health and SRH, while only 4 % were livelihoods and life skills services. The remaining 37 % of services monitored during the coverage exercise catered to counseling or mental health, sports and recreation, education, food and agriculture, and other program areas not defined in the study (Weiner 2011). This suggested a heavy bias towards health and SRH programs, possibly at the expense of other critical areas that help young people build their social and human capital.

Results of the coverage exercise were disseminated to various stakeholders and motivated local NGOs (including those who had participated in the coverage exercise as well as other AGWG members) to begin concentrating resources on reaching the marginalized youth in their areas. This approach was one step towards ensuring young people expanded access to programs. Additional activities, as described in

---

[15] In Liberia, coverage exercise study data were used with the 2007 DHS to identify populations of young girls who were underserved at the youth services that participated in the study. This analysis provided the evidence for the design of the three programs for specific populations of vulnerable adolescent girls, which are discussed in Step 4 below.

Step 4 below, helped service providers establish more holistic programs, based on the premise that young people require more than just SRH information to minimize exposure to high-risk situations and to develop the skills needed to become more autonomous decision-makers, capable of obtaining safe and respectable work to support themselves.

Step 4: Establishing Program Examples
The evidence generated and disseminated gave rise to more informed advocacy for holistic program approaches addressing the needs of young people under-represented in current youth initiatives. In July 2009, further training was received by representatives from six AGWG-member organizations, along with the service providers of a World Bank-supported initiative called the Economic Empowerment of Adolescent Girls (EPAG). The training covered a range of topics: programming essentials for adolescent girls, procedures to identify vulnerable groups, ways to involve the young participants' gatekeepers and to keep program graduates engaged in ongoing activities, program monitoring, and community outreach. Participants were also provided technical assistance on the development of a proposal for a pilot program targeting specific youth subgroups, which they would later submit to potential donors. By mid-2010, three of the six participating organizations had received small seed grants to launch pilot programs. A fourth NGO founded by a young woman leader of the AGWG later obtained funds to expand a mentoring program to adolescent girls aged 10–14. The promising initial experiences of three of these programming initiatives are reviewed briefly below:

(1) THINK (Touching Humans In Need of Kindness), a local NGO that has worked since the end of the civil conflict with former female child soldiers, launched an innovative project in a small fishing community on the outskirts of Monrovia. THINK staff participated in the July 2009 workshop, analyzed the profile of girls normally reached by their programs, and targeted their proposal at younger adolescents in the King Grey community of Greater Monrovia. This population was identified to be at high risk for transactional sex, STIs, and early school dropout. The resulting intervention was a 'safe spaces' program designed for girls to build their social network; increase SRH knowledge and literacy skills; and provide opportunities for receiving health care as well as assistance to those out-of-school who were interested in returning to school.[16] THINK is now one of the lead local NGOs working to mainstream an agenda for adolescent girls into the national policy environment. THINK has also partnered with UN agencies to include additional targeted interventions for young females.
(2) The Children's Assistance Program is a local NGO that has been working for two decades to assist boys and girls from the slum areas in the Old Road community of Monrovia. Its participation in the July 2009 workshop led to the

[16] A 'safe spaces' program is based on providing a girls' only space where participants can build their social capital, acquire skills, share with their peers in a non-threatening environment, and receive mentoring from older adolescent females (Brady 2003).

design of a small business development program integrated with SRH and general health information for single, out-of-school mothers. The intervention uses the safe spaces model to provide these young mothers with opportunities to develop critical business skills, expand SRH knowledge, and tap into a community savings group with other young women from the community.

(3) The Planned Parenthood Association of Liberia (PPAL) began working in the mid-1950s and was an early associate member of the International Planned Parenthood Federation (IPPF) in Africa. It assumed a strong role in the AGWG. After participating in the July 2009 workshop and reviewing the services it had resumed after the civil conflict had ended, PPAL decided to include a targeted safe spaces program for out-of-school 10–14 year-olds at a site where it already provided services as part of a joint UN program. PPAL sought to replicate this targeted intervention at other sites; however, this has proved more challenging than anticipated.

The high profile of the AGWG and its members' multiple activities has attracted considerable domestic and international attention from donors, research groups, and other stakeholders. The growing body of presented evidence, several program examples, and the attention garnered by the World Bank's new EPAG initiative have all contributed to a growing momentum to attract agencies willing to actively engage this ongoing dialogue.

Step 5: Developing a Research Agenda
The last step in this process consists of interested parties working together to develop a research agenda to establish a more comprehensive body of evidence on the lives of Liberian youth. From the outset of the project, Population Council staff members had engaged the national statistics office (the Liberian Institute of Statistics and Geo-Information Services, LISGIS), as well as UN agencies and relevant NGOs, as key partners to provide evidence for the support of policy and program design. The goal was to engage local stakeholders to define the types of data that support planning and decision-making. This included AGWG members and the various institutions involved in the ongoing targeted interventions. The confluence of expertise on local data, youth programming, and policy and research helped establish a growing body of evidence spanning from the national to program levels. Along with examples of research projects from other countries, this set the stage for the sharing of ideas on a national research agenda focusing on vulnerable young people.

Adolescent surveys similar to those conducted by Population Council in other countries provide valuable, detailed data on specific aspects of young people's lives and the relationships of different factors that lead to vulnerability.[17] These studies fit

---

[17] For example, comparable work has been conducted in Ethiopia (Erulkar et al. 2004a, b). The case of Ethiopia is exemplary of the linkage between research and a programmatic response, one of the objectives of the Liberia project (See also footnote 12 above).

into a larger research agenda for promoting evidence-based programs and policies for young people and serve as a foundation for the design of targeted interventions. The launch of these types of studies, however, requires a serious commitment of resources from both donors and local partners, something absent in Liberia at the time.

15.4.4 Ongoing Challenges

It proved very challenging to advance all the steps described above and to maintain momentum to keep a large number of diverse players engaged. Large lag times between activities and staff changes within the partner agencies had created gaps in the knowledge and skills required for integrating data into the decision-making process to implement evidence-based strategies. These gaps have proved difficult to close. Changing institutional priorities have, at times, side-tracked efforts to design new programs for newly identified subgroups of young people.

As of this writing in mid-2012, the various stakeholders were working with project donors and other partner institutions to strengthen project coordination within the AGWG. This would ensure project sustainability and effectiveness, and help fortify communication channels between Liberian and international partners. The success of a more integrated approach to developing targeted programs clearly requires a strong coordinating body from the beginning, with dedicated funding to support staff changes and potential shifts in the priorities of partners.

Advancement of project goals has also been impeded by shifts in the priorities of key donors and local leaders. Liberia has been a priority country for many donors following the cessation of civil conflict and the 2005 election of President Sirleaf, as evidenced by the amount of official development assistance (ODA) received.[18] However, it has proved difficult to find donors willing to continue committing to a project that takes multiple years to develop local capacity to reach the point where partner organizations can scale up the targeted evidence-based interventions, such as those pilot programs described in this chapter.

This project has sought to establish a process for generating data and integrating such evidence into decision-making so as to expand and improve programs targeted at vulnerable young people. Presently, however, there is still no mechanism established to measure the impact of the activities described in this chapter at the institutional level (such as more informed, evidence-based decision-making or increased programmatic attention devoted to specific populations of young people) in order

---

[18] According to Aidflows (a source of global data on aid funding from the World Bank Group and the Organisation for Economic Co-operation and Development, OECD), net ODA disbursements to Liberia rose steadily from US$286.9 million in 2006 to US$717.4 million in 2007 and US$1220.9 million in 2008, before decreasing to US$512.6 million in 2009. In 2010, however, net ODA disbursements spiked to US$1425.1 (see www.aidflows.org, accessed April 26, 2012).

to report any data-based successes. To do this, parties involved since the launch of the project need to design a study to measure the impact of the process, including the programs to which it has given rise.

15.5   Discussion

A number of local service providers from the AGWG (and the new EPAG initiative) involved in the project since its launch in early 2008 have taken specific steps to include more holistic strategies to address adolescent SRH needs by integrating topics such as livelihoods, literacy, and business development into their project curriculums. The AGWG has seen a steady increase in participation from local and (more recently) international NGOs interested in expanding service delivery to adolescent girls and other vulnerable subgroups. Its significance as a network for information exchange with the potential for greater involvement in future research and programmatic effort has not been lost on others. This includes several government ministries that have shown a greater willingness to review their internal policies as they relate to adolescent girls, to support the AGWG in their respective activities, and to strengthen institutional capacity to deal with issues related to vulnerable youth. Indeed, at the time of writing, the Ministry of Youth and Sports included a line item in its operational budget to support the AGWG in addressing the needs of adolescent girls in their work.

The Ministry of Gender and Development has also taken significant steps towards ensuring that the policies and programs it supports are more evidence-based and targeted at vulnerable groups of adolescent girls. As the lead government ministry for the World Bank's EPAG project, it has received a considerable amount of institutional strengthening and resources to support an expanded agenda for adolescent girls. In 2010, the Ministry formed the Adolescent Girls Policy Advocacy Team to influence decision-makers in formulating policy to enhance the social and economic empowerment of adolescent girls. As the Ministry's role within the EPAG project has expanded, its staff has taken a more active role within the AGWG to increase awareness of new opportunities, inform the community of the availability of data, and facilitate networking opportunities to help strengthen the participating agencies' methods for delivering targeted interventions.

The activities described in this chapter were aimed at generating evidence necessary to inform the design of targeted interventions that use a more holistic approach to build the social and human capital of vulnerable young people. In most settings, including Liberia, programs for youth abound. But who are the actual beneficiaries of these programs? Are they the intended beneficiaries? And who are the programs not reaching? Coverage exercise data help NGOs and other stakeholders answer these questions and can provide valuable information to program planners. The first coverage exercise study was conducted in 2003 for 13 participating programs in Ethiopia. It showed that 78 % of beneficiaries aged 10–24 were in school, with over 90 % in school for three programs. However, the 2000 Ethiopia DHS showed that only 17 % of rural girls were in school, as were 66 % of all boys and 52 % of urban boys (Mekbib et al. 2005). The triangulation of the data showed an over-representation of in-school youth at the local participating programs and suggest a greater need for more targeted interventions for out-of-school young people as part of their portfolio of services. Researchers in Ethiopia responded by conducting two adolescent studies in high priority areas to obtain a more in-depth understanding of the circumstances in which they live.

This included a 2004 survey conducted to identify the needs of over 1,000 young people living in a slum area of Addis Ababa. A high proportion of this population comprised rural migrants, many of who were neither in school nor living with their parents and were holding low paying jobs such as domestic workers (Erulkar et al. 2004a). Thus, Ethiopian agencies participating in the process launched the Biruh Tesfa ("Bright Future") program in this area to provide the migrant girls and young women with SRH and health information on HIV prevention, sexual exploitation, and abuse, along with literacy, life skills, and opportunities to minimize social isolation through establishing a network of friends (Erulkar et al. 2011). The process used to generate the data for informing intervention design was similar to that recommended for Liberia.

In Liberia, the coverage exercise proved a valuable source of information for programs seeking to reach vulnerable youth and highlighted that only 4 % of services monitored during the time of the study were for livelihoods and life skills. THINK used these data to identify a specific group of adolescent girls (those aged 10–14 and out-of-school) who were largely underrepresented in the programs assessed during the coverage exercise study. The coverage exercise data, coupled with the local NGO's experience working with the target community, helped it develop the case for a program integrating SRH services, livelihoods training, and educational support for vulnerable girls. It obtained funding needed to launch the program in 2010. THINK staff have been active in the AGWG since its inception and participated in both the coverage exercise study and the July 2009 workshop on developing evidence-based programs. This led to the development of the targeted program described in this chapter. The agency has now assumed a prominent role in a new Adolescent Girls Advocacy and Leadership Initiative, which campaigns for girls' rights at the national level in a number of countries around the world.

For various reasons that included donor and in-country partners' priorities, the project played out in Malawi in a very different way. Donors ascribed less priority to Malawi than to Liberia and dedicated fewer resources to putting together a multisectoral coalition to help carry the project through its various stages. In November 2008, three Malawian NGOs attended a workshop held in Nairobi similar in design to the July 2009 programming workshop later held in Liberia, with participants designing a targeted program for a specific group of adolescent girls. Later that year, the UNFPA/Malawi country office launched a coverage exercise study to gather evidence to support its local implementing partners and provide data for advocacy campaigns, such as one to end child marriage. Despite this initiative, no programs similar to those launched in Liberia ever took hold at the time of writing, possibly due to the lack of significant momentum such as that created by the AGWG and its partners, to continue pushing forward the agenda for targeted interventions for vulnerable young people. However, much of the data collection and analysis in

Malawi has been used to support a strong, multi-sectoral campaign to end child marriage and press legal changes for such purpose. This highlights the flexible nature of the phased approach to support local initiatives on high priority issues.

It is likely that project uptake on such a wide scale in Liberia was facilitated by the high level of donor interest and the widely acknowledged need for more innovative service delivery in a post-conflict setting. A movement was built from the bottom up with support from government ministries and UN agencies. The circumstances were quite different in Malawi, but data linking the outcomes with the different stages of the project in each country are lacking for a true cross-country comparison. However, the differences in both process and outcome are noteworthy particularly for thinking about the application of this integrated approach in other settings.

15.6   Conclusion

Providing equitable access to programs and services that build young people's social and human capital in a meaningful way is a key responsibility of the development community. The circumstances that lead to vulnerability will be more effectively mitigated by holistic programs that build the skills and knowledge required by youth to stay in school, obtain gainful employment, avoid high-risk sexual encounters, and delay marriage and childbearing. Poor SRH outcomes are linked with poor educational outcomes and limited opportunities for safe work. Nevertheless, high quality programs are not enough if they are accessible only to young people with greater social and economic resources. In post-conflict settings such as Liberia, expanding the evidence-base to deepen understanding of the complex relationship between the well-being of vulnerable youth and a country's development goals is crucial to developing meaningful interventions. Establishing a systematic process to address the needs of the most vulnerable and marginalized young people will ensure that local partners (from NGOs to government ministries or UN agencies) are sufficiently capable to play their respective roles in development efforts.

Acknowledgement   The authors would like to thank Eric Green (Duke University) for his helpful comments on an earlier version of this paper and Judith Bruce (Population Council) for her vision and passion regarding efforts to ensure the well-being of adolescent girls in the developing world.

References

Brady, M. (2003). Safe spaces for adolescent girls. *Adolescent and youth sexual and reproductive health: Charting directions for a second generation of programming-background documents for the meeting* (pp. 155–176). Available at: http://www.popcouncil.org/pdfs/AYSRH/7.pdf

Bruce, J. (2003). Steps in building evidence-based programs for adolescents. *Adolescent and youth sexual and reproductive health: Charting directions for a second generation of programming-background documents for the meeting* (pp. 29–42). http://www.popcouncil.org/pdfs/AYSRH/2jb1.pdf

Bruce, J. (2007). The girls left behind: Outside the box and out of reach. *Global AIDSLink* (101), 14–15. http://www.globalhealth.org/publications/article.php3?id=1597

Ellis, S. (2006). *The mask of anarchy updated edition: The destruction of Liberia and the religious dimension of an African civil war*. New York: New York University Press.

Erulkar, A. S., Mekbib, T., Simie, N., & Gulema, T. (2004a). *Adolescent life in low income and slum areas of Addis Ababa, Ethiopia*. New York: Population Council.

Erulkar, A. S., Mekbib, T., Simie, N., & Gulema, T. (2004b). *The experience of adolescence in rural Amhara region, Ethiopia*. New York: Population Council.

Erulkar, A. S., Semunegus, B., & Mekonnen, G. (2011). *Biruh Tesfa* provides domestic workers, orphans, and migrants in urban Ethiopia with social support, HIV education, and skills. *Promoting healthy, safe, and productive transitions to adulthood* (Brief No. 21). New York: Population Council.

Esiet, A. O., & Whitaker, C. (2002). Coming to terms with politics and gender: The evolution of an adolescent reproductive health program in Nigeria. In N. Haberland & D. Measham (Eds.), *Responding to Cairo: Case studies of changing practice in reproductive health and family planning* (pp. 149–167). New York: Population Council.

Hallman, K. (2007). Nonconsensual sex, school enrollment and educational outcomes in South Africa. *Africa Insight, 37*(3), 454–472.

ICF Macro. (2011). *MEASURE demographic and health survey country region geodatabase*. Date downloaded: May 12, 2011.

Knowles, J. C., & Behrman, J. R. (2005). *The economic returns to investing in youth in developing countries: A review of the literature*. Washington, DC: World Bank.

Kruk, M. E., Rockers, P. C., Williams, E. H., Varpilah, S. T., Macauly, R., Saydee, G., & Galea, S. (2010). Availability of essential health services in post-conflict Liberia. *Bulletin of the World Health Organization, 88*(7), 527–534.

LISGIS. (2009). *2008 population and housing census final results*. Monrovia: Liberia Institute of Statistics and Geo-Information Services (LISGIS).

LISGIS, Ministry of Health and Social Welfare [Liberia], National AIDS Control Program [Liberia], and Macro International Inc. (2008). *Liberia demographic and health survey 2007*. Monrovia: Liberia Institute of Statistics and Geo-Information Services (LISGIS) and Macro International Inc.

Lloyd, C. B. (Ed.). (2005). *Growing up global: The changing transitions to adulthood in developing countries*. Washington, DC: National Academies Press.

Lloyd, C. B. (2006). Schooling and adolescent reproductive behavior in developing countries. Paper commissioned by the United Nations Millennium Project for the report *Public choices, private decisions: Sexual and reproductive health and the millennium development goals*. New York: UN Millennium Project.

Macro International Inc. (2011). MEASURE DHS STATcompiler. http://www.measuredhs.com. Accessed 4 June 2011.

Mekbib, T., Erulkar, A. S., & Belete, F. (2005). Who are the targets of youth programs: Results of a capacity building exercise in Ethiopia. *The Ethiopian Journal of Health Development, 19*(1), 60–62.

Population Council. (2009a). *The adolescent experience in-depth: Using data to identify and reach the most vulnerable young people: Liberia 2007*. New York: Population Council.

Population Council. (2009b). *Momentum December 2009: Adolescent girls*. New York: Population Council.

Republic of Liberia. (2008). *Poverty reduction strategy*. Monrovia: Republic of Liberia.

Solà-Martín, A. (2011). Liberia: Security challenges, development fundamentals. *Third World Quarterly, 32*(7), 1217–1232.

Swidler, A., & Watkins, S. C. (2007). Ties of dependence: AIDS and transactional sex in rural Malawi. *Studies in Family Planning, 38*(3), 147–162.

Twerefou, D. K., & Kawar, M. (2008). *Towards decent work in Liberia: A labour market and employment assessment*. Geneva: International Labour Organization.

UNAIDS. (2010). *UNAIDS report on the global AIDS epidemic: 2010.* Geneva: Joint United Nations Programme on HIV/AIDS (UNAIDS). Available at: http://www.unaids.org/globalreport/default.htm

UNICEF. (2005). *Early marriage, a harmful traditional practice. A statistical exploration, 2005.* New York: United Nations Children's Fund.

Wamoyi, J., Wight, D., Plummer, M., Mshana, G. H., & Ross, D. (2010). Transactional sex amongst young people in rural northern Tanzania: An ethnography of young women's motivations and negotiations. *Reproductive Health, 7*(2), 1–18.

Weiner, A. (2010). Geographic variations in inequities in access to sexual and reproductive health services. *Studies in Family Planning, 41*(2), 134–138.

Weiner, A. (2011). Assessing equity of access in youth programs. *Promoting healthy, safe, and productive transitions to adulthood* (Brief No. 28). New York: Population Council.

World Bank. (2010). *World development indicators 2010.* Washington, DC: World Bank.

About the Authors

Philip Baba Adongo, Ph.D., is senior lecturer and head of the Department of Social and Behavioral Science, School of Public Health, University of Ghana. Previously, he was Principal Research Fellow at the Navrongo Health Research Centre where he served as an investigator on the collaborative team that led the Navrongo Community Health and Family Planning Project (CHFP). This project provided the service delivery model adopted and implemented nationally as the Community Health and Family Planning and Services (CHPS) Initiative. As a program specialist with UNICEF Ghana, he coordinated the planning and implementation of an operations research study on the Intermittent Preventive Treatment of malaria in Infants (IPTi) using sulphadoxine-pyrimethamine (SP). This study was also implemented in Malawi, Benin and Madagascar. Additionally, he has investigated cross-border migration and HIV/AIDS in Ghana, Togo, and Burkina Faso. Dr. Adongo holds a doctorate in epidemiology and population health from the London School of Hygiene and Tropical Medicine.

Alaka Malwade Basu, M.Sc., is a professor in the Department of Developmental Sociology, Cornell University, and is currently visiting professor at Jawaharlal Nehru University, New Delhi. For 6 years, she was also the Director of the South Asia Program at Cornell University. She has taught at Delhi University and Harvard University. She is a social demographer with strong interests in public health. Alaka Basu's expertise and research is predominantly in the areas of reproductive health and family planning, gender and development, child health and mortality, and the context and politics of population policy. Professor Basu was the chair of the IUSSP (International Union for the Scientific Study of Population) Scientific Committee on Anthropological Demography. She has also been a member of the Committees on Reproductive Health and on Population Projections of the National Research Council at the U.S. National Academy of Sciences.

Colin D. Baynes, MPH, is a program manager at the Heilbrunn Department of Population and Family Health, Columbia University, where he was earlier an Allan M. Rosenfield Scholar for Sexual and Reproductive Health. He has worked in the

A. Kulczycki (ed.), *Critical Issues in Reproductive Health*, The Springer Series on Demographic Methods and Population Analysis 33, DOI 10.1007/978-94-007-6722-5, © Springer Science+Business Media Dordrecht 2014

Upper East Region of Ghana on studies that evaluated the Community-based Health Planning and Services (CHPS) program, the long-term impact of community-based distribution of family planning, and maternal and infant care-seeking practices. He works for the Heilbrunn Department in Tanzania on a trial of a community health worker strategy to reduce child mortality and improve maternal health. He has also worked on related issues in Uganda, Namibia, Pakistan, Thailand and Ecuador.

Stan Bernstein, MS, earlier co-ran a Population and Development training program at the University of Michigan and supported related projects in Asia and Africa funded by the ILO (International Labour Organization), UNFPA, and USAID. In 1991, newly at UNFPA, he led estimation of the requirements needed to implement the population and reproductive health measures set out at the ICPD. He then served for 10 years as principal researcher, writer and coordinator of UNFPA's "State of World Population" report, addressing multiple population and development themes. He co-managed the "ICPD+15" effort and advanced UN collaborative projects, including inter-agency publications on heath and the development of tools for costing requirements for achieving MDG 4 and 5. On secondment to the United Nations Millennium Project, he led production of "Public Choices, Private Decisions: Sexual and Reproductive Health and the MDGs" (2006) and promoted adoption of universal access to reproductive health as an MDG target. He has since retired from the UN and is a partner in ReGeneration Consulting LLC.

Neil Datta, MA, is Secretary of the European Parliamentary Forum on Population and Development (EPF), a network of European Members of Parliaments committed to protecting and improving women's sexual and reproductive health and rights (SRHR) across the developing world. For the past 12 years, he has been observing, assisting and coordinating the work of MEPs committed to SRHR issues across the continent. A political scientist by training, as the founding member of EPF he has helped create a strong network of all-party parliamentary groups on population and development in over 28 Parliaments in Europe. He is also the co-chair of the Resource Mobilisation and Awareness Working Group of the Reproductive Health Supplies Coalition and serves on the advisory board of the Women Deliver initiative. Previously, he coordinated the Parliamentary Programme of the International Planned Parenthood Federation European Network.

Suzanne Dhall, DrPH, recently received her doctorate in maternal and child health from the University of Alabama at Birmingham. Her dissertation focused on fertility enhancing drugs, assisted reproductive technologies, and their maternal and infant outcomes. She is interested in using available population-based sources to explore these issues further, as well as in assisting persons struggling with infertility. She is training to become a certified health education specialist (CHES) to counsel individuals and couples coping with infertility. In this work, she would like to enhance communication between those considering treatment options and the health care providers who offer them.

Laneta Dorflinger, Ph.D., is distinguished scientist and vice president at FHI 360. She directs its Preventive Technologies Agreement, a global program to develop and introduce microbicides and oral pre-exposure prophylaxis (PrEP) using antiretrovirals. She also directs a USAID-funded award to develop biodegradable contraceptive implants, and is a technical leader for several contraceptive development activities including Sino-implant (II). Before joining FHI 360, she worked for 7 years in the Office of Population at USAID focusing on contraceptive technology. Dr. Dorflinger has received several noteworthy awards, including the Science and Technology in Development award from USAID. She has authored or co-authored numerous articles on contraceptive technology and microbicides. She received her undergraduate degree in chemistry from Lafayette College, her doctorate in physiology from Yale University, and did post-doctoral training at the Harvard School of Public Health.

Karen Hardee, Ph.D., is senior fellow and deputy director of population and reproductive health for the Health Policy Project at the Futures Group and has been visiting senior fellow at the Population Reference Bureau. She is also president of Hardee Associates LLC. A social demographer for 25 years, Dr. Hardee has focused her career on issues related to family planning and reproductive health, population and development, HIV, gender integration, climate change, evidence-based policy, and monitoring and evaluation. Dr. Hardee began investigating the relationships between reproductive health and climate change when working as Vice-President for Research at Population Action International, including through fieldwork in Ethiopia. She holds a doctorate from Cornell University's population and development program.

Dennis Hodgson, Ph.D., is a professor of sociology and anthropology at Fairfield University. He received his doctorate in Sociology from Cornell University's International Population Program. His areas of specialty are social demography, policy formation, and the history of population thought. He is the author of a number of articles on the interplay of demographic thought and international population policy formation that have appeared in *Population and Development Review*. His articles include treatments of how the relationship between feminists and population controllers has changed over time, as well as an examination of the consequences of defining family planning in a way that excludes induced abortion. His long-term research interest is in tracing America's changing population priorities from colonial times to the present.

Roy Jacobstein, M.D., MPH, has been the clinical director of the RESPOND Project and its predecessor ACQUIRE Project, managed by EngenderHealth, since 2002. Previously, he was an independent consultant to the World Bank, USAID, Save the Children, and other organizations. He also served as Chief of the Communication, Management and Training Division of the Office of Population at USAID/Washington. He has worked in over 20 countries worldwide, including Bangladesh, Bulgaria, Ethiopia, Ghana, India, Indonesia, Kenya, Malawi, Mexico, Nepal, Pakistan, Rwanda, and Turkey. Dr. Jacobstein serves as an expert technical advisor to WHO on its *Medical Eligibility Criteria for Contraceptive Use, Selected Practice Recommendations for Contraceptive Use,* and on community-based access to injectable contraception. He co-chaired USAID Working Groups that developed the Implants Toolkit and the IUD Toolkit, electronic resources on these family planning methods. He has authored many papers and briefs on a range of family planning/reproductive health subjects.

Andrew B. Kantner, Ph.D., has longstanding interests in international demography, reproductive health, and social medicine, with special expertise in program monitoring/evaluation (M&E). He is currently serving as a Technical Adviser to the Policy Division of the United Nations Population Division in New York. During the last decade, he has participated in USAID and UNFPA project evaluations in South and Southeastern Asia, Eastern Europe, and sub-Saharan Africa. From 1990 to 1999 he was a senior fellow in the Program on Population, East–west Center, Honolulu, Hawaii, and provided administrative and technical support for population and reproductive health projects in the Asia-Pacific region. Earlier, he served with USAID/Indonesia as an adviser to the Indonesian National Family Planning Coordinating Board (BKKBN), and was a reproductive and child health research manager with USAID/Bangladesh. He also provided field-based technical support to UNFPA projects in Bangladesh, China, Egypt, and Nepal. He recently co-authored the book entitled *International Discord on Population and Development* (Palgrave Macmillan, 2009).

Andrzej Kulczycki, Ph.D., is associate professor in the Department of Health Care Organization and Policy, University of Alabama at Birmingham (UAB). He links public health with the social and policy sciences to study and advance population and reproductive health issues, policies, and programs. He has broad international experience in research, teaching, and consulting in multiple areas of reproductive health. His interests also include demography, maternal and child health, health systems and services. His current research includes expanding barrier contraceptive choices, investigating biomarkers of semen exposure, examining fertility behavior and population and health policy, and designing provider-based strategies to increase HPV vaccination coverage and adherence. Dr. Kulczycki is Chair of the Population, Reproductive and Sexual Health section of the American Public Health Association, and serves on several CDC working groups to assist completion of the National Action Plan for the prevention, detection, and management of infertility. His publications include *The Abortion Debate in the World Arena* (Macmillan and Routledge, 1999). Earlier, he was a faculty member at the American University of Beirut (AUB) and a research associate at the University of Michigan.

Elizabeth Lule, M.Sc., is manager of operations services at the World Bank and responsible for quality assurance and effectiveness of operations in Africa. She recently worked on developing the World Bank Africa Strategy *"Africa's Future and World Bank Support to it."* Earlier, she was manager of the AIDS Campaign Team for Africa, responsible for policy direction, implementation and coordination of the World Bank's HIV/AIDS work in Africa including overseeing the implementation of the US$2 billion multi-country HIV/AIDS program in over 30 African countries. Before 2006, she was the World Bank's adviser for population and reproductive, maternal and child health. Additionally, Elizabeth was Africa regional vice president for Pathfinder International and had previously worked with USAID in Nigeria as program coordinator for the health, nutrition and population program and as technical adviser of the Family Health Services Project. She completed her graduate studies in medical demography at the London School of Hygiene and Tropical Medicine and the London School of Economics. As this book went to press, Elizabeth was about to move to a new position at the Bill & Melinda Gates Foundation, where she will direct its family planning portfolio.

Maja Micevska Scharf, Ph.D., earned her doctorate in economics from Claremont Graduate University, USA, and has since been affiliated with universities and research institutes in several European countries. She was affiliated with the Netherlands Interdisciplinary Demographic Institute (NIDI), where she led a large-scale research project monitoring resource flows for reproductive health. Currently, she holds professorship appointments at Webster University, Leiden and Roosevelt Academy, Middelburg (the Netherlands). Her main fields of research are in development economics and population economics.

Reid Miller, MPH, recently graduated with her MPH from the University of North Carolina's Gillings School of Global Public Health and now works with the WHO's Department of Reproductive Health researching *mHealth*, the use of cell phone technology for health interventions. She provides technical support for *mHealth* projects in Africa and Southeast Asia, which work to improve the ability of community health workers to deliver maternal and reproductive health services through the use of mobile devices. Together these projects will contribute to global guidance on *mHealth*. Earlier, from 2008 to 2010, Reid was a Peace Corps community health and HIV/AIDS prevention volunteer in Togo, West Africa, where she developed and implemented a program to train village women to be community health volunteers.

Hosam Moustafa Abdel Hafez, MBBCh., an Egyptian physician, is from the town of Kafr el-Sheikh and graduated from Al-Azhar Medical School. He also has training in Islamic jurisprudence, with a particular focus on Islamic interpretation of new medical technologies. In 2008, he started working with Lisa L. Wynn on a project investigating local interpretations and representations of reproductive health technologies in Egypt. He is currently completing postdoctoral surgical training in Germany.

Derek H. Owen, Ph.D., is a scientist in the clinical sciences group at FHI 360 specializing in drug delivery systems. He is a chemical engineer who, in graduate school, studied changes in cervical mucus properties and how those changes influence sperm motility. Dr. Owen spent 12 years as a research professor in Duke University's Department of Biomedical Engineering. There he studied the material properties of drug delivery gels, particularly microbicidal gels for the prevention of HIV transmission, and the properties of the vitreous and drug delivery to the eye. Since joining FHI 360, he has worked mainly on projects involving drug delivery to the female reproductive tract. In addition to his quality assurance work on Sino-implant (II), he has managed programs to develop erythromycin as a method of non-surgical sterilization and a clinical trial of a biodegradable female contraceptive implant.

Daniel E. Pellegrom, M.Div., has headed three organizations during his four decade long career in reproductive health. For 26 years, he was president of Pathfinder International, the longest tenure of any head of a reproductive health organization, increasing its annual budget from $8milion to $100 million. In 1996, Pathfinder became only the second U.S.-based organization to receive the United Nations Population Award. Dan is widely respected for his experience in management and advocacy. He was awarded the Union Medal by Union Theological Seminary in New York City, its highest honor, in 2011. Dan has served on various boards of directors including the Guttmacher Institute, Planned Parenthood, World Neighbors, and is a past board chair of both the Brush Foundation and InterAction, the largest coalition of U.S.-based humanitarian organizations working abroad. He has written op-ed pieces for *The Boston Globe*, *The New York Times*, and other influential newspapers, as well as provided testimony at Congressional hearings and other public forums.

James F. Phillips, Ph.D., is professor of clinical population and family health, Columbia University Mailman School of Public Health, where he conducts research on health systems and policy issues. Dr. Phillips collaborated with the Ghana Health Service in designing, implementing, and evaluating the Navrongo Experiment, a study that provided conclusive evidence that family planning services can lead to fertility decline in a traditional African societal setting. Improvements in maternal and child health associated with the project represent the most rapid declines in maternal and childhood mortality ever recorded for a rural African population, with project service systems becoming the model for a national program. Dr. Phillips has developed and tested methods for accelerating the pace of scaling-up initiatives around the world. His current research is based on exchanges of health system innovations between Tanzania and Ghana, two countries at the forefront of health development in sub-Saharan Africa.

Kate H. Rademacher, MHA, has over 10 years of experience in family planning and reproductive health program design and management. She currently works on the research utilization team at FHI 360 where she helps accelerate the translation of research findings into policy and practice. She has expertise in several technical areas including increasing access to long-acting methods of contraception; continuation of injectables use; integration of family planning and MCH services; media literacy and sexual health; and social entrepreneurship. Ms. Rademacher manages a research utilization portfolio on family planning and immunization integration for the USAID-funded PROGRESS project, and serves as the strategic partnership manager on the Sino-implant (II) project, an initiative designed to increase access to implants in resource-constrained settings. Ms. Rademacher has an undergraduate degree from Wesleyan University and a master's of Healthcare Administration from the University of North Carolina at Chapel Hill.

Ahmed Ragab, M.D., Ph.D., is a professor of reproductive health at Al-Azhar University. He has worked and conducted research on reproductive and sexual health in several countries including Egypt, Kyrgyzstan, Syria, and the Darfur camps in Eastern Chad and Somalia. He has also worked as a consultant for a number of national and international organizations including UNICEF, the Egyptian Family Planning Association, Save the Children, and the Ford Foundation. In addition to writing several books on research methodologies in sexual and reproductive health, he has published a number of journal articles and policy reports in both Arabic and English. His research interests and activism center about reducing maternal mortality, female genital mutilation, and gender-based violence.

Jill Sheffield, MA, is the founder and president of Women Deliver, an international not-for-profit initiative dedicated to achieving MDG5. Jill completed advanced degrees at Columbia University, Teachers College, where she was later recognized as a distinguished alumna, and she also received the American Public Health Association's Lifetime Achievement Award in 2008. She founded Family Care International in 1987. Twenty years later, after she "retired," Jill founded Women Deliver, believing a global organization focused on MDG5 was needed to secure international and national political support and resources. Women Deliver has become a leading advocacy organization, noted especially for its global conferences. Though she has devoted her career to maternal and sexual and reproductive health, Jill believes her true education came when she worked in the family planning/reproductive health outpatient clinic of Pumwani Maternity Hospital in Nairobi, Kenya.

John Stanback, Ph.D., is a health services researcher with 25 years of experience in family planning program research. Dr. Stanback leads a team of US- and Africa-based researchers at FHI 360 whose work focuses on improving access to family planning for the underserved. An adjunct professor in the Department of Maternal and Child Health at the University of North Carolina (UNC) at Chapel Hill, John Stanback completed his doctorate in health policy and administration from UNC and a master's degree in economics from Duke University. In 2004, Dr. Stanback led the first study of safety and feasibility of community-based distribution (CBD) of injectables in Africa, which took place in Nakasongola, Uganda. That study showed community health workers can safely provide injectable contraceptives, and served as the basis for scale-up of this practice within Uganda and other African countries.

Markus J. Steiner, Ph.D., MSPH, has worked at FHI 360 as a senior epidemiologist for the past 23 years, primarily focusing on studies concerned with contraceptive effectiveness. He has extensive experience conducting research around the world (Brazil, Cameroon, Chile, China, Ethiopia, Ghana, Hungary, India, Jamaica, Kenya, Ghana, Malawi, Sri Lanka, Thailand, the Dominican Republic, Turkey, and Zimbabwe). He has published over 70 peer-reviewed articles and serves as an ad hoc reviewer for a number of scientific journals. In 2001 he was named adjunct professor in the Department of Epidemiology, School of Public Health, University of North Carolina at Chapel Hill, where he received his doctorate in reproductive epidemiology in 1999. Currently, Dr. Steiner leads a multi-year initiative funded by the Bill & Melinda Gates Foundation to provide technical assistance to a manufacturer of a low-cost contraceptive implant, Sino-implant (II).

Marleen Temmerman, M.D., MPH, Ph.D., was appointed in 2012 as Director of the Department of Reproductive Health and Research and the UNDP/UNFPA/ WHO/World Bank Special Programme of Research, Development and Research Training in Human Reproduction. She is also professor of obstetrics and gynaecology (Ob/Gyn), Ghent University, and founding director of its International Centre for Reproductive Health (ICRH) which implements research, training, and service delivery projects in Europe, Latin America, Africa and Asia. As a Belgian senator, she has been a member of the health and foreign affairs committees, chair of an advisory group on HIV/AIDS, and collaborated with the European Parliamentary Forum on Population and Development (EPF). She started working in Kenya as a young Ob/Gyn and STI/HIV researcher in the mid-1980s. Since then, HIV/AIDS and sexual and reproductive health and rights have been at the top of her agenda as a practitioner, a politician and a private person.

Heather L. Vahdat, MPH, has over 10 years of experience in biological, clinical, and public health research. Her specific areas of research experience include: uterine fibroids, non-surgical sterilization, emergency contraception, contraceptive efficacy, and adherence to antiretroviral therapy in developing countries. Ms. Vahdat serves as project manager for the Bill & Melinda Gates Foundation-funded Sino-implant (II) initiative. She is also one of the key scientists involved in developing FHI 360's Mobile for Reproductive Health (m4RH) text messaging program, including conceptualization and implementation of strategies to utilize text messaging for promotion of contraceptive use, uptake, and continuation. Ms. Vahdat received her MPH from the University of North Carolina at Chapel Hill.

Hendrik P. van Dalen, Ph.D., is a full professor of macroeconomics at Tilburg University and CentER, and a senior research associate at the Netherlands Interdisciplinary Demographic Institute (NIDI) in The Hague. He was previously affiliated with the Erasmus University Rotterdam, the Tinbergen Institute, the Scientific Council for Government Policy and the Dutch Council of Economic Advisors. His research interests cover the economics of aging, pensions, migration, and population aid and policy.

Adam Weiner, MA, is a consultant to the poverty, gender and youth program of the Population Council, where he was previously a staff associate. He has played a variety of roles in the implementation of targeted, evidence-based adolescent programs as part of a larger effort to engage government, non-governmental and UN agencies to mainstream the needs of the most vulnerable subgroups of young people, particularly girls. He serves as technical advisor to various in-country partners on capacity building projects and on the development of evidence-based strategies for policy analysis and program design in Liberia, Malawi, Pakistan, Guatemala, Nicaragua, El Salvador and Belize. He holds an MA in international political economy and development from Fordham University.

L.L. Wynn, Ph.D., completed her doctorate in anthropology at Princeton University and subsequently held two postdoctoral research appointments in Princeton's Office of Population Research. In 2007 she joined Macquarie University in Sydney,

Australia, where she is senior lecturer in the Department of Anthropology. Her first book, *Pyramids and Nightclubs: A Travel-Ethnography of Western and Arab Imaginations of Egypt, from King Tut and Colonies of Atlantis to Sex Orgies, Rumors about a Marauding Prince, and Blond Belly Dancers* (University of Texas Press, 2007), was also translated into Arabic. A second book, *Emergency Contraception: The Story of a Global Reproductive Health Technology* (Palgrave Macmillan, 2012), is co-edited with Angel M. Foster. Her current research is funded by an Australian Research Council discovery project grant, and it examines new reproductive health technologies in Egypt.

Index

A

A Better World for All: Progress Towards the International Development Goals (OECD, 2000), 230

Abortifacient, 85, 88–90, 92, 98, 245

Abortion, 7, 8, 10, 28, 29, 31, 216–218, 227, 228
  legal, 153, 155, 156, 158–161, 163–167, 174, 228
  medical, 228
  policies, 8, 153–174
  spontaneous, 140
  unsafe, 136, 138, 140, 158, 228

Abortion Policies: A Global Review, 155

Abuja Declaration (2001), 239

Accelerating Contraceptive Use Project (Afghanistan), 277, 278

Accountability, 228

Accra Agenda (2008), 239

Acquire Project, 250, 252–257, 259, 260

Adaptation (to climate change), 9, 177, 180–182, 185–190

Addis Ababa, 316, 324

Additionality, 185

Adolescent Girls Working Group (AGWG), Liberia, 315, 319–324

Adolescents, 16, 17, 308–310, 313–316, 319–321, 323, 324

Advance Family Planning project, 235

Advocacy, 223, 224, 226, 227, 252, 253, 255, 258, 261, 315, 316, 319, 320, 323, 324
  efforts, 12, 226, 227
  groups, 54

Advocates, 11

Afghanistan, 277, 278

Africa, 2, 4, 5, 8, 14–16, 59, 60, 63, 64, 154, 157, 158, 160, 161, 169, 173, 184, 237, 239, 243, 265–282, 307, 310, 311, 313, 314, 321
  Central, 130, 137, 147, 149
  Eastern, 130, 137, 147, 149, 243, 267, 276
  Northern, 243
  Southern, 135, 147, 267
  Western, 130, 137, 147, 149, 310, 311

African American, 111, 112

AIDS. *See* HIV/AIDS

Al-Ahram (Egyptian newspaper), 90

Al-Azhar Islamic, 87

Al-Azhar University, 93

Alma Ata Declaration (1978), 238

Amenorrhea, 280

American Society for Reproductive Medicine (ASRM), 104, 109, 121, 122

Anemia, 245

Antenatal care, 4, 36, 44, 48, 49, 134, 138, 139, 198, 207, 230
  coverage, 48

Anti-choice/anti-abortion groups/lobbies, 166, 222, 223

Antinatalist, 153, 154, 156–162, 167, 168, 172–174

Anti-retroviral (ARV) treatment, 3, 10, 141, 267

Apgar scores, 115, 117–119, 121, 122

Arab countries, 4, 6, 36–39, 41, 51, 52, 54

Argentina, 169, 171

ART. *See* Assisted reproductive technology (ART)

Artificial insemination, 105, 109, 111, 114

A. Kulczycki (ed.), *Critical Issues in Reproductive Health*, The Springer Series on Demographic Methods and Population Analysis 33, DOI 10.1007/978-94-007-6722-5, © Springer Science+Business Media Dordrecht 2014

Development assistance, 9, 131, 143, 201,
202, 206, 220, 238
Development assistance for health (DAH), 238
Development community/planning, 9
DHS. *See* Demographic and Health
Surveys (DHS)
Diabetes mellitus, gestational (GDM), 113,
114, 118–120, 122
Diagnostic protocols, 3, 4, 22
Diaphragm, 219
Diarrhoea, 221
Diffusion of innovations theory, 247, 272, 273
Disability adjusted life years (DALYs), 235
Disparities, 236, 237
DKT-Egypt, 86–89, 91, 92, 95, 98, 100, 101
Dogmas, 224
"Do no harm" (*primum non nocere*,
or non-maleficence), 249
Donor(s), 132, 134, 138, 143, 145, 148, 228,
265, 272, 273, 276, 280
assistance, 134, 143
policies, 9, 145, 205, 207, 238–239
Douche, 85
Durbar (community gathering), Ghana, 62
Dysmenorrhea, 26

E
Earth, 229
Eclampsia, 114, 118–120, 122
Ecological balance, 223
Economically active population, 136
Economic Empowerment of Adolescent Girls
(EPAG), Liberia, 320, 321, 323
Economic well-being, 1
ECP. *See* Emergency contraceptive pills (ECPs)
EDHS. *See* Egyptian Demographic and Health
Survey (EDHS)
Educational attainment, 113, 117, 131, 132,
310, 311, 313, 315, 319
Egypt, 4–6, 35–54, 85–101, 129, 130, 133,
137, 140, 141, 145–147, 240
Ministry of Health, 89–91, 100
Service Improvement Fund, 147
Egyptian, 227
Egyptian Demographic and Health Survey
(EDHS), 36–39, 41–43, 50–52
EIM. *See* European IVF Monitoring program
(EIM)
EMA. *See* European Medicines Agency (EMA)
Embryo, 104, 105, 107, 108, 121
transfer, 104, 108, 122
Emergency contraception, 3, 5, 6, 85–101, 228
local interpretations, 85–101

Emergency contraceptive pills (ECPs), 5, 86
Emergency obstetric care, 134, 138, 139,
146, 149
Emergency obstetric services, 143
Emotional/mental health, 23
Empowerment of women, 11, 12, 40, 43, 45,
54, 130, 134, 230, 233, 236, 239
Engender Health, 252, 253, 256, 261
Ensoulment, 29, 94, 95
Environmental hazards, 104
EPAG. *See* Economic Empowerment of
Adolescent Girls (EPAG), Liberia
Epidemic, 236
Equity, 12, 14, 237, 239, 240, 255
ESHRE. *See* European Society for Human
Reproduction and Embryology
(ESHRE)
Ethical perspectives, 107
Ethiopia, 15, 181, 187, 276–277, 314, 316,
318, 321, 323, 324
Europe, 6, 8, 11, 36, 132, 138, 140, 142–144,
154, 158, 163–166, 168–170,
172, 278
Central, 165, 166
Eastern, 138, 140, 165, 166, 172
Western, 132, 144, 172
European Court of Human Rights, 165
European IVF Monitoring program (EIM),
108
European Medicines Agency (EMA), 286
European Parliamentary Forum on Population
and Development, 224
European Parliament, member (MEP), 11, 221
European Society for Human Reproduction
and Embryology (ESHRE),
107, 108
European Union (EU), 10, 165, 221, 222
Evangelical Christian organizations, 92
Exemption Scheme (Ghana), 66
Experimental design, 61–63

F
Faith-based Organizations, 15
Fallopian tubes, 245
Family Health International (FHI 360), 270,
272, 275, 279, 286, 287, 290–296,
298–301
Family Health Model (Egypt), 147, 148
Family-life education, 227
Family planning, 1, 2, 5, 7–15, 59–63, 65,
68–80, 131–138, 141–145, 147–150,
219–227
methods (*see* Contraceptive methods)

Printed by Printforce, the Netherlands